Building a Legacy

Jones and Bartlett Series in Oncology

Building a Legacy
Voices of Oncology Nurses

Brenda Nevidjon, RN, MSN

Associate Chief Operating Officer for Nursing Services
Duke University Medical Center

Editor, *ONS News*

Jones and Bartlett Publishers

Boston   *London*

Editorial, Sales, and Customer Service Offices
Jones and Bartlett Publishers
One Exeter Plaza
Boston, MA 02116
1-800-832-0034
617-859-3900

Jones and Bartlett Publishers International
7 Melrose Terrace
London W67RL
England

Library of Congress Cataloging-in-Publication Data
Building a legacy: voices of oncology nurses / Brenda Nevidjon.
    editor.
      p.   cm.
    ISBN 0-86720-727-2
    1. Cancer—Nursing. I. Nevidjon, Brenda.
    RC266.B85   1995
    610.73'698—dc20   95-4063
                                                                      CIP

Acquisitions Editor: Jan Wall
Production Editor: Anne Noonan
Manufacturing Buyer: Dana L. Cerrito
Editorial Production Service: WordCrafters Editorial Services, Inc.
Cover Design: Hannus Design Associates
Printing and Binding: Edwards Brothers

Printed in the United States of America

99 98 97 96 95 10 9 8 7 6 5 4 3 2 1

For oncology nurses past, present, and future . . .

the voices which are silent,
the voices making a difference every day,
the voices yet to be heard.

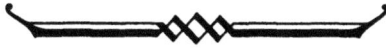

Contents

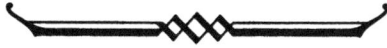

Foreword

A legacy is a personal gift, freely given, for the benefit or pleasure of another. *Building a Legacy: Voices of Oncology Nursing* is an authentic gift beyond measure. History and hope are bundled exquisitely and shared generously to enrich our lives with purpose, passion, and persistence. By capturing the rich stories of nurses who have excelled in diverse roles and shaped the specialty of oncology nursing, the book honors all cancer nurses and celebrates the twentieth anniversary of the Oncology Nursing Society.

Builders agree that foundations must be constructed soundly to support the structure and keep secure what is housed inside. Foundations may extend several feet below the ground and can be overlooked. Just as foundations are not always visible, voices are not always heard. *Building a Legacy* shows us how strong the foundation of oncology nursing is. It addresses not only the past but teaches us which values are the cement of the foundation.

Nurses face unprecedented challenges as health-care reform threatens workplace stability and access to cancer care. Professional organizations are working to assist members with educational and skill development needed for future roles. In oncology, this means insuring that there are oncology nurses prepared to provide a continuum of services from prevention to rehabilitation. Many of the authors in this book describe the incredible learning experiences they have had through association with other oncology nurses and as a benefit of being part of an organized specialty group.

As ONS celebrates its twentieth anniversary, this book provides an answer to the question, "What is the role of the specialty organization in supporting oncology nurses throughout their career?" Founders of ONS describe the early days of their efforts to establish an organization to unite nurses who cared for people with cancer and to meet the educational needs of the rapidly increasing number of nurses in the specialty. Many authors describe how invaluable the organization has been in their development as cancer nurses and in their careers.

It is the intimate accounts of the authors' experiences with patients and families that remind us about what nursing's foundation is: making a difference in the lives of others, doing good. It is equally apparent that the authors have learned valuable lessons from their patients which have influenced their lives. They allow us to see moments of sadness and celebration. They reveal professional and personal choices made coincidentally, easily, or with difficulty. They are gracious in thanking those who have mentored them. It is a book in which you can recognize yourself.

We all share the experience of family and friends asking, "What is it that you do?" Now, administrators, legislators, and insurers ask tough questions about what we do, demand measurable outcomes, and challenge us to describe how we make a difference. As oncology nurses, we know our worth and we know our foundation is strong. This book captures for us the essence of oncology nursing, vividly depicting the tangible and the intangible in our lives. It is our legacy.

Linda Burnworth Johnson, RN, MS, OCN
President, 1994–1995
Oncology Nursing Society
and
Nursing Staff Development Specialist
Arthur G. James Cancer Hospital and Research Institute

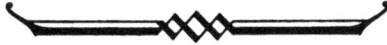

Preface

My memory of wanting to be a nurse reaches back to a very young age. I have explored several times the influences in my life which kept me on the path to nursing. How and why people chose certain careers has always fascinated me and I have found storytelling to be educational as well as entertaining. Storytelling was an integral part of my childhood with my father's stories of what it was like to grow up on the farm, my mother's stories of meeting and marrying my father, and my grandmother's stories of her youth in England. To have served as the editor of this book has been a gift.

The origins of the book are rooted in two ONS activities. The ONS Membership and Public Relations Committee, as it was then known, began exploring the question of what is the life cycle of an oncology nurse. That question was posed by then president Deborah Mayer and executive director Pearl Moore. The Life Cycle Task Force was created and charged to identify the essential concepts that represent major influences throughout an oncology nurse's life. Co-chaired by Karen Kane McDonnell and Betty Ferrell, the task force generated a multisite study led by Marlene Zichi Cohen to examine qualitatively the concepts from interviews with nurses. The personal stories were compelling.

In 1991 at the annual ONS Congress, a special symposium titled "Legacy of Leadership: Pioneers, Prophets, and Proteges" was held. Pamela J. Haylock conceived of that special symposium as a method for looking at questions such as: Which nurses made early contributions to the specialty? Who had the vision and laid the foundation for ONS? Evaluations indicated that participants wanted more stories about oncology nursing.

As a result of the high interest in learning from others' stories, a recommendation was made to the ONS Board to publish a book of stories. I remember a conversation with Karen Kane McDonnell about the results of the Life Cycle Task Force and how to communicate information through the *ONS News*. We briefly discussed the idea of a book. I mentioned some recent books of nurses' stories I had read. I also mentioned how very pleased I would be to help with the project in whatever way. When the time came, she remembered my interest and I appreciate her connecting me to this project and the ONS Board for approving my editorship.

The process of obtaining stories for this book was designed by a talented Advisory Committee. I would like to thank Teresa Coluccio, Jeanne Erickson, Julie Jackson, Linda Burnworth Johnson, Jan Kinzler, Karen Kane McDonnell, and Steve Wagner for their help in taking a germ of an idea about stories of oncology nurses, giving it focus, and designing the process.

A group of authors were invited to share their stories. These were oncology nurses who the Advisory Board believed had important roles in the development of oncology nursing practice or in the establishment of ONS. A call was then issued to the oncology nursing community for nominations of stories. Many responded for themselves or by nominating a colleague. Thanks to the assistance of Teresa Caluccio and Jeanne Erickson, a list was generated from the nominations to round out the book.

I have had the privilege to read these stories several times. In fact, I had to read each several times before I could make any editorial suggestions. They are filled with emotion. Many a colleague heard my laughter at some of the humor and my respect for the courage and creativity in these stories. My husband also heard my tears as I read him particularly moving passages.

My work has been assisted by a number of people: Shelly Yanek at ONS; Jennie Simpson, Sauda Zahra, and Beth Barnhill at Duke; Jim Keating and Jan Wall at Jones and Bartlett; and Laura Cleveland at WordCrafters. I have appreciated their talent and support. I extend a special thanks to Tracie Jones who helped in many urgent situations and willingly stayed longer hours with my son.

ONS has been an important part of my career as an oncology nurse. I will be forever grateful for the opportunities I have had as a member and, in particular, the role in preparing this legacy.

Brenda Nevidjon

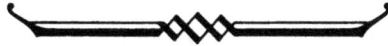

Contributors

Kathryn Marie Ahne, RN, BSN,
  OCN
Nurse Clinician III
Texas Oncology, PA

Karen Angstadt, RN, OCN
Staff Nurse
North Florida Regional Medical
  Center

Joyce Arena, RN, MSN, OCN
Oncology Clinic Nurse Specialist
Bridgeport Hospital

Susan B. Baird, RN, MPH, MA
Director of Nursing and
  Patient Services
Fox-Chase Cancer Center

Jeanne Q. Benoliel, DNSc, FAAN
Professor Emeritus
School of Nursing, University of
  Washington

Jeannine Brant, RN, MS, OCN
Oncology Clinical Nurse Special-
  ist/Pain Consultant
St. Vincent Hospital & Health
  Center

Cynthia Cantril, RN MPH
Cancer Consultant/Educator

Sandy Creamer, RN, MS, OCN
Coordinator of Oncology/Hema-
  tology Services
Saint's Memorial Medical Center

Karen Hassey Dow, RN,
  PhD, FAAN
Director of Education
Geffen Cancer Center and
  Research Institute

Coni Ellis, BSN, MS, C, OCN,
  CETN
Outreach/E.T. Instructor, Nurs-
  ing Staff Development
University of Texas M. D. Ander-
  son Comprehensive Cancer
  Center

Betty Ferrell, PhD, FAAN
Associate Research Scientist
City of Hope Medical Center

Rosemary Ford, BA, BS
Outpatient Nurse Manager
Fred Hutchison Cancer Research
  Center

Juanita Garrison, RN, BS
Clinical Nurse Oncology Coordi-
nator
University of Kentucky Medical
Center

Mary Gerbracht, RN, MSN, OCN
Cancer Center Program Coordinator
St. Paul Medical Center

Elaine Glass, RN, MS, OCN
Clinical Nurse Specialist
The James Cancer Hospital

Janith Griffith, RN, BSN, OCN
Staff Nurse
Cancer Care Center
St. Luke's Hospital

Mary Magee Gullatte, RN, BSN,
MN
Nurse Manager
Emory University Hospital

Shirley Gullo, MSN, RN, OCN
Oncology Clinical Nurse Specialist
The Cleveland Clinic Foundation

Pamela J. Haylock, RN, MA
Cancer Care Consultant

Laura Hilderley, RN, MS
Clinical Nurse Specialist
Radiation Oncology Services

Renilda E. Hilkemeyer, RN, BS,
PhD(Hon) Doctor of Public
Service
Retired Nurse Oncologist

Ryan Iwamoto, ARNP, MN
Radiation Oncology Clinical
Nurse Specialist
Mason Clinic

Judith Johnson, PhD, RN, FAAN
Oncology Consultant

Susan A. Leigh, BSN, RN
Cancer Survivorship Consultant

Jean Nelson Lonergan, RN, BS,
OCN
National Bone Marrow Trans-
plant Consultant

Deborah Mayer, RN, MSN, OCN,
FAAN
Oncology Clinical Nurse Specialist
Princess Margaret Hospital

Ruth McCorkle, PhD, FAAN
American Cancer Society Professor
School of Nursing, University of
Pennsylvania

Christine Miaskowski, RN, PhD,
FAAN
Associate Professor and Interim
Chair
Department of Physiological
Nursing
University of California, San
Francisco

Pearl Moore, RN, MN
Executive Director
Oncology Nursing Society

Catherine O'Brien, RN, BS, MS
Ambulatory Oncology Nurse
Coordinator
Cancer Institute
Mary Immaculate Hospital

Kim Parylovich, BSN, MSN
Oncology Clinical Nurse Specialist
Sunrise Hospital & Medical
Center

Karen Pfeifer, RN, MSN, CNA, OCN
Doctoral Student/Graduate Teaching Assistant
Texas Woman's University—
College of Nursing

Joan A. Piemme, RN, MNED, FAAN
HIV Coordinator
VA Medical Center Martinsburg, West Virginia

Nita Kay Schulz, RN, BSN, OCN
Ambulatory Care/Adult Hematology-Oncology Nurse
Peter S. Kennedy, MD

Judith A. Spross, PhD (Candidate), RN
Clinical Nurse Specialist
Braintree Hospital

Shirley Stagner, MSN
Director, Community Affairs
The Memphis Cancer Center

Debra Thaler-DeMers, BSN, RN, PHN
Good Samaritan Hospital
Oncology Department

Adynel (Andi) Wood, PNP, RN
Pediatric Nurse Practitioner in Hematology-Oncology
St. Jude Children's Research Hospital

Connie Henke Yarbro, RN, BSN
Director of Nursing Resource Development
Regional Cancer Center
Memorial Medical Center

1

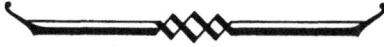

Kathryn Marie Ahne

"It's not what we hoped it would be. . . ." Those were the words of my trusted breast surgeon to me, age 31, following my unanticipated breast biopsy. Little did I realize at that time the impact they were to have on me, the breast oncology nurse.

I first became interested in oncology nursing while in school, where I had the option of taking an elective, Oncology Nursing. Since I came from a family with a strong history of cancer, I thought I could benefit from the course. The instructor was very dynamic and impressed me so much that I signed up to do my adult nursing clinical rotation with her and subsequently did my final senior management rotation with her. The entire rotation was on an oncology unit where we were each teamed up with a staff nurse who acted as our role model and mentor. I was paired with Mary. I'll never forget her calm, quieting, and professional demeanor.

Mary showed a genuine caring attitude toward her patients. She treated them with respect and dignity. She was also a true team player on the unit. I never saw her engage in gossip or heard her say anything detrimental concerning another staff member. She was an excellent example to try to follow. Over the course of those months I had the privilege to care for one man in particular several times. Dick was the first patient to whom I grew attached. It was very difficult for me when he died. I remember cutting his death notice out of the paper thinking I would save it to remember him and his wife. Little did I realize at that time that I wouldn't need to look at that piece of paper to recall Dick's courageousness and perseverance.

When I finished nursing school, I was able to secure a position on a busy oncology unit. Now the learning really began. I worked on the inpatient unit for three years. By the end of that time, I needed a change. Long hours, heavy patient loads, politics, and overall stress started to weigh me down. I was having trouble maintaining a positive attitude.

A position had opened up at the same hospital in the Outpatient Oncology Ambulatory Clinic which sounded like the change for me. I began working primarily with an oncologist who specialized in breast cancer, managing his patient load and administering blood products and chemotherapy.

Relationships with patients now took on a different tone. In the outpatient setting, it was now an ongoing relationship with them, from the shock of initial diagnosis, to chemo, follow-up, recurrence, and dying. I got to know the patients and their families on a much deeper level than I had on the inpatient unit.

For me the nurse/patient boundary question has always been present. Patients undoubtedly become interested in your personal life and frequently ask questions like, "Aren't you married yet? What's he waiting for?" They come to rely on you and want to know what's going on when you're not there. Ironically enough, my patients were some of the most supportive people to me when my own mother was diagnosed with cancer.

I had always thought she was a walking "time bomb." She was overweight and had a major smoking history. Her cigarettes and my oncology roots clashed many a time. She died four and a half months after being diagnosed with an unknown primary tumor. Her cancer did not respond to chemo or radiation; it aggressively just took over her body.

While she was sick and even after she died, I dealt with her illness as a nurse and not as a daughter. My sister, a physician, and I became the "bad guys" in the family as we spoke about a "Do Not Resuscitate" order for Mom. We explained her poor prognosis and that compressions on her chest during CPR could crush her bones. I tried in vain to discuss my mother's wishes with her, but she could not bring herself to discuss it. I showed my family how to try to make Mom more comfortable with pillows, pain medicines, and other comfort measures every oncology nurse tries. I hate to admit it, but I even tried to get Mom to drink nutritional supplements, not realizing that was the last thing she wanted.

I remember the support I received from my own patients during that time and when she finally passed away. They understood. They cared. They sent me cards, books, flowers, and knew just what to say. I also became acquainted with the staff nurses on Mom's floor, whom I ran into at the ONS Congress that year. I learned how much it means to families to have confidence in their oncology nurse and what it's like to feel that your loved one is in competent hands. Ironically enough, Mom was on the same oncology unit where I had spent my senior school rotation.

When my Mom died, I realized how important it was for me to be with her when she actually passed on. One by one, each of us six kids arrived from various parts of the country. The last family member, my brother, made it to her bedside 15 minutes before she died. I know he would never have forgiven himself if he had not made it in time.

I have always felt the need for closure in my relationships with my patients. When I worked on the inpatient unit, I felt closure with my patients by taking care of their postmortem needs. I treated their bodies with respect in getting them ready to leave our floor. If I was particularly close with a patient, I attended his or her funeral as well. It meant a lot to me, and I know it meant a lot to the family for me to go. I still send at least a card and/or attend a memorial service when a patient dies.

My own experience with cancer took me quite by surprise. I am an active American Cancer Society volunteer and when Breast Cancer Awareness Month rolled around, I agreed to do a radio interview in which I stressed the importance of breast self-exams and mammography. Shortly after that, I was asked to do a breast self-exam class for employees at a local company. I try to do breast self-exams on a monthly basis, but actually only end up doing them every three months. Feeling somewhat hypocritical, I went home and examined my breast.

Much to my surprise I noticed dimpling on the outer portion of my right breast which hadn't been there before. I felt extensively and failed to find any abnormal lumps, but I do have fibrocystic breasts. I tried not to be alarmed. With my oncology background, every time I have an ache or pain, I think that I have metastatic disease that just hasn't been diagnosed yet. I was seeing my gynecologist two weeks after that for my annual exam so I decided to show it to him. He examined me thoroughly and found nothing. I asked him if I could get a mammogram due to my family history, even though I was only 31. Several family members had been diagnosed with breast cancer. My gynecologist said I could have a mammogram, and asked that I send him a copy of the report. Since I had been seen by him, I guess I felt a false sense of reassurance that everything was O.K. I did not get my mammogram for five or six weeks. Much to my surprise there were two areas of microcalcification on the films. The mammogram was done in my own office, and I knew what I saw on those films. I obviously was concerned and showed them to the oncologist with whom I worked. He said, "I'm no radiologist, but who do you want for your breast surgeon?"

Thus began several months that would shed a totally different light on everything I do. I did get in to see the breast surgeon at the next available appointment. She told me there was a 50–50 chance that this could be malignant. With my background, I knew that all breast lumps were not malignant, but I was concerned that there was a 50–50 chance that the results would be positive. I began to notify my family members that I was about to undergo a breast biopsy, but I tried to play it down. I didn't tell many of my close friends because I did not want to cause any alarm.

My breast surgeon explained that I would undergo a needle local-ization followed by biopsy. I immediately went home and began digging through my oncology books to find out more specifics about needle localization. I was in an information-seeking phase and read just about everything I could get my hands on.

I never really realized what people went through before they even stepped into our medical oncology office. I just knew they went through biopsy and/or surgery. I didn't realize how much they already had survived. I was quite apprehensive about the needle localization proce-dure. I am embarrassed to say that I actually passed out during the procedure. I remember telling the tech, the nurse, and the physician that I was starting to feel very lightheaded. Next thing I knew, I was lying flat on a stretcher with several people around me. It was very frightening. They told me that I had just passed out and I was O.K. I had just had a vasovagal episode. Shortly after I realized what was going on, I remember thinking, "My God, are the needles still in place?" I wanted to be sure that I didn't have to go through that procedure again. They re-X-rayed, and determined that the needle localization wires were still where they needed to be, and the procedure ended a short time later.

I was very grateful to the nurse in the breast center when she insisted on accompanying my boyfriend and me over to the Surgicenter. When I got to the Surgicenter, I asked for the nurse I knew, and she came out to see me, quite surprised that I was undergoing a breast biopsy. When I got into the O.R. and lay down on the table, I recognized another nurse whose husband I had taken care of several years before. She stated that he was doing well and said she would tell him that she had seen me. The nurses made a big difference in my emotional comfort.

The next thing I knew, I was in a recliner in the recovery room with my boyfriend sitting close by. Shortly thereafter, my breast surgeon came by and broke the news to me. I remember feeling as if somebody had just punched me hard in the stomach. I wondered if I was really there or dreaming this, and just kept hoping that this wasn't true. This couldn't be happening to me; I was a breast cancer nurse! I was too young. I was a health professional, and these things didn't happen to us. I remember going home that evening totally dreading breaking the news to my Dad who was anxiously awaiting my call. I felt so badly having to tell him, and found myself reassuring him as well as trying to reassure myself that everything was going to be all right, even though I didn't know what was in store for me.

I saw the breast surgeon again the next morning and found out that I did not have clear margins from my biopsy site. Therefore, I would require a re-excision and possibly a mastectomy. Thus began the agonizing decision of whether to go with the lumpectomy and axillary dissection or a mastectomy. If I went the mastectomy route, I then had to decide whether or not to undergo immediate reconstruction. A day after the biopsy, I saw the breast surgeon, radiation oncologist, and a plastic surgeon, and had a bone scan and chest X-ray done for staging studies. The bone scan was the last thing I had done that day. While I was lying there on that table, the whole impact of everything just caught up to me: "My God, we're checking to see whether I've got metastatic disease. . . . I've got cancer!"

The tech who did my bone scan stands out in my mind as being such a kind man who treated me like a human being. When I started crying, he was very supportive and allowed me to talk, and to cry. I hadn't let myself do it yet. Fortunately, the radiologist waited and was able to give me an immediate verbal report that my bone scan and chest X-ray were clear. What a relief!

I learned the importance of having someone designated to communicate with family and friends. I didn't feel like I should ask my boyfriend, so I did it myself. I must have explained lumpectomy versus mastectomy hundreds of times—to family, to friends, to co-workers. The hard part was that no one could make the decision for me. I wanted to evaluate all of my options, but the final decision was quite difficult to make. I was perplexed after seeing the plastic surgeon and radiation oncologist. I finally decided to leave it in God's hands. We would go with the re-excision and axillary dissection and see if we could get clear margins at that time. If we weren't able to get clear margins, then I would proceed with a mastectomy at a later date.

My oldest sister came the week after my biopsy to be with me for my surgery. It really helped to have her there. By then, my boyfriend's parents were also back from their vacation trip. What a shock it was for them to hear the news. My boyfriend and his mother came along with me to the surgery also. I woke up in the recovery room, lying on a stretcher. I remember feeling pain like I had never felt before. I felt like a wimp asking for pain medicine; however, they were generous in giving it to me. The familiar faces of the staff really helped once again.

We had decided to do the axillary dissection and the excision as an outpatient procedure, so I was to go home at the end of the day. I remember lying there in the recovery room thinking, "My gosh, why did I decide not to do this in the hospital?" I was so afraid to move my right arm because it hurt badly when I moved it. One of the recovery room nurses put me in my place by reminding me that I shouldn't be afraid to use it and in fact needed to use it like a normal arm. The homecare nurse came out that night to check my dressings and showed me how to do wound care. My sister helped me with that as well as stripping the JP drain tube.

I saw the breast surgeon the morning after my surgery. I was so consumed with knowing if I had clear margins and if I would need to undergo a mastectomy, that I didn't even think about my nodal status. The surgeon thought that she had gotten pretty good margins, with the exception of one questionably involved positive margin remaining. She felt that radiation would take care of this. At least I knew that I didn't need any further surgery at that time. But never had I even thought that I would have any positive nodes. Surely we had caught this thing early enough! Well, apparently not. I was told that I had 3 out of 29 positive axillary nodes—another kick in the stomach. Now I would need chemotherapy for sure.

After my biopsy, I had discussed my options with the oncologist with whom I work. It had really helped to use him as a sounding board to help make my decision. I had already discussed chemotherapy options. If I was node-negative, I would go with one protocol, and if I was node-positive, I would go with another protocol. Now I knew which one I was going to go with.

The next step was seeing the medical oncologist. The natural option would have been to see the oncologist with whom I work. However, I felt that this was just too close to home. Ironically, just a couple of months before all of this happened, another nurse and I had discussed who we would comprise on our "dream team" of physicians should we ever need them. I then made my own appointment with the medical oncologist of my choice, who was also in my office. We discussed various options, from four courses of 5-Fluorouracil, doxorubicin, and cyclophosphamide to six courses of treatment followed with an autologous bone marrow transplant. He was the first to mention a bone marrow transplant and got me very concerned over my situation. In the end we decided to go with an investigational protocol using four courses of FAC +/−, the growth factor GM-CSF. I felt that higher dose chemotherapy was the best option available to me at that time and was agreeable to participate in a study. Unfortunately for me, we knew that I must be on the placebo arm of the study and not getting any growth factors because of my blood counts. Naturally, I knew all the horrid things that could happen when blood counts are very low. I imagined that I was spontaneously hemorrhaging into my brain when my platelet count was so low, and every little headache I had made all the difference in the world to me.

I was determined not to let any of this slow me down, and probably did myself more damage than good. I continued working my normal hours except that I worked a half day following my treatment and six hours the day after that. I was able to do a Cancer Survivors Day 5K walk when my hematocrit was 26. I did have to slow down on the inclines because I became short of breath. Although I was fine going up the stairs, once I got to the top I was quite winded. When all of this started happening, I was quite upset being reminded that I wasn't "normal" anymore.

As an oncology nurse, I have volunteered for the American Cancer Society and facilitated the local "Look Good, Feel Better" program. We always discussed changes in physical appearance that made a difference in the psychological well-being of the oncology patient. Never had I known how true that was. I remember attending a Young Adult Support group 10 days after my first chemo treatment and running my fingers through my hair. Getting those first few strands of hair caught in my hand gave me the same feeling in my stomach as when my surgeon told me that I had breast cancer. To me, the hair loss was the worst part of the whole experience.

A friend and I went wig shopping on Christmas Eve, the week prior to my first chemo treatment. I had always recommended several different wig shops to patients based on feedback I received from other patients. Now, for the first time, I was going to check these places out myself. I found that price as well as service varied greatly among the various shops. This helped me realize how important it is that we know about services we recommend to patients.

Some days I thought I was doing well just to get myself out of bed. Prior to starting chemo I felt that I knew everything that I could expect. After all, I did patient teaching all the time on this. Little did I know until I actually went through it! I had a primary oncology nurse and talked to her at least three times weekly regarding my blood counts and other concerns. She knew the ins and outs of everything I went through. I kept wondering if everyone went through all of these different side effects, since several of those I had had never been reported before. I could now inform patients of other symptoms they might expect and what to do to minimize them.

My emotions were truly tested twice when two of our patients, both in their 30s, developed recurrences. Both were on the same study that I was on. I tried constantly to remember that every situation is different. I found myself looking through their charts to see how many lymph nodes they had involved, their receptor status, and ploidy status. Dealing with these two patients brought things closer to home than ever. I was still trying to make it through initial treatment, and now I had to deal with the thought of recurrence. During the time that the first of these patients had a recurrence, I really started to wonder if the treatment plan I had chosen was going to be good enough to take care of my own cancer. I talked with my oncologist about getting six treatments instead of four. We finally compromised and decided that we would wait and see what happened with my blood counts. Each treatment had to be delayed by a couple of days. However, after the fourth treatment, it took five to six weeks for my blood counts to come back up, so that decision was made by itself. I know at this point that I did everything I could have. If I had gone with higher doses or additional doses of the chemotherapy, I would have been running the risk of cardiac damage from the adriamycin.

The next step was radiation. I remember my first appointment with the radiation oncologist who actually said that he was flattered that I had picked him. In my mind, there wasn't anybody else. When the radiation oncology nurse was teaching me about my treatment, he treated me like he would any other patient. I appreciated this because radiation wasn't my area of expertise. I remember that the Radiation Department staff called me Ms. Ahne, and I had to repeatedly tell them that they could call me by my first name. I appreciated the respect they showed by not presuming to use my first name.

I had just started getting over the side effects from the chemotherapy when I started radiation. I was starting to settle into a routine and to get accustomed to not having a hair on my head. I could finally look in the mirror without crying. Radiation very abruptly reminded me that I was under treatment for breast cancer. I got my marks put on, which limited my wardrobe if I was going to continue to try and disguise my situation. I didn't realize how many V-neck shirts and blouses I had until I couldn't wear them. Fortunately for me, the most distinctive markings were able to come off once I started treatment. The ones I had to leave on for treatment were hidden under my clothes.

Radiation was a whole new experience for me. I quickly came to trust my tech, and when she wasn't there, I was suspicious of anyone else. I understood the importance of trying to be consistent with patients. Since I wasn't as familiar with radiation, I was really in the hands of the techs. I had difficulty thinking that anything was even happening since I couldn't actually see anything, and only heard the high-pitched noise of the cobalt machine. I was instructed just to lie still while the tech and her assistant ran out of the room and closed the heavy glass door behind them. Talk about feeling isolated!

The only thing I didn't appreciate about my radiation experience was that while I was lying on the table unable to move, various people came into the room and didn't identify themselves. More specifically, I was disrobed from the waist up. Although my modesty had gone away since all this had begun, I was conscious of unannounced staff in the room. It would have helped if they had excused themselves for interrupting, or had explained who they were or what they were doing there. I felt my privacy was not being respected.

As stated earlier, closure with my patients has always been important for me. In our office we try to make a big affair about a patient's last chemotherapy treatment by celebrating with confetti, hugs, and clapping. I received my last treatment after hours one workday with only the nurse administering my chemo and my boyfriend. I just walked out the door and that was it. Much to my surprise, about three weeks later, my coworkers had a party for me. It was then that I was able to realize that chemo was finally over. I think I surprised everyone when I took my confetti-laden wig off my head just to shake it out, which was so much easier than trying to shake it out with it on my head.

The end of radiation was pretty anticlimactic. I just walked out the door and that was it. On some days it's hard to believe that everything is over, and on other days it feels as if I didn't go through anything. I have started to get my stamina, my motivation, and my hair back. Once my eyebrows and eyelashes were completely back in, everyone stated that I looked so much better, but little did they know it was just because of the fact that I had hair on my face again. I still plan to have a final "I'm done with my cancer treatment" bash. I feel that this is important for me to officially finish this whole experience.

Through this entire experience, I would say that people's *presence* made the difference. Every card, every phone call, every note of encouragement made all the difference in the world to me. It is very easy to detect when someone was talking *at* me instead of *to* me. Eye contact and touch became very important; presence became very important. I could tell when people were there doing their job and when someone was there who genuinely cared for my well-being. I remember a nurse patting one of my hands and holding onto my arm while giving me my chemotherapy in the other. That small gesture made me aware that she was there for me. Everyone identified themselves by name and told me what their position was; even the O.R. nurse introduced herself prior to surgery. She stated that she would be with me for the duration of my surgery. I was comforted to know who was going to be with me while I was under anesthesia. I have a much better understanding of what patients have experienced before they come to our office.

When I was first diagnosed, the doctor with whom I work told patients that I had cancer. I didn't mind this at first. However, word of my diagnosis spread quickly through the city's support groups, and several of my patients found out about it that way. I confirmed my diagnosis when they asked me, but eventually I asked the physician to stop publicizing this. I have selectively disclosed my diagnosis and have been able to assist those having a particularly difficult time.

The veteran patients were very supportive of me. I now understand the anxiety of having a new ache or pain. In my nursing career, it has always been "us," the health professionals, and "them," the patients. I am still adjusting to the fact that now I am one of "them." There is a fine line separating me from that identity. I still find myself struggling with that on a daily basis.

I learned how much of an impression the office leaves on someone. Everything from physical appearance to the personalities of the employees makes an impact. It's amazing how much one can hear or see going on in an office while sitting in the waiting room. I also have become aware of the importance of timeliness with which phone calls are returned and test results are obtained. I make it a point to tell patients to call us back the following day to get their test reports, and if they haven't, I call them. I now understand that they may be reluctant to call because of fear of what the results may show. I know that if you are waiting for a doctor's office to call back, you may be doing little of anything else but waiting.

At times I think it would have been easier not to have been a health professional, especially an oncology nurse. My sister, who is an anesthesiologist in another part of the country, found this to be true as well. When I was first diagnosed, she spoke with her colleagues in surgery and oncology, and got as many different opinions as people she talked to. She found the whole experience confusing and frustrating. I have realized how important programs like "Look Good, Feel Better" can be for someone's morale while undergoing treatment changes. I personally found it difficult to attend support groups because I had facilitated so many, and I wasn't ready to run into my own patients.

Balancing my personal and professional lives has always been a struggle for me. I tend to be an overachiever and try to attend as many inservices, conferences, and meetings as possible. I never minded coming in early or staying late on the job; I did whatever was required to get things done to my satisfaction. Since being diagnosed, I have had to make more of an effort at taking care of myself. This has meant taking breaks during the workday and limiting the extra hours I work. I found that all of my energy was going into my job, and I had nothing left for me at the end of the day. For probably 80 to 90 percent of my treatment, I continued to work extra hours trying to convince myself that I wasn't going to let this slow me down. It finally caught up with me when I was almost finished with all of my treatments and I finally broke down. I now realize how important it is for us to advise patients to rest and to balance their activities.

I can visualize the long-term impact on how I can make a difference both in my patients' lives as well as in helping in the prevention and early detection of breast cancer. Having a nursing background and breast cancer specialization, I have the knowledge and the ability to make this work for others. I have stayed in oncology nursing all of these years for the same reason I went into it. I felt then, as I do now, that you can't change the fact that patients have been diagnosed with cancer; it is a life-threatening and very scary disease. The difference we can make in patients' lives through small interventions will have a major impact on their overall experience with cancer. I intend to make an even greater impact now through my experience dealing with this disease personally as I continue my oncology nursing career.

Endnote

I would like to thank Helen McCracken for being a special friend and support through this all, and for providing her secretarial support for this project.

2

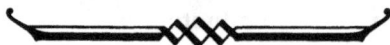

Karen Angstadt

Ever since I can remember, I have wanted to be a nurse. As a child, I can remember thinking that nurses exuded such an air of authority in their crisp, white uniforms and their unique hats. I so wanted to wear one of those wonderfully stylish hats. I was very disappointed to learn that nurses as a rule did not wear them anymore. As I grew older, I still wanted to be a nurse, except now for all of the clichéd reasons, such as to help people and perhaps to make a difference in someone's life. I also discovered that I really liked to read anything medical and majored in science in high school. I went as far as taking Latin, as it was a requirement at the time.

Although my career choice had always been to be a nurse, due to extenuating circumstances, I had to delay further education. My plans were further waylaid when I met someone with a beautiful smile and gorgeous blue eyes. After having three sons, I still had not gone back to school. However, I guess childhood dreams die hard. I talked so much about being a nurse that my husband strongly encouraged me to go back to school. Actually, I believe what he said was for me to go back to school or stop talking about it.

I was very worried and scared. I was 34 years old and 16 years out of high school. I had been a housewife that entire time, interacting and conversing mostly with children. I did not know if my brain had atrophied from disuse and if it could be revived and would still function with some semblance of intelligence. To be honest, I had a headache for the first week of school, before it occurred to me that it was probably my brain protesting all of the new activity. Nursing school was hard, but made easier by the making of some very good friends. We helped each other study and gave each other encouragement. My husband and children were an immeasurable help, from understanding about the time I was gone, to helping with the housework and cooking their meals. They even helped me study. However, it was so easy to get discouraged. I can remember one time when my best study buddy and I were particularly down. My husband surprised us with T-shirts that said, "Endeavor to persevere." We wore those shirts for inspiration for a long time. I cannot describe fully the elation I felt in a dream realized, and how proud I was of myself when I finally graduated. I thought it would never happen, especially after getting married and having three sons. I will always be grateful to those who encouraged and helped me through those rough years of school, but I am especially appreciative to my husband.

As long as I can remember, I have heard the word *cancer* mumbled in hushed tones along with the words *pain* and *death*. I would hear family members and friends discuss someone with cancer as if they were already dead. I would hear about bald, emaciated people who were constantly throwing up and in constant pain. No wonder I, like most people, thought of cancer as awful. This distorted view of having cancer was no more evident than in my discussion with one of our patients recently. She is my age and has a problem that required numerous surgeries and an uncountable number of hospitalizations. She has become a friend. During one of her recent stays, she was discussing the frustrations and problems of being in the hospital again. She said to me that at least she did not have cancer, as she knew that I had had cancer. I was really floored, because I had always thought that despite my cancer, at least I did not have her perpetual problem. This scenario, however, does demonstrate the fear and death-sentence mentality still associated with cancer.

In nursing school I learned that one of our assigned units was the oncology unit. I envisioned my fearful picture of a cancer patient and I counted my lucky stars when I was assigned to another unit. When I graduated from school, I wanted to work at a particular hospital. The only unit that wanted to hire me was the oncology unit that I had managed to avoid in nursing school. What irony, my one big fear come to life! I guess some divine justice could be found in the situation. The head nurse was reluctant to hire me because my mother and aunt had had breast cancer two years before. I told her I did not think it would be a problem and I thought I might have more insight into the problems encountered by cancer patients. My intentions were to work there six months and then transfer to another unit. But after eight years, I am still on the cancer unit by choice.

I started on the night shift right out of school. I was so scared, scared that I would make a terrible mistake and hurt, or worse yet, kill someone. For six months, I had a tension headache by the end of every shift and was going to quit every day and begin early retirement. But with time and a lot of patience and encouragement from my fellow nurses, and my husband saying, "Oh, no, this was your dream" (my words come back to haunt me), I stayed in my chosen profession. Most nights I am very glad of my choice. The night shift staff who oriented me were very intelligent and conscientious nurses. They taught me to take pride in what I did and how to do it correctly the first time. I graduated from school with all of the book learning, but there are a lot of things not taught in books, some common sense things that only experience teaches. Eventually I developed a sense, an intuition, for potential problems with patients even before their vital signs or other symptoms make it apparent. I still work with the same charge nurse and I have learned a lot from her. She is not much older than me, but we just helped her celebrate her 30th year in nursing. You can imagine the knowledge she has and the stories she can tell of "the good old days." I really admire this nurse. She is tough, but has kept her sense of humor and has a heart of gold. She shows a tremendous amount of compassion and understanding for her patients, their families and her coworkers. She is never too busy to listen. I am very glad and proud to have her not only as a charge nurse, but also as a good friend.

I have worked nights for eight years by choice. I like the pace. I like the feeling of a little more autonomy. Working nights, I have had to learn what to do in certain situations, such as when is it O.K. to call the doctor at 3 A.M. (trust me, the doctor does not want to hear about constipation at this time). There is the erroneous assumption that all of the patients sleep during the night shift. Wrong!! Have you ever had a particularly nagging problem and could not sleep? Just imagine the diagnosis of cancer as the problem and all of its ramifications. No wonder a lot of these patients cannot sleep at night. As a night nurse, you have to physically and psychologically help these patients sleep; whether it involves giving a sleeping or pain pill or letting them vent their concerns and frustrations. Sometimes shared problems do not loom so big. In order to contend with the day's problems and tests, these patients need to be afforded a good night's sleep.

I did not realize the full responsibility encountered in nursing. I guess I thought when I was dreaming of nursing that I would walk around in my starched white uniform and hat and dispense medicine with a smile and go home. I now realize that was a very naive picture. It is very sobering to realize that I am responsible for everything I do and for everything that happens. It is very awesome to know that some patients' lives depend on me.

I have had many pleasant surprises as an oncology nurse. For instance, with the ever-changing treatments and the increasingly complicated technology, I found that I could keep all of the skills I learned in nursing school and acquire many more. It seems as if our unit is always busy; thus time goes by fast and there are very few slow nights. If an oncology patient has one IV, they have numerous. There always seems to be a lot of medicines to give. The patients also have a lot of problems, whether physical or psychological, that have to be dealt with. Oncology patients who are hospitalized are generally very sick or dying; thus they require a great deal of time. I like the feeling of being needed and the self-fulfillment I experience in taking care of these patients.

I found early on in my nursing career that I needed, as a nurse and as a person, to deal with the suffering and dying that I was witnessing. To see people my own age and even younger have cancer and even die, is to have to in some way come to terms with my own mortality. I had always envisioned myself as growing old, old and healthy, but I had to rethink that naive assumption. I had to incorporate my belief in God and the hereafter with the unfairness that fate brings. A patient would die and I would know that I had done all that I could and that they would not suffer anymore. On the other hand, someone else would die and I could not help but think that the uniqueness of that person would not be seen on earth again. All they were or could be is lost, but for their memory. I thought that when someone died or gets well and went home, I would never forget them. I have found to my dismay that since there are so many, I can see their faces and maybe even remember some of their stories, but not their names. I only hope that their families and friends keep something of that person in their hearts and memories.

In the field of oncology, the same patients come in numerous times bringing their family with them. As an oncology nurse, I have learned to care for these patients and their families as people, to know them aside from their diagnoses. In nursing school, I learned not to be personal with patients and to use therapeutic questions and answers. But all of these patients and their families touch your heart as a person. With time, these patients learn to know you as a person, as a friend, and ask questions about your family, about how you are feeling, and what you have been doing. Everyone knew when I went to Germany to see our first grandchild and they all wanted to see my pictures. Of course, I very proudly showed them to any and all who wanted to see. I think their interest and curiosity in their nurses is for two reasons. First, asking about others takes some of the focus off their problems, and for a while at least, they do not have to think about cancer. Second, the patients want to know us as people, to feel close to us. When they come in for care, they want to feel that they know us and that we are in essence an extended family with all of the loving and caring that comes with familial intimacy. A rapport, a trust is established with these patients and their families. I try not to get emotionally involved, but the patients will not allow this distancing. They want to feel close to their nurses. All of this sharing of intimate knowledge of each other makes it very hard emotionally if the patient receives bad news or dies. It is very hard to watch a friend die, because by now these patients are friends. I know in my heart of hearts that we have done all that we could do, and that they are better off leaving this world.

I have learned a lot from these patients and their families. I have learned the absolute importance to one's well-being of family and friends. I have seen them deal with adversity with courage, with humor, and with anger. I have learned that all patients act differently and that there is no right way to act, and that no matter how they act, it is just good, honest emotion.

I observed these patients and wondered how I would act if I was ever told I had cancer. Since my mother and her sister had breast cancer, I knew my chances were great. My mom and aunt were both diagnosed in their 60s, so I thought I could deal with it down the road. What I had not anticipated was being diagnosed with breast cancer one month shy of turning 42. After five years of oncology nursing and with my family history of cancer, I thought I understood the diagnosis—cancer. I quickly found a new and intimate understanding when a very compassionate surgeon told me I had breast cancer, after I had been told that they were just benign tumors. I had always wondered what I would do. I found out. I stopped breathing and heard nothing else the doctor said after the word *cancer*. It felt as if someone had sucker punched me and robbed me of my ability to breathe. For some reason, it was important for me to keep my composure and not to cry. I was at the doctor's office alone and I wondered how I was going to get home. I was devastated and felt as if I had just been handed a death sentence. I have often wondered if doctors and nurses are aware of how the diagnosis of cancer can affect a patient, of how mind-numbing it can be. I will always be grateful to the doctor and his office staff. They made all of the arrangements while I was still in the examining room and told me not to worry, to just leave. I am so glad I did not have to deal with any of the appointments or anything as mundane as money. They told me to just walk straight through the waiting room and out.

I went to see my head nurse to make arrangements for more time off. She knew where I had been, took one look at me, and said, "Oh, shit," and closed her office door. She just held me, no clichés, no words of encouragement, just held me in a silent expression of empathy, while I cried. I know first hand that sometimes there are no words, but the only expression of sympathy and understanding needed by a patient or family member is someone to hold their hand or to offer a shoulder to cry on. My head nurse's simple gesture of caring impressed me and I now feel more comfortable being with patients and not feeling the need for verbal communication. That awful day I was told I had cancer stands out in my mind for obvious reasons, but also because the day was made easier by the thoughtfulness and compassionate concern expressed by some very special people.

With a great deal of reluctance and terror, I had surgery when my oncologist assured me that anything less would jeopardize my life. I was very angry and withdrawn in the hospital and even after I went home. I was angry at fate, angry that it had to happen, angry because I thought I was too young. I was particularly upset about the disfigurement from surgery, and—no offense to my surgeon—I felt mutilated. I was so angry that I did not want to talk to anyone. I am still embarrassed to this day to think that I even refused to see the pastor of my church. I withdrew into myself and did not want to go out or talk to anyone, but luckily my family and friends would not allow my retreat. With their attention and encouragement, they helped me accept what had happened and rejoin the world. I received cards, phone calls, and presents nearly every day. Most of my good friends are oncology nurses, so they had some understanding of what I was going through, and they proved to be faithful friends. Who else has a friend they can call at midnight, crying, and in the course of an hour be reassured by that person that they are not going to die and, yes, the doctor had told them everything. I had such a friend, my charge nurse, my voice of reason one lonely night.

I never asked the proverbial question, Why me? Because, why not me? I am no more special than anyone else, even though I would at times like to think so. The anger kept me going and kept my fighting spirit alive. When I would get depressed, I would remember how mad I had been and how this thing called cancer was not going to beat me. Do not get me wrong, I am still scared even after three disease-free years that it will come back. My mother says that even after ten years there is always that terror-filled thought that maybe with this check-up they will find it has come back. Every so often I think, "Oh, my God, I have had cancer," and I worry about a "what if" scenario. However, I cannot let paranoia ruin my life. Sometimes it is hard to keep a positive attitude when I see all of the patients that come in with recurrences. My heart drops to this day when I see the diagnosis "recurrence or metastatic breast cancer" on a patient's Kardex. My oncologist knows of my fear and never misses an opportunity to reassure me of my good prognosis.

The disfigurement was always hard for me. I knew I should keep a positive attitude and that I had a good prognosis, but it was always hard to look down on my body where there used to be a "D" cup and which was now flat. At first, I was worried about what my husband would think and how he would accept the new me. I voiced my concerns to him one day that I just did not feel sexy in my clothes anymore. He reassured me in a special way that he still loved me and found me special. He arranged a romantic evening at a motel room. Now that is acceptance and told me more than words could ever have conveyed. To be honest, the disfigurement always bothered me because I could never forget. It was always there. When I took off my clothes, there it was in the mirror (or, I guess as the case should be, was not).

The prosthesis was never comfortable. It was hot and heavy. Even though it was supposed to be the same weight as my natural breast, it always felt ten pounds heavier. It would never stay put in my bra and no matter how I tried, it tended to wander, so sometimes I would look down and I would be a little off center. Despite the discomfort, there were some funny situations with the prosthesis. For instance, one of our nurses was not feeling well and I felt so badly that she had to work knowing that she felt ill. I went over to tell her how sorry I was that she was sick and she leaned her head on my chest. She then proceeded to squeeze my breast, exclaiming that it felt so real and wasn't it amazing what medical technology could do. I was momentarily tongue-tied, but then said that it was my real breast she was squeezing. We have had so many good laughs over that incident. Another time I was swimming and my prosthesis side started feeling very heavy and I discovered that there was a tiny pinhole in it and I had been taking on water. Naturally, this was the start of my vacation, so I spent the rest of the week with a slightly heavier breast.

I have never dealt with pain very well. My husband says that I do not "do pain" at all. I admit it, I hate to hurt and will take something in a heartbeat. After my surgery, I hurt from one thing or another for about six months. I really have a new insight into how chronic pain affects one physically and mentally. To get up every morning or have sleep interrupted due to pain and know that you have to face another day of pain to whatever degree is very discouraging and drains one of the energy and determination to fight. Luckily, I had an oncologist who believed in a pain-free state.

After a great deal of soul-searching and strong advice from my oncologist, I did something that as an oncology nurse I said I would never do, I started chemotherapy. I guess "never say never" would be the appropriate thought here. I guess one of my main reasons for not wanting to take chemotherapy was that I did not want to lose my hair, any of it. I have few vanities in my life, but my hair is one of them. I had one patient's wife tell me that the hair loss was the hardest part for her husband. Every time I pulled a handful of my hair out, I cried. I cried a lot with my hair loss, even though I never had to wear a wig. Luckily, I have a tremendously thick head of hair. I felt badly about myself until my hair started to look like it did before the chemotherapy.

The doctor told me that statistically speaking my odds were better with chemotherapy. I really hate statistics, but no more so than when I was that one in the one out of ten women who will get breast cancer in their lifetime. The doctors can quote the statistics dispassionately and most of them sound great, until that moment in time when you are the one. I had eight chemotherapy treatments and I hated every one of them. I tried to be positive about the treatments and think of them as life-saving. It was a little hard to be positive when I was watching someone run poisons into my body. After my first treatment, someone said to me, "Now, wasn't that easy?" I was really taken aback, as this was someone who should have known how hard it was. I told this person that if she thought it was so easy, let me start an IV on her and let me run poisons into her body and then give her the added worry about the long-term effect of these drugs. This person really looked surprised at this information. I hope if nothing else, I made her rethink her impression of the ease of receiving chemotherapy. The drugs always made me feel a little ill, like with morning sickness (oh, great, morning sickness again). It got to the point that the mention of chemotherapy or even the sight of the nurse who gave me chemotherapy would give me that nauseated feeling. I felt badly that every time I saw the nurse who gave me chemo, a wave of nausea would overcome me. It was not easy and every time it got harder emotionally. I would cry for three days before each treatment and even at times went into the office for my chemo still boo-hooing. There were some days I felt so sick and such a tiredness of body and soul that I wanted to chuck it all and take my chances with the odds. However, with the encouragement of family and friends, I finished my treatments. I felt a jubilation of the soul and a great sense of accomplishment when I finished my last one.

I received my chemotherapy in the doctor's office. His office nurse and other staff members are wonderful and tried to make everything easier. They were friendly and had a bright, cheery room set up for chemotherapy with a TV, VCR, numerous books, and hard candy available. I sat back in a very comfortable recliner with my legs up and told the nurse to give me my Lorazepam first. I am afraid I was not a very cooperative patient. I did not want to join any support groups nor interact with other patients. I just wanted to come in, get my chemotherapy, and leave without much talking. It sounds odd, harsh when I think back now, but it was how I had to do it, and the nurse and the other staff members respected my wishes. Maybe it was selfish of me, but since I had to deal with cancer patients at work and at the office, I just wanted to concentrate on myself.

After the quoting of more statistics (my favorite thing, again), I also decided to have radiation. After the initial shock of the necessity of more treatments, I did not expect this to be a big deal. When the doctors started talking about doing the radiation in such a way as to miss my heart and lungs, they had my full attention and participation. I knew I would have radiation burns, but I also knew they would heal because I had seen "before" and "after" pictures. It was, however, now my body that was burned and they seemed so much worse than any pictures I had ever seen. It was also quite uncomfortable. I knew what to expect, but the first time I lay on the table, I was so scared. Everyone left the room and the machine started to hum and my heart proceeded to race out of my chest. I wanted to get up off the table and race out the door. Coming in for treatments every weekday for 33 times is so exhausting, plus I had the added effects of the chemotherapy. The entire staff at the radiation center, from the doctors to the nurse, the office staff, and the technologists, were very accessible and were always willing to answer questions. In fact, they encouraged questions and expressions of feelings and problems.

Six months ago, I underwent reconstruction. A long time ago my husband had made me realize he loved me for who I was. I had also learned as a nurse and as a mastectomy patient that with time and support the human spirit can be very adaptable. I thought long and hard before I decided to proceed. For reasons of comfort and to improve my self-awareness, I had surgery. I am so glad about the surgery and feel better about myself. I even had the other side made smaller and the *pièce de résistance* was a tummy tuck. I obviously have a lot of scars, but am still very happy with the results.

Dreams and aspirations keep the spirit alive and fresh, and the realization of one's dreams is food for the soul. I feel very lucky to have realized my dream of becoming a nurse. I am doing what I love and I get a great deal of personal satisfaction from it. I am a staff nurse and deal with patients every day. For now that is what I want to continue to do. Maybe down the road I will go back to school and do something different, such as research.

I got into oncology nursing very reluctantly. I am proud that I have passed my OCN certification twice. I stay in oncology nursing for two reasons. First, the nurses in oncology are special. They work very hard emotionally and physically and are the dedicated and caring nurses I envisioned as a child. They go out of their way to help their patients. Second, I stay because of the patients. I like getting to know these patients so personally. I admire them for their courage and humor.

Seeing the fragility of life as a nurse, and after having had cancer myself, I appreciate and cherish good health. I hate being sick, as do most people. I rejoice every day I get up and feel good. I have learned never to take good health for granted. It is, by the same token, very hard to remember that I *have had* cancer, as opposed to *having* it. One week I had five doctors' appointments, but everything was negative, so I concentrate on the *having had* part of cancer. Being an oncology nurse and experiencing cancer has reinforced what is important in life—family and friends. All have been a great help during my nursing school days and even more so while I was ill. If it had not been for everyone, especially my husband, I do not know if I would have made it through. After having cancer, the small problems of life pale in comparison. I try not to let them bother me, because frankly, I am just so glad to be here, doing what I dreamed of and in good health. I take the time to appreciate the hearts of life, such as my husband and children, our first grandchild, and the wonders of nature. Life is too short. Find the work you love, take that long-planned vacation, do activities with family and friends, and stop to listen, see, and hear.

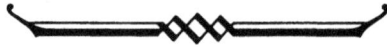

3

Joyce Arena

The big "C" diagnosis was out. I was told to keep it under my hat, but there was no way I was going to deal with cancer by keeping quiet. As I waited to hear my name called over the loudspeaker in the Radiation Medicine Department of Montefiore Hospital in the Bronx, I thought about nursing as a way of dealing with this silence. I always wanted to be a nurse. At the time, I didn't perceive having cancer as fate, but it was. At least for me I saw it as a new beginning. So in the depths of the winter of 1969, I learned I could be diagnosed with, treated for, and survive cancer. Surviving treatment was only the first phase of my surviving cancer.

Adapting to life after cancer was one thing, but becoming a cancer nurse was the real challenge. Cancer had transformed my life, changed me, and gave me the opportunity to pursue a lifelong dream of becoming a nurse. I had to say goodbye to the old me and get acquainted with the new me who had this desperate need to help people, like me, with cancer.

In 1969, you didn't talk about cancer. Emily Post still hasn't come up with the proper etiquette for telling people you have cancer. Those of us being treated were isolated in the bowels of the hospital or in the basement where many radiation therapy departments are and have to be. Most of the patients being treated at this time didn't know they had cancer. I remember my doctor tried to pull a fast one on me too. He tried to use a fancy name: a lymphoproliferative disorder that required some treatments. He didn't expect me to ask what the name of that disorder was. When he said Hodgkins disease, I said the word *cancer* for the first time. His eyes welled up with tears as did mine and the bond between us would never be broken. I didn't know it at that time, but at some point during my nursing career I would be his nurse.

At the time of my diagnosis, I was working as a junior accountant, a job I was good at but didn't enjoy, so I resigned. I learned early on to take risks. It was really hard to get anyone to talk to you about cancer, let alone give you any answers to your questions. I loved my nurses but I felt sorry for them at the same time. They just weren't prepared to help. There were no oncology nurses in 1969, at least not in my community hospital. The nurses thought I was going to die and so did I. I almost did, of outdated information. The very first thing I read about Hodgkins disease was in the 1959 edition of the Merck Manual and Hodgkins had a poor outlook.

They say courage is grace under fire. Well, it took all the grace I had to make it through my first visit to Montefiore. The waiting room was packed with all sorts of people who looked like characters out of a Steven Spielberg movie: purple markings all over them and few hairs left sticking out from their heads. I witnessed one woman having a seizure. I wanted to run out of there but knew I couldn't. I soon came to love all of those people as I became one of them: purple markings all over my body, sprigs of hair left.

Some days our trips to Montefiore from Westport, Connecticut, were ordeals and there were several problems to solve. The *we* was either my father, and my husband, or my sister and me. The first problem we encountered was the snow. It seemed to be the worst winter in years, and we always got behind someone doing 15 miles per hour. Battling the snow, depression, and my fatigue turned me into a less-than-nice person. I'm sure if you ask my family which problems were the hardest they would reply differently. But since it's my story, this is gospel. One day on the way home, tired physically and mentally, I asked my husband and sister to let me out on the side of the road—you know, like they do for the Eskimos when they're dying. Thank God they knew this feeling would pass. I thank God for my sister, Dorene, who always had the gift of making me feel so worthwhile. Another problem was parking. I remember telling the other patients in the waiting room not to talk to me because my father was circling the block and I couldn't lose my turn. I think it was toward my last few treatments that we figured out there was a patient parking lot. So much for the informed patient. My dad was the chauffeur most days which was much more dangerous than my cancer. My father is not the greatest driver and has this tendency to fall asleep at the wheel. I would be exhausted and dozing off when I would look over to see that dad was too. I would yell out, "Dad! One of us has to stay awake and I think since you're driving it should be you!"

My mother kept the fires burning at home and welcomed us with words of encouragement always. I don't know how she did it. Somedays I tortured them all. Midway through treatments I could barely swallow my own saliva but was so hungry. I would do anything to eat. One night my family was in the kitchen eating and I was in the living room feeling sorry for myself. The smell of the food was so good. I yelled into the kitchen, "I hear you eating in there!" Everyone got up from the table choking as they swallowed, feeling sufficiently guilty with poor me in the other room unable to eat. I didn't think they would react that way. When I saw their faces I knew what I had done and realized at that point I didn't have to worry about surviving cancer—they were going to kill me. I came to know my family in a different way and we became a different family. Cancer can bring you together or tear you apart. Not very demonstrative, we kissed and hugged for the first time. Surviving has a lot to do with the people that surround you. I don't know who said this, but I'll quote it anyway. "Rich is not how much money you have; it is measured by the people you have beside you." Markings, blocks, big machines, little machines, changes in markings, hair loss, weight loss. All of this was overwhelming to me, not to mention nausea, sore throat, or fatigue. I learned when my treatments were completed that they didn't tell you those side effects for a reason. They feared you wouldn't show up if you knew the treatments were the cause. Have we come a long way! Now when patients sign a consent form for radiation therapy they are told everything.

I'm one of the nurses who values the importance of patient education. I learned to ask my patients how they like to receive information and how much. I think not knowing is much more stressful than the truth, but one of my very first patients always asked me to place a brown paper bag over her head during her Doxorubicin therapy. She told me if she didn't see the bright red color she wouldn't get sick. For her, it was much more stressful to watch.

Had I been diagnosed today, an oncology nurse would help me cope. Then, no one was comfortable with this topic but me and other cancer patients. Sometimes I found other cancer patients weren't willing to talk about it either. I soon learned that asking questions and learning about my cancer was my way of coping. I also learned early on that young people have a sick sense of humor. At least I did. I tortured my family with this humor. Somehow the things I did that I thought were funny were not perceived in quite that way. Today, I have a special love for young people with cancer who react the same way I did. When I teach nurses about caring for cancer patients, I emphasize the lonely hours of the morning. Our Dog, Tammy, slept by my side and helped me feel safe. Oncology nurses know how to make you feel safe too. Nothing technical. A hand held out or sitting by your side, just like Tammy did for me. I had to have some relief from the desperate isolation I was feeling. There were no nurses who felt comfortable teaching me about cancer and I tried to rationalize their treatment of me. They just didn't have the answers to my questions and didn't know how to get me the answers. I knew for certain that my age (24) was too close for comfort.

More and more my thoughts turned to my lifelong dream of becoming a nurse. Even though I hadn't wished upon a star, it is the time when you're feeling tired and blue that fate steps in and sees you through. I guess you could say Jiminy Cricket was one of my first oncology nurses. When I could no longer bear the isolation, I decided I needed to talk with someone who had experienced the same diagnosis. Another valuable lesson I learned to follow. Patients often tell you what they need if you can't help. My cousin had Hodgkins disease ten years before and was willing to share some of her experience with me. Then another friend of the family came forward as did a few more. I asked so many questions, bombarding these poor people with my need to know what was to be. We now have ACS programs all over the country where cancer patients visit other cancer patients. I wasn't so far off in my idea to help myself.

Armed with my dreams and ridiculous sprigs of hair, I was off to nursing school. I bargained a lot with God, but my requests were always small. I started out in an LPN program. My promise to the Lord, if he would let me live through the year, was that I would be the best nurse ever. I vowed to take care of cancer patients the way they needed to be taken care of. After all, who knew better than I. It turned out to be a very long year with a lot of studying. I practiced a lot on my husband. He still remembers who Lillian Wald is and I don't. Only once did I sweat or doubt graduation. I got the flu and of course they thought I had a bowel obstruction. Thank God my sister came forward to say she had the flu too. She saved me another exploratory laparotomy. My capping ceremony after four months in the program was the first good moment in my life after my treatment. I wore my cap to bed that night. It was hard to give it up when the nursing profession decided that hats did not make the nurse.

I graduated in 1970, the only student not needing to make up, and I scored one of the highest grades on the LPN boards. During that year I had to learn everything so I had little time to concentrate on cancer, let alone mine. I learned so much about life, too. I also developed my sense of humor which has carried me through some of the roughest times in my life. After graduation, I chose to focus my energies toward cancer patients. I landed a job at Norwalk Hospital on a unit where my oncologist admitted most of his patients. I had to face my cancer right up close: the treatment, the threat of recurrence, and my role as a nurse. My battle with cancer had stripped me down to the bare essentials, leaving my priorities and values a little rearranged in the process. I was afraid I would be robbed of the time due me and, if cancer was my wake-up call, what I would do now that I was awake. I was driven. I found that surviving a life-threatening illness left me with a great sense of obligation and a feeling of guilt for having survived. I was given a second chance and wasn't sure why. It left me with the gnawing feeling that I had to do something worthwhile, so cancer nursing was to be my contribution. I can remember my very first weeks working as a nurse. I would comb the halls looking for cancer patients. I found great comfort in this for a while but soon it was too much for me. I began seeing myself in the bed. I wondered how I would die. I found it hard to distance myself because I thought no one could take care of these patients the way I did. I believed I had the power to keep them alive. Patients saw something different in my care; I sat and listened; I gave information about tests and explanations for care.

Limited and frustrated as an LPN, I knew what I had to do. In order to do more for patients I had to get my R.N. So I made another bargain with God. I was smarter this time. This bargain didn't have a time limit. I just asked for my R.N. In the early 1970s, I took an office job with my medical doctor and applied to Norwalk Community College. I received my A.D.R.N. in 1975. Working full time and attending school full time was quite an experience but I loved every minute of it. I also learned a lot about medicine. Dr. Falsone was a great teacher and saw me as a good student.

I was still visiting cancer patients on special request but I wasn't working as a cancer nurse. My presence was the help I was offering and I learned that sometimes that is what is needed. Some visits to patients were very painful learning experiences for me. I said too much one time and the patient complained to her doctor: I remember he screamed at me. I barely slept that night worrying about what I had done. It took me a long time to realize it wasn't only what I had done, it was the doctor's error also. He had shared information with me that he had not shared with his patient. This was a real lesson in the skill of providing information. Getting feedback from patients is so important. It is important to check and recheck for what is undertstood and what is heard. Dealing with this was hard. I realized I needed to learn more about this communication game. I attended any and all programs for nurses that involved taking care of cancer patients.

At one meeting I met the executive director of the American Cancer Society, Southern Fairfield County Unit, Justine Perry. I expressed my wish to do something for the American Cancer Society and along with millions of other Americans I developed the addiction of volunteerism. You feel so good about yourself. I have been a volunteer for over 25 years, serving as chair of the nursing committee and the service and rehabilitation committee. I became one of the first facilitators of the first patient support group in Connecticut. I can still remember the training sessions with Hank Mandell and Michele Webber, from the Center for Death, Dying, and Bereavement in New Haven. Both were social workers. Hank was an adjunct professor at Yale. This is where I met Tish Knopf and she helped me to see that I had more to offer than just my personal experiences. She saw in me something I had not been able to see. A light went off when I realized my experience led me to nursing but my talent kept me there.

My first group experience was an experience. I had to fight with the doctors about the group. They feared patients would compare notes. I learned early on that not just anyone can facilitate a group because the control is not in our hands but in the hands of our patients. They can choose if they want to hear us, if we have been helpful or if we have said the wrong thing. I have continued to lead a support group for nearly 25 years.

I don't wonder anymore how I made it through those first groups; I know I prayed a lot. But God alone wasn't my only help; I counted on the Oncology Nursing Society. It was at the annual meetings that I began to build my knowledge base. When I was in nursing school there was no cancer nursing curriculum. I had to rely on articles from the *Oncology Nursing Forum*, round table discussions, research reports, and my peers.

I decided to leave the safety of the doctor's office and applied for the position of cancer nurse clinician at Norwalk Hospital. I would be working with my oncologist which was risky but I would also be working with an oncology nurse. I was to start work in September of 1978. That March, Melinda Cade and I began to talk about what we thought oncology nursing was. To my surprise we felt the same way. We were also attending the same university and in some of the same classes. I was elated to have found a colleague who thought about cancer nursing in the same way I did. This was really going to be the turning point for me. She was the kind of nurse that I would like to have take care of me. I was excited about my new role, but at the same time I was scared. I knew I'd have to prove what I had been talking about. I'd have to be as good as I said cancer nurses should be and deal with my high expectations. Although I was afraid I would fail, patients loved me: I was great at instilling hope and confidence and could explain what treatment was really like, but I had no experience as a cancer nurse. Melinda and I became partners. We learned that working together successfully was the result of some very hard work. In 1978 I received the ACS Courage Award for the State of Connecticut. I was the second recipient ever. The first recipient, Mark Santangelo, lost his leg to osteogenic sarcoma and was a skier and a golfer. I felt inferior to him and the award had an unsettling effect on me. I felt guilty about surviving. I wasn't dying and living was great. I didn't know at the time that surviving cancer meant that living should be great. I was being honored for my work on behalf of cancer patients. When I received the award, I was given a standing ovation. I realized for the first time that I deserved to be applauded. I survived cancer and managed to turn it into a positive experience. My second chance at life was a gift, and it had taken me all this time to accept myself.

Prior to the award, I had not felt well and I continued to feel that something was going on. Melinda and I were studying for a chemistry exam one night and I started getting chest pains. I asked her if she remembered how to do CPR. She couldn't count my pulse and I couldn't breathe. A sense of doom came over me. I thought, "What if this is the end and I spent it studying for a chemistry exam?" I wanted to go to Bloomingdales but instead Melinda called an ambulance. I guess I had confused her by yelling for help and then saying I didn't want to go to the hospital in an ambulance. Melinda called my oncologist and my doctor and they all arrived at the same time. I had postradiation-induced pericarditis and myocarditis. When I got to the hospital, besides wondering about the number of people accompanying me, they asked me for some data, hooked me up to a monitor, and admitted me. I rationalized this event as a payment for my survival. They didn't really think it was related to the cancer treatment. This complication wasn't described in the literature yet. I went through a lot of guessing games because medicine had not caught up with the treatment side effects of Hodgkins disease. In the 1980s, Vincent DeVita presented a 10-year follow-up study outlining the long-term side effects of treatment, but this information was not yet widely disseminated. I remember when I became hypothyroid from the treatments, I had to convince the endocrinologist that this in fact was a risk associated with treatment for Hodgkins disease. To this day when he makes this diagnosis on a patient with a prior history of radiation therapy for Hodgkins disease, he gives me credit for his knowledge.

In the fall of 1978 I said my goodbyes and left the safety of Doctor Falsone and the patients who came to love me as much as I loved them. I had to leave. I began my career officially as a cancer nurse. I attended my first Oncology Nursing Society Congress in 1979. What an experience; I was overwhelmed. I think I attended every lecture I could feasibly cram into a day. I asked so many questions of the presenters. I was so exhilarated and renewed. I still get this feeling year in and year out. I have only missed one Congress since then due to illness. It was at the ONS Congress that I learned for the first time that cancer nursing was alive and flourishing. I was not alone as a cancer nurse. I learned that although these nurses didn't have cancer, they knew exactly how I felt. I saw an opportunity to use my experience better. I knew there were very few cancer patients that were cancer nurses and I was ready for the challenge.

From 1978 to 1982 I worked at Norwalk Hospital. I gave it my all, but it turned out to be a very difficult experience for me. As I learned to be a cancer nurse, I had to find a way to weave being a cancer patient into my practice in a productive way. The oncology team had enough cancer patients to take care of, they didn't need me with CANCER tattooed on my forehead. I could not bear what I perceived as terrible injustices and deficits in the care of cancer patients. The first time I screamed at a nurse for not medicating a patient, the head nurse on the unit told me I couldn't come there anymore. The head nurse was right. I had to learn that my message was good but the way I was delivering it was awful. My anger at the nurses' inability to treat the patient's pain was my own hurt and I had to get over this if I wanted to make a difference. It was the patient in the bed who was in need of pain management, not me. Mrs. Lopat helped me to learn this and we became great colleagues and great friends. She taught me patience, something you lose along the way being held hostage in waiting rooms.

I worked very long hours and saw patients in their homes. I was beginning to make a difference and see change in the way nurses cared for cancer patients. During this time I was caring for a young man with colon cancer and his family. Lenny and Rose were very angry at the surgeon because they were told after his surgery that all the cancer was removed, but now he had a recurrence. He underwent chemotherapy, but the cancer continued to grow and he became weaker. His reason for being alive was to walk his daughter down the aisle. He was in a great deal of pain and I taught Rose how to give him injections for pain. I continued to make visits to their home to see how they were doing. This was in the early 1980s and there was no hospice. For the first time in my career I learned how to support a patient and a family through a crisis. Their eldest daughter's wedding was coming up and I enlisted the troops to get Lenny strong enough to walk his daughter down the aisle. The next day he experienced a psychotic episode. Rose called me to tell me he was next door because he thought she was poisoning him. I talked Lenny back to the house where he described the letdown in knowing that the one thing that was keeping him alive had taken place. It wasn't too long before Lenny slipped into a coma. The entire family was there to celebrate Lenny's life and derive comfort from the end to his suffering in his death. I thought then and still do that this was a good death—getting one final wish, having your family surround you with love. What a triumph for them and for me.

I was both sad and joyful at Lenny's death. I never worked so hard and loved every moment of it but this was the first of many cases like this. I was learning a lot but I was experiencing burnout. It really got to me and I began to have trouble sleeping. I just couldn't figure out the way to develop a balance. I studied at Sloan-Kettering, Yale, M.D. Anderson, but there was no course to help me with my intense need to do it all. Paul Schulman, M.D., my boss and oncologist, taught me well about cancer and its treatment. We read every X-ray, every slide, and went to the O.R. with as many patients as possible. I attended over two hundred autopsies. I was very sound in my knowledge base and found I knew a lot more than most nurses.

What I hadn't learned yet was how to be a cancer nurse who had experienced cancer herself. During this time I met Connie Engelking at Westchester County Medical Center while studying for my bachelor's at Pace University. She was just beginning her role as clinical nurse specialist. She was so energetic and taught me many things. She became and is still one of my mentors. We talked about taking care of cancer patients. I also was taking a course on death and dying. We wrote a journal for this course. I was always giving everyone credit for my surviving cancer and for my work on behalf of cancer patients. My professor wrote back that I deserved the recognition I received. From then on I graciously accepted my dual role as an oncology nurse and a cancer survivor. In 1982 I went to work at Danbury Hospital and I met Catherine Corbelli who taught me how to give my gifts to my patients. I came to her burnt out and worn out. She worked the pants off me and I never experienced burnout again. I learned how to teach other nurses to care for cancer patients. This was the key to really feeling like I was using my experience to help others with cancer. The more cancer nurses I could train the better the care would be. I developed competency-based training programs utilizing the Oncology Nursing Society standards of care. I worked at Danbury from 1982 through 1987 when Cathy left to come to Bridgeport Hospital. I had developed the staff of the cancer unit and was so proud to be a part of that team. Cathy asked me to come to Bridgeport. Although I had mixed feelings, I loved working with her and I packed up five years of cancer nursing materials and headed for Bridgeport. At Bridgeport Hospital, I met Susan Fisher. We became great friends and great colleagues. Learning from each other, respecting each other's gifts. After several years, Susan began to notice that I could no longer keep up with her. She was my exercise guru and watched over me during aerobics class. She taught me the value of exercise as a stress reducer. What she didn't know was that I was never awake. She made me go to the 6 A.M. class. I knew there would come a time when I would have to deal with the side effects of my therapy and it had almost escaped my awareness because during this time my mother-in-law was diagnosed with lung cancer in Florida. It couldn't have come at a worse time in my life. I was finishing up my thesis in graduate school. I knew I had to put it on hold and take care of her. We put a hospital bed in our living room where all the activity was, in front of a bright picture window. She loved it. She had wonderful care. I used to call her "Mrs. Astor from the Pain in the Astors," but I couldn't have asked for a better patient. She had a wonderful sense of humor as do I and we got on famously.

I learned a valuable lesson from this experience. Now I had to be the daughter-in-law, not the cancer nurse nor the cancer patient. It was very hard and very frustrating. I used to tell families how wonderful it was to take their loved ones home to die. I'm not too quick to say that anymore. It is wonderful but very hard on everyone concerned and you really need a lot of support and help. It has to be a family decision. Her friends showered her with flowers and company until the day she died. I learned a valuable lesson from Lucy. Sooner or later we will all experience something we thought was entirely different. Her death left me feeling empty for a while.

I finally completed my masters degree in nursing from Western Connecticut State University. Working at Bridgeport Hospital has been the best part of my career. The oncologists—Drs. Rosman, Folman, Malefatto, Berger, Kopelson, and Dunbar—and support team demonstrate to me every day why I survived. I have had the opportunity to be a part of the training for a wonderful group of nurses. I have come of age; practicing as an oncology clinical nurse specialist has allowed me the privilege of so many rich experiences. Just when I learned to put the fear of recurrence down a couple of rungs on my ladder, I was diagnosed with atrial fibrillation. I was experiencing heart rates of 300–400 beats per minute. I was exhausted and began to look like that sick person again. My colleagues were whispering and wondering about the status of my health. At this low point, I received a call from Genevieve Foley that I had won the Lane Adams Award, 1991. What a thrill. It made facing the uncertainty more bearable. I had learned to make peace with this concept over the years. After all, life is a terminal illness. My granny had taught me, "Life is grim but not necessarily serious."

I'm a little slower now but I have figured out that I have a *why* to live. As Friedrich Nietzche says, with the why all figured out you can bear almost any how. I had won an award for doing something that I loved. I had finally figured this out. I was happiest when caring for cancer patients and teaching nurses how to care for cancer patients. It took me all these years to realize that I would have done this anyway. Being a cancer nurse is the overall best thing that has happened to me since my cancer diagnosis. Some things late, not never . . .

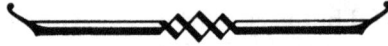

4

Susan B. Baird

In February 1994 I received a letter from the Oncology Nursing Society: "I am pleased to announce that you have been selected to receive the 1994 Linda Arenth Excellence in Nursing Administration Award for your contributions to oncology nursing." I was shocked—thrilled but shocked in the most pleasant of ways. Imagine my further shock when I received a second letter from ONS in March 1994 in which ONS President Sandra Schafer related, "Congratulations on being selected to receive the 1994 Distinguished Service Award." There had to be a mistake, I thought, this just could not be. Two prestigious awards in one year. I reached out to phone the ONS national office to double-check but I stopped before dialing. I stopped because a tidal wave of emotion totally knocked me off my moorings and left me awash—relationships, discoveries, initiatives, growth, connections, caring, love, and losses. With tears flowing readily, I felt as though I was being hugged by every patient, nurse, and author I'd ever had the privilege to be with.

How could this unbelievable recognition be coming to me, a nurse for 30 years who has often been asked, "Don't you miss *real* nursing?" My own mother has asked at various points in my career, "Now, what is it you *really* do?" Here is an oncology nurse who has to confess reluctantly that she has never given chemo except at home to a very close friend. Am I a *real* oncology nurse? But, perhaps this is jumping too far ahead. I'm going to back up a bit, about 30 years.

My Roots in Nursing

I came into nursing at a time when girls from middle-class families could be teachers, nurses, or secretaries—at least according to my guidance counselor. Having worked several years as a candystriper under the watchful eyes of the Sisters of Charity who helped me believe that my presence there and the tasks I was assigned (folding diapers, packaging rubber gloves, feeding patients, and "terminally" cleaning units) were totally indispensable to the hospital and the welfare of its patients, I felt fixed on becoming a physician. My parents, although not thrilled about the choice, found it preferable to my entering the convent, a possibility they envisioned being subliminally processed during the hundreds of hours I spent at the hospital. During my junior year at high school, I applied to college under an early admissions program for pre-med, was accepted, and felt so secure while the rest of my friends were waiting midway through their senior year to hear from schools.

I was assigned to the pediatric unit often then (folding diapers and feeding) and witnessed the downward course of Tommy, an eight-year-old with leukemia. Deeply inscribed in my memory of this brave boy and his family is the frustration I saw in his caregivers who knew how little treatment there was to offer then. The frustration is balanced in my memory by how lovingly he was cared for and supported. It is a purple memory—gentian violet was frequently swabbed onto his open lesions, leaving a white and purple body swathed in white and purple bed-clothes. Mention gentian violet, and I see Tommy. It might be nice to say that Tommy helped me make a decision about oncology, but that is not true. I had no idea then what kind of physician I would be. But, perhaps he planted a seed.

Then my guidance counselor again began her chorus about girls from middle-class families. What was I doing to my family? Didn't I want to become a wife and mother? Could I point to one woman physician who was successful as both a physician and homemaker? Remember, it was 1960.

So, I panicked and ran around looking at nursing schools. If I was going to be a nurse, I was going to the best school I could find. "Real nurses go to diploma schools!" I was told, and so I did. I went to The Johns Hopkins Hospital School of Nursing in Baltimore and, although I had some rocky times while I was there, I've never regretted my choice. I think I held some sort of record for calling my trunk up from the storage room; thinking about packing up and leaving was my knee-jerk response to tough times. I squeaked through anatomy and physiology and microbiology but excelled in clinical practice and leadership experiences. Perhaps some messages were there for me even then. During a particularly down time in training (surely everyone has at least one), I wrote a disdainful editorial in the school paper about the down side of nursing. It raised wrath within the nursing school office and my editorial stint was abruptly ended, at least for then.

My three months with the Baltimore City Health Department were my very best experience. We carried our own home-care caseload. Babies in bureau drawers, nipples on Coca-Cola bottles, and taking thermometers outside to read because of nonexistent lighting were commonplace as you fought with the cockroaches for a clean place to put your bag (on newspaper you brought with you, of course). For patients at home with cancer, odor and pain prevailed.

I remember little about oncology at Hopkins; there was no cancer center then, no oncology units. Patients were integrated on the various services and we learned about cancer as one of many diseases within body systems: breast diseases in med-surg and prostate cancer in urology. Patients with breast cancer stand out most in my memory. Most had radical mastectomies; Halsted's classic approach was developed at Hopkins. These women stayed in the hospital for 14 days then! For those who have only seen old pictures of pulleys over doors for exercising and hands gingerly climbing up walls, it may surprise you to know we were right there teaching patients as this was a nursing and not a physical medicine responsibility. The treatment options were still limited and we saw far too many cases of late disease. Cancer as an area of specialization was not in evidence at Hopkins and I don't remember it being of particular importance in our curriculum. That recollection was reinforced several years ago when I sorted through and discarded my class notes from Hopkins. I had moved them from house to house, state to state, along with my textbooks as though the notes or the books had some sacred value. They did not.

I do continue to move a small brown box that contains my nursing caps. They touch the sentimental part of me but, more importantly, they remind me of two deep nursing roots that are Hopkins-bred. One is the nurse's obligation to preserve patient dignity. The other is that Hopkins nurses are trained to lead. You heard both tenets so often that when you graduated you believed the first to the depth of your soul and the second to the core of your intellect. You also knew you were good, *really good*. That confidence of being *really good* faded after a few years, but the memory of it is wonderful. Ask any Hopkins nurse.

Life always seems simpler when looking backward. Hopkins students were frequently engaged as juniors, married right after graduation, boards taken and initial jobs begun, and first babies a year or so thereafter. I followed that path and our small family embarked on a variety of interesting adventures. Nursing was my job and I did it well wherever I went. But, as did many wives at this time, I followed my husband. He had a *career*. I knew I could and did get a job anywhere we went. After the interview, they wanted you to start by the next shift. These were great years to be in nursing and that's where I always was except for a few years running a hotel and owning a guesthouse and then a restaurant. They always told us those diet kitchen experiences would serve some useful purpose!

American Cancer Society

Most of us recognize certain pivotal events in our professional lives and mine has had many. A major one was the American Cancer Society's First National Nursing Conference held in Chicago in 1974. I remember it so well. I was director of inservice education at a small New Hampshire hospital when I got a call from the state division shortly before the conference. "Would you like to fill in for someone who can't go at the last minute?" the woman asked. She told me they would pay my expenses and that they hoped I would "do a little volunteer work" for ACS in return. I was elated at the opportunity and that "little bit of volunteer work" has spanned 20 years, included wonderful associations with the national organization and three divisions, and offered an opportunity to edit the sixth edition (1991) of the *Cancer Source Book for Nurses*. In 1990, I received the Distinguished Service Award of the American Cancer Society. It was a beautiful and deeply moving tribute, an overwhelming demonstration of caring by my colleagues, yet also a constant reminder to me that I have received far more than I have given in these associations.

The Chicago conference was a real turning point for me with two aspects standing out in my mind. One was listening to Virginia Barckley, then head of nursing activities for ACS. This tiny woman, with both hands grasping the sides of the podium as if to help her see over its top, delivered a powerful message about the opportunity for nurses to make a strong contribution to cancer care. Her distinctive voice and wonderful story-telling ability are still with me and I know how privileged I was to have come into cancer nursing during her era and to have benefited from her experience and commitment. The other major event was a luncheon lecture by Dame Cecily Saunders, the driving force behind the development of St. Christopher's Hospice in London. Hospice, as we know it now, was a newly emerging concept then and her presentation of it was so compelling that had she asked for ten volunteers to follow her to London, we would have killed one another trying to get to her side. Attending that conference prompted a definite decision that I would find a way to become more involved in cancer nursing.

Shortly afterward, ACS again offered me an outstanding opportunity. I was to be one of several New Hampshire nurses to go to Memorial Sloan-Kettering (MSK) for its training program. We stayed at the Barbizon Hotel for Women—before it was rehabilitated! It was like being in a dorm; the housemother was ever-present and we were forever being told we were too noisy. We got high on New York cheesecake and the theater, but it was our daily experiences at MSK that were truly unbelievable for nurses from small rural hospitals. We were astounded at the radical surgery being done: hemicorpectomies and radical head and neck procedures were things we had read about, but seeing them was a totally different experience. For some reason, the observational experience in the recovery room stands firm in my memory. I was so impressed with the work the nurses were doing there. I remember thinking, "If they ask me to stay, I just will." They didn't. It was, however, a tremendous experience to be with nurses who were contributing to the early development of cancer nursing as specialty practice, to catch their enthusiasm and dedication, and to benefit from their experience.

I have had more wonderful experiences with the American Cancer Society than I could ever relate here. A special event was the Nursing Research Conference in Hawaii in 1985. I was presenting a paper on my research, entitled "The Effect of Cancer in a Parent on Role Relationships with Nurse Daughters." I had just left the NIH and without good funding, but ACS came through again. The Maryland Division's Nursing Education Committee, under Linda Arenth's leadership at that time, awarded me one of their travel scholarships. ACS's regional representative put me in touch with Graceanne Ehlke, then a doctoral student at Catholic University in Washington, D.C., but Hawaii born and bred. She offered to let me stay with her at her father's house for the conference. One of the most memorable trips and precious friendships I have ever had began with that meeting. Graceanne's life ended just days after the 1992 ACS Research Conference. With Trish Greene's help, I was able to bring Graceanne to the conference for a few hours, a final opportunity to be surrounded by her colleagues and to feel their compassion and love.

Indeed, ACS has been very good to me. I went from a chance attendee at the first national conference to keynote speaker for the Fifth National Conference, and to their award recipient in 1990—a long and wonderful road.

Cancer Administration

Almost every position I have ever had in nursing has come serendipitously and, believe me, I have been the recipient of some excellent serendipity. Not long after that first ACS conference, I was asked to be on the education committee of a large grant at Dartmouth Medical School, the Breast Cancer Network Demonstration Project (BCNDP). Dr. Donald Catino, a local internist on the committee, thought there should be some nursing input, and I credit him for getting me started in a project that eventually turned into a full-time position as education director and, in its last six months, project director. "If money were no object, what could we do to reduce the morbidity and mortality of breast cancer among New Hampshire women?" was the prevailing question the project asked. We may never again work under such a platitude, but the challenge continues. It seems hard to believe today but our major efforts in that grant (1975–1980) were to improve the quality of mammography (few hospitals had dedicated mammography units or radiologists adequately prepared in interpreting them), reduce the number of radical surgeries, and increase the knowledge level of women and their care providers.

That project took me to every nook and cranny of New Hampshire as well as to NIH to give my first major presentation. At home during practice, my speech took thirteen minutes, but I was so nervous I delivered it in about nine and never skipped a word. I also began to commute to Boston for a MPH degree. I knew if I was going to continue in cancer control, I needed a lot more background in research methods and chronic epidemiology. Two-and-one-half hours each way, twice a week, I felt I lived in my car. During this time, I was named to the faculty of the Dartmouth Medical School. As an instructor in the Department of Family and Community Medicine, I helped teach what I was just learning. I was the *first* nurse appointed to the medical school faculty; several others followed.

As the BCNDP began to wind down, I was selected to be the Associate Director for Cancer Control of the Norris Cotton Cancer Center at Dartmouth-Hitchcock Medical Center (DHMC). I had to interview with Dr. Ross McIntyre, then director and at home with a ruptured disk. Imagine sitting in a chair for a very important interview when the person interviewing you is lying on the living room floor in his pajamas! We began a wonderful working relationship initiating projects in cancer control, writing grants, and continuing our outreach education. I had the most wonderful secretary, Vera Bergen. She made so much possible—but more on Vera later.

I was asked to be on the DHMC search committee for a person to direct the development and implementation for New Hampshire's first hospital-based, home-care department. The person would also be an Assistant Director of Nursing at DHMC. I loved the search committee work but got so carried away with the idea of the project that I resigned from the committee and became a candidate. I had worked in home care right after graduation and thought this was every home health nurse's dream—to start an agency from scratch. I felt very reluctant to leave the Cancer Center but knew I would still be involved in a number of ways. Getting things rolling was no problem but I did find it difficult to adjust from oncology to a very diverse patient population. The Home Health Supervisor once said to me, "You know, some people find CHF important." "Important, yes," I replied. "But also boring."

"Could you come to NIH to do some consulting for the Cancer Nursing Service at the Clinical Center, NIH?" That beginning eventually led to my going to the NIH in 1981. Our family was ready for a move from winter and, for the first time, the move was made for *my career*, not my husband's. The Clinical Center was a wild place—the term "government bureaucracy" took on new meaning. I had little patience with the rules, mazes, and paper trails, but I marveled at the staff. I had never witnessed such skilled clinicians and I truly admired their dedication to quality patient care and to oncology research. Given today's financial constraints and challenges, it seems almost impossible to believe that we had only to comply with an FTE quota and a travel and education budget. Supplies and equipment abounded. Construction and redesign were everywhere with wonderful features and furnishings. We had a computerized patient record system that I would give anything for today. If I had patience with the government system, I found I was able to hire wonderful people and build a great team. Judy Spross, Marguerite Donaghue, Barbara Farley, and Joan Piemme were among the "brightest and the best." Judy and Maggie convened the first invitational meeting of oncology clinical nurse specialists. Their efforts resulted in a planning document well used by CNSs across the country. I learned a great deal at the Clinical Center and have very fond memories of working with such dedicated oncology nurses as Kathy Gorell, Rosie Smith, Rachel Brown, Donna Huffer, and Mary Fraser.

The final great serendipitous position I want to include here is my current one, Director of Nursing and Patient Services at the Fox Chase Cancer Center in Philadelphia. Jim Lynch, administrator of the hospital at FCCC and a former colleague from Norris Cotton Cancer Center, called in 1990 and told me they were recruiting for a new director. I knew I was definitely *not* interested; I was already fully and overly committed to the *Oncology Nursing Forum*, editing two books, trying to do a history of ONS, and also being a doctoral student. He pursued and arranged a meeting with Medical Director Bob Comis and himself at a downtown hotel. We had a great meeting but I was very firm about one thing—I was not interested. I told them I would, however, help them with a search. Dr. Comis said, "We've done our search, you are it, now how can we make it happen?" Meeting with the managers and CNSs helped convince me to give this more serious thought—they were tremendous, very knowledgeable, full of energy. Two former medical colleagues from NIH were at FCCC as well, Dr. Robert Young is FCCC President and Dr. Robert Ozols was at that time Chairman of Medicine (and is now Medical Director). I finally reasoned that if they had worked with me in the past and still wanted me, and I had worked with them in the past and knew we could work well together that it had to be a good thing.

I came to Fox Chase in December 1990 and it is a wonderful experience. This is a beautiful facility and, since we treat only cancer, everyone who works here wants to work with cancer patients. It makes a huge difference not to have to compete with other services for space, staff, or focus. The staff is top-notch in every way. Their care is excellent and, in addition, they lecture, publish, accomplish Herculean tasks through committees, participate in research, and have babies. They are very good at having babies! Over the past year, I have been asked to take administrative responsibility for several other departments. This is typical among my administrative colleagues and, far from detracting from nursing, enhances collaboration across disciplines. I could not do all this without the help of a wise and knowing secretary, Wilma Mackle, and the expert contributions of my assistant and colleague, Joanne Hambleton.

When I came to FCCC, I heard that the administrators, finance, and public relations people from NIH-designated comprehensive cancer centers met regularly for networking. "When do the nursing administrators meet?" I asked. "They don't," Jim Lynch told me. "They will," I thought. After a few quick calls to nursing executive colleagues Sharon Krumm at Hopkins and Joyce Yasko at Pittsburgh, the first meeting was scheduled. It started as a half-day, open-agenda meeting and is now an important day-and-a-half meeting held twice a year at rotating sites among cancer centers. Jim's encouragement for that first meeting meant a great deal in setting the precedent for individual centers to sponsor the ongoing meetings that yield so much in terms of information sharing and support.

Oncology Nursing Society

The earliest applications for ONS membership required a letter of reference. I worked hard on my application, hoping I would be accepted as membership was not automatic. Similar to the beginnings of most specialty organizations, initial membership requirements were more exclusionary than inclusionary. It seemed an interminable wait to get that membership card. I was not in the formative group for ONS, nor was I a charter member, but I was in soon thereafter. ONS has been a major and positive force in my professional life ever since.

I attended that first "real" meeting in Toronto (1976) and listened to the initial presentation of the ONS Bylaws by Pearl Moore. Should it be cancer nursing or oncology nursing? Long debate ensued among the early leaders. I attended the meeting in Boston (fall 1976) and heard about the planning for the 1977 Congress in Denver. Tish Knobf from Yale was Congress Chair. Having had experience planning educational efforts through our breast cancer grant, I volunteered to help, never imagining I would actually be asked to do so. Anyone attending a recent ONS Congress has *no* idea of those early ones. Registrations were sent in to a committee member who kept track of the checks for the treasurer, name tags were written by hand, and all handout materials were prepared by the speaker or the committee members themselves.

After the Denver meeting, ONS President Lisa Begg asked me to go to San Diego for ONS and select the hotel for the 1980 Congress. It was like being Queen for a Day—I was escorted around by the Convention Bureau, staying a night here and a night there to try out the major hotels. My family enjoyed free passes to all major San Diego attractions, leaving me to decide what amenities would be most important to the attendees. I fell in love with the Del Coronado, its grandness and history. But it was not convenient and seemed then to run out of hot water at predictable times each morning. I settled on the Sheraton and signed the contract—hard to believe a single member had that much responsibility back then—confident we would never fill the facilities I had booked. We did, and then some.

I served on the Congress Committee for several years, chairing the 1979 Congress in Washington, D.C. We were still doing most everything ourselves. Joan Piemme was the local arrangements person and took care of all the hotel dealings. She also stored all the Congress materials in her garage and we had to lug them over ourselves to the hotel the day before. ONS and DHMC shared the expenses to bring my secretary, Vera Bergen, with me to the Congress. Vera handled registrations and assisted with anything and everything—what a lifesaver! The committee had decided to start commercial exhibits that year. When we were shown the exhibit hall, we were overwhelmed. Nothing ever looked bigger or emptier! I had to tell the manager that what we had in mind was about six tabletop displays, not fire engines and airplanes. Linda Rickell was in charge and had to cajole vendors into coming. One publisher would send a display, but not a sales representative. Linda actually had to unpack the books they sent, take the orders, and repack the materials for return. The exhibit hall as it exists today was not even imaginable! Susan Hubbard wrote all of the name tags for that record crowd of 1,200. Hotel registration was a mess—they had no room for our keynote speaker! But, as is true at most weddings, no one but family knew how it was really supposed to be.

I subsequently served on Congress committees chaired by Connie Yarbro, Jeanne Rogers, and Kay O'Connor. Each chairperson brought her own special touch and addition. When educational exhibits were added in Connie's year, everyone was really naive—the committee for not knowing the attendees would take anything not nailed down (including the one and only copy of the Duke Oncology Nursing Procedure Manual) and exhibitors for bringing their only copies of many materials. But, each Congress was another step forward in meeting development and in providing an opportunity to demonstrate the continuing evolvement of the specialty. Each Congress has had its own tote bag and I had a complete set until recently when I decided they would never become collector's items. Newer Congress Committee members do miss out on one special routine—the collating of handouts and the filling of the bags. Round and round the tables we went, more rounds and more hours each year and now only a memory.

In 1979, I ran for ONS president. Looking back, I don't know how I ever had the courage to do so. I had little national-level experience, but few people had at that point of ONS development. Simultaneously, the ONS board of directors was seeking a journal editor to carry on the fine beginnings of Daryl Maass. No one wanted the job. The board approached my opponent, Connie Yarbro, and myself to see if whoever lost the election would agree to take over the journal. The rest, as they say, is history. During the opening cocktail reception, the nominating committee called us both outside and told us that Connie was the new president. As we convened for the Annual Business Meeting, New Hampshire colleagues brought forth a gorgeous corsage for me to wear while seated at the podium. "But I lost," I said tearily. "You're a winner to us," they replied. Then I really cried.

Both Connie and I have agreed many times that the ONS members knew what they were doing in that vote. Connie was an outstanding president and I found the editorship of the journal the most rewarding experience in my career. I had the good fortune to inherit the journal in its infancy and to grow with it. Early on I made contact with Jannetti, Inc., to handle the journal advertising. Tony Jannetti and his staff have been wonderful friends and supporters of ONS, handling *Oncology Nursing Forum* advertising and Congress display space. Steve Gray, new to Jannetti's then, was our advertising sales rep. He came to editorial board meetings and we developed a long and lasting relationship. I learned so much from Steve and Tony and from their art director, Jean Hernandez. Most of all, I have always felt supported professionally and personally by Tony and Steve as well as by Eleanor, Tony's wife. Tony has sent me flowers more often than any other man in my life! He sent me lovely yellow roses in Cincinnati for my ONS awards; to express her own personal congratulations, Eleanor sent fragrant peach roses a few hours later. These are wonderfully giving and loving people who continue to be special to me even though our work associations through ONS are over. Several years ago, Eleanor was at FCCC for treatment and continues to celebrate her survival through follow-up here. Steve's father, Jim, is currently in treatment here, enabling me to give back some of the caring they have all shown me.

How do you convey the essence of *Oncology Nursing Forum*'s development in the 11 years I was editor (1979–1990)? I will never do justice to the devotion of its reviewers and editorial board members, the dedication of its authors, or the continued support from ONS board members and committee chairs. There were lots of victories—from quarterly to six issues a year, from saddle-stitched to perfect binding, from almost no advertising to a very healthy advertising picture—each a hurdle. Our early editorial board meetings were held in Etna, New Hampshire, at Moose Mountain Lodge, a tiny piece of heaven where ideas were as abundant as the home-baked bread and fires in the hearth. We walked to the huge working beaver dam for inspiration and drove down the mountain to the Dartmouth Printing Company to see how and where "our" journal was printed and shipped. I can still picture Bobbie Scofield sitting in the kitchen exchanging recipes with our innkeeper.

In the early years, I did the whole journal, from overseeing the review process to laying out the pages. I used to say, "If you liked paper dolls as a child, you'll love layout." At first I did it at the kitchen counter, and then moved to better office space as the journal and my time grew with it. I was helped for many years by Exa Murray, one of the best secretaries in the whole world. She was as devoted to the journal as anyone could be; nothing I asked of her was ever too much. When the operations end of the journal moved to the ONS office in Pittsburgh, Exa's work with the journal was ended, but our friendship remains. She is indeed one of the most beautiful people I have worked with.

There is no way I can begin to mention any one editorial board member without doing injustice to the number I can't mention but who will always be in my heart. Every success for the journal came from their dedication to the needs of its readers. They worked unbelievably hard to be creative and practical in their features and in looking ahead to the information demands of oncology nurses everywhere. Starting the *ONS NEWS* was another special achievement, intended to move the news of the organization out of the journal, reaching members more often, and perhaps (we hoped, we prayed) increasing our chances of getting into *INDEX MEDICUS*. This final goal was achieved after several attempts, assuring increased accessibility and prestige. The announcement was celebrated poolside during a blistering hot Arizona meeting of board and committees. The newsletter, meanwhile, has developed into a wonderful communication of its own under the great leadership of Karen Hassey Dow and now Brenda Nevidjon.

The *Oncology Nursing Forum* arrived at my house in 1979 in one small cardboard carton. It left in two stages: first in a moving van to Pittsburgh when the operations shifted to Annette Sullivan. It was hard to give up those big-girl paper dolls and all that went with them, but I guess it was time and I respected her experience and commitment to quality. I liked working with Annette, Vicki, and their great crew but, nonetheless, it was very sad. The final move of the journal came in 1990—some going to Pittsburgh and the rest to Rose Mary Carroll-Johnson in California, the new editor.

The *Oncology Nursing Forum* will always be with me. The journal remains in thoughtful gifts I have received from the editorial board and staff over the years, in the tremendous ONS staff, in a wonderful scrapbook of letters from editorial board members, in two commemorative resolutions, and in a beautiful glass and wood tribute from the board of directors. Just this past year, the writing awards were retitled to include my name—an overwhelming tribute. There are also wonderful memories of editorial board meetings and connections with absolutely the best people—their work, their lives, their babies, and their graduations. It remains in memories of sharing the pleasure of new authors as they see their work develop into a polished product. What makes *ONF* such a wonderful collage of memories for me is that I have never had even the slightest of regrets about passing on the helm. I enjoy the journal's continuing development and marvel at its value as a resource and as a reflection of the continued emergence of oncology as a nursing specialty. I know in my heart-of-hearts that it was time and that it was good.

Sharing Experiences

Three major routes for sharing my experiences in cancer nursing have been writing, lecturing, and networking. I am a better editor than writer, I think, but I have had good opportunities to convey my thoughts in the literature. Writing editorials for the *Oncology Nursing Forum* gave me frequent opportunity to climb on my soapbox. I got tremendous feedback on my editorials and was well repaid for the agony I often went through in their creation by the comments that they had proven useful to others, having been posted or quoted elsewhere. My first book, *Decision Making in Oncology Nursing*, was part of a series on decision making. The physician series had been in existence for quite some time, but the nursing series was a new idea. The book was to be totally comprised of decision trees. Each chapter was two pages—one the tree and one the explanatory notes. I chose nurses who really knew their symptom management but it is impossible to imagine the challenge of condensing their vast knowledge into the key points on the tree. I credit them all for their perseverance; Judy Spross, Joan Piemme, Maggie Donoghue, and Debbie Mayer were among those creative people.

Working with Ruth McCorkle and Marcia Grant on *Cancer Nursing: A Comprehensive Textbook* was somewhat like climbing a mountain in the dark with bare feet, but we have been a great working team and managed never to all be down at the same time. The first edition won an *American Journal of Nursing* Book of the Year Award and each hard-working author deserves part of the prestige.

I have enjoyed helping others with their writing through workshops and one-on-one consultation. I enjoy helping people who don't even ask for or want my help. My staff knows I never read anything without editing as I go. They take it with good humor or at least they humor me into thinking so. I believed for a long time I could only write with a #3 Ticonderoga pencil and a new white-lined pad. Now, don't ask me to write anything longer than two sentences without a word processor.

Being on the lecture circuit off and on for several years has resulted in adventures that could be their own book. I once arrived for a three-day conference with suits picked up at the cleaners on the way. Imagine my dismay to find I had jackets but no skirts! I once got settled on a plane to Los Angeles only to have the pilot talking about arrival time in Ontario as we taxied down the runway. As we soared upward, I steeled myself not to get unnerved. Calmly I asked the cabin attendant where the plane was headed. "Don't you know?" she gasped. Then I learned Ontario was a smaller airport outside of Los Angeles. I once left my speech in the seat pocket when I deplaned.

I always put a small clock on the podium when I speak because I tend to talk fast but have a lot I want to include. I've left countless clocks on hotel podiums in most major cities of the United States. Speaking has taken me almost everywhere—there are only five states where I have not spoken. When I do those, I'm retiring. I think I've spoken in every town in Ohio with more than two nurses, but Ohio folks are always very good to me and it is sort of like a second home. I've met some of the most wonderful nurses in the whole world on speaking engagements and had fascinating adventures. On one trip to the University of Iowa, we got stranded because of storms. I ended up going home with a young dentist and his wife, spending the night with them after all of us had dinner at the house of another stranded physician. Of course the dentist called the Program Chair where I had spoken to have her verify that this was Iowa and it was indeed safe. On another trip, I had a couple of days at a Montana horse ranch at a time I needed the rest the most.

A few trips were extremely special. Tish Knobf arranged for me to speak at the European Cancer Nursing Conference in the Netherlands. What a treat! From there I went to London to do some consulting for the Royal College of Nursing's oncology newsletter. They said they were not able to pay me but asked what they could do. I asked them to arrange time for me at St. Thomas with the Nightingale memorabilia (this was premuseum). My nurse-cousin Jane, who was living in London at the time, accompanied me on this wonderful historical exploration, followed by lunch with student nurses from Guys Hospital. I have never felt closer to the roots of our profession than I did in the Nightingale chapel.

Through a wonderful continuing education/travel program, I had trips to Russia, China, and Switzerland. As education director for each of these trips, I got to choose a teaching companion. Imagine the sheer ecstasy of calling someone and saying, "How would you like a two-week expense paid trip to ———?" Judy Spross went with me to Russia. Having dreamt about the trip for so long, we stood on Red Square that first morning asking each other over and over, "Is this real? Are we actually standing here?" On my first trip to China, I asked Connie Yarbro to go and tactfully tried to tell her that we would probably be without amenities (irons, curling irons, etc.), since China was then not used to tourists, and that she would have to be prepared to dress casually and look less than great. I have to tell you that Connie looked terrific, as always, everywhere she went. Our visits were extremely successful; we were so welcomed by the Chinese wherever we went. Want a really great trip? Have Jeanne Rogers and Pat Klopovich go along. They added tremendously to every aspect of my first China trip. Jeanne could win an award for the "most complete suitcase." She had everything—even printed tissue paper to use as gift wrap for a present to our tour guide. To Switzerland and later on a second trip to China, Pearl Moore was the second instructor. Eager for a special Swiss confection, we convinced the tour guide it was Pearl's birthday (it was not) and were rewarded with a marvelous cake. In China we both fought intestinal problems and found that under pressure we could lecture on each other's subjects. Whoever could stand up, get dressed, and show up gave the talk! I know many other oncology nurses had similar opportunities and adventures with these travel tours and we share unbelievable experiences we will never forget.

Finally, the opportunities to network about issues of common concern and to profit from one another's experiences is perhaps the most valuable part of specialty nursing. Sometimes I think about the hundreds of wonderful nurses I know and realize that had I never ventured into this specialty and gotten involved in so many ways over time, my life would be far emptier. I am a person who takes real pleasure in the growth and accomplishments of others. I like to see people rewarded. I like to see people get in touch with the resources they need, whether it is locating an oncology nurse close to where a relative needs help, or a letter of reference. I don't know, for example, how many letters of reference or support I have written for people for their school applications, positions, promotions, grants, or awards. I love to do them because it is such a simple way to pay back the many kindnesses people have shown me throughout my own career.

Summing It Up

Oncology nursing has been very, very good to me. I have had opportunities I could only have imagined and adventures that have made my life fuller and richer. I have been recognized for many achievements, but I also live with some sadnesses. I was chosen to write a history of the Oncology Nursing Society and put in a tremendous effort to do the necessary research and develop a workable framework. I have been unable to pull it all together and it is a very deep sense of failure that I carry for that despite a very benevolent response from the ONS board of directors. I began a doctoral program in the History and Sociology of Science, intending to focus on nursing history by looking at the work of cancer nursing and how it has or has not been influenced by technological advances. I did some great beginning work and enjoyed the challenge of changing fields at the doctoral level. I was helped tremendously by an American Cancer Society Doctoral Scholarship. I had to opt out of the program at the master's level and try to find solace in the fact that I learned a lot, that I enjoyed what I learned, and that I can pick it up again formally sometime, maybe.

I have had tremendous support from family and friends throughout my career. I have a great group of nurse friends who vacation together—Judy Spross, Joan Piemme, Mavis Ferguson, Alice Longman, and Shirley Girouard. We find renewal in our adventures together and love and support that continue throughout the year. Some of us talk of retiring together. We will read all the journals we never quite got to and compare our CVs. We will wonder if it was all worth it and whether indeed we did make a difference through our individual practices and contributions. I will quit asking if I was a "real" oncology nurse and be content that my life in nursing was abundantly rich and bountifully blessed. It should be more than enough.

5

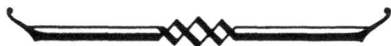

Jeanne Q. Benoliel

As I begin this story, I am in the second month of my 74th year. A lot of changes have taken place during my 56 years as a nurse. As I think back, I realize that my life in nursing consists of many interlocking stories and themes.

Early Life

Born into a Navy family in 1919, I spent the first 18 years of my life in San Diego. I was not one who "always wanted to be a nurse" but made the decision during my last year of high school. In 1938 I enrolled for study in a hospital school of nursing in San Francisco. This was my first time being away from home, and I went through a period of terrible homesickness.

When I began nursing, specialization was defined in functional terms (teacher, supervisor) and in clinical fields (tuberculosis, mental illness) for which patients were sent to special hospitals often located on the outskirts of town. In those days the work of nurses in hospitals centered on hygiene and comfort measures for patients in combination with carrying out medical orders for treatment. In the hospital where I trained, the bulk of nursing care was given by students, and the work included assignments, often alone, on the evening and night shifts. My first assignment on nights occurred soon after capping. I can recall being very afraid that I might make a mistake.

I completed my program of studies in the fall of 1941, passed the state board examination for the R.N. license, and became a staff nurse at the San Diego County Hospital. Shortly after I began work, the bombing of Pearl Harbor took place. I worked at the tuberculosis pavilion for 20 months before returning to school to work toward a degree mainly because I had a scholarship to be used before the end of 1943. At that time the pressures on young nurses to enroll in the military were great. After one quarter of study at UCSF Berkeley, combined with part-time evening work in a local hospital, I enrolled in the Army Nurse Corps in October 1943. I spent 21 of my 27 months of army duty in the South Pacific on the islands of New Guinea, Biak, and Luzon.

After the War I went to college, supported by the G.I. Bill of Rights, and was awarded a B.S. in Nursing Education in 1948. In retrospect, I wonder if I would have returned to school without that financial support. I was not a nurse who was "dedicated" to nursing. Like the majority of women of my generation, I was committed to the idea that work was something women did until they married and had a family.

In 1948 I became an instructor at a hospital school of nursing in Fresno, California, where I remained for five years. On my first day at work I was told that I would be teaching a course, Drugs and Solutions, starting the next day. That assignment pushed me into a rapid self-study program—to stay ahead of the students. Fortunately, math was not a problem area for me, but it certainly turned out to be the case for many students.

A Decade of Change

In 1949 I married. In 1951—during the week of our second wedding anniversary—I became aware that something was wrong with my husband. I was unable to communicate with him. The doctor diagnosed the problem as paranoid schizophrenia. Without much money, I faced the painful task of having him committed to a state mental hospital where he was in and out several times over the next two years.

At the time of diagnosis and commitment proceedings, I was so upset that I had trouble eating. In six weeks I lost 30 pounds, and in so doing, became aware of having lumpy breasts. In fantasy I could see myself having to have bilateral mastectomies. I was so frightened that it took me two weeks to make an appointment for a check-up. I cannot remember whether I was told I probably had fibrocystic disease. But that experience started me on a regimen of monthly breast self-exams and yearly examinations by a surgeon.

In 1953 I chose to leave my marriage out of a feeling that I slowly was being destroyed. In 1954 I enrolled for graduate study in nursing at UCLA, receiving the M.S. degree in 1955. During that year of graduate study, I moved into depression (I am sure in the aftermath of leaving my husband) and began therapy—thanks to a discerning and sensitive teacher (not in nursing, I might note).

I joined the faculty of the UCLA School of Nursing in 1955 and stayed there for four years. During that period, my youngest sister died unexpectedly of a brain hemorrhage (1956) while eight months pregnant with her fourth child. In 1957, my mother had gall bladder surgery, and in July of 1958 my father died of stomach cancer. I often thought that my father never recovered from my sister's death. It seemed to be one of the factors triggering his own dying.

Just two months prior to my father's death, I went for a regular breast check-up. I had noticed no changes myself, so I almost went into shock when the surgeon said, "I think we ought to do a biopsy." I was really scared and phoned my mother for support. Heavily involved in caring for my dying father at home, she cut me off sharply, saying that everything would be all right. Later I could understand her inability to be supportive, but at that particular time I needed something she could not give.

The biopsy was performed in a hospital in Santa Monica, and the diagnosis of fibrocystic disease was confirmed. But what I mainly remember is the terrible feeling of wondering if I would wake up without a breast. That experience had a powerful effect on me, and I am sure it served as a stimulus to my growing interest in understanding how people adjusted to what I called mutilating surgeries.

While all of these changes were happening in my personal life, I found myself becoming bored with the everyday tasks of faculty life. I enjoyed teaching and especially the RNB students, many of whom resented having to return to school. Yet teaching alone was not enough. Fortunately, an opportunity arose for me to enroll in an experimental research training program for nurses, conducted at UCLA for two years (1959–1961). That choice initiated my movement into a research career.

A Shift into Research

My two years in the experimental research training program were important for two reasons. I was introduced to the language and procedures of research and statistics, with emphasis on physiological studies. I was provided the oppportunity to write a proposal to study the adjustment processes of women during the first year after mastectomy. Ironically, I was stimulated as well to ponder whether I wanted to stay in nursing, study for a Ph.D. in neurophysiology, or work as a statistician.

The mastectomy proposal was submitted to NIH through the School of Nursing at UCLA. In 1961 we learned that the study had been approved and funded by the National Institute of Mental Health. I had just taken a position as statistician in the School of Public Health. Shortly after, I found myself holding a dual research appointment in both schools, and faced with the enormous task of implementing the research plan.

The mastectomy study (1961–1963) was a turning point in my

professional career. Through it I began a journey into the intellectual world of social science in combination with the everyday world of women struggling to make sense out of their changed lives. Through it I also met Anselm Strauss who invited me to join him in San Francisco on a sociological investigation of dying patients and hospital personnel. During those five years I learned a great deal about field research under his mentorship. I began to be known in nursing and other fields for my writings about the impact of death, dying, and life-threatening illness on patients, families, and nurses.

My experiences in these two areas of research taught me much about the realities of doing research and the political nature of team relationships. These experiences contributed a great deal to my development as an autonomous person, but not without pain—as I have described in some detail elsewhere (Schorr & Zimmerman, 1988). These experiences also influenced me to obtain a doctoral degree—the so-called "ticket to the union" to remain in academic life.

It is worth noting that, though interested in what I was doing, I was not committed to nursing on a 24-hour-a-day basis. Rather, I was involved in many kinds of social and community activities and with many different people who were not in the health care business. I was still committed to finding the right man to marry and hoped to have children (but only if I married by the age of 40). In both Los Angeles and San Francisco I met a lot of fascinating people and had a lot of exciting adventures.

Movement into Oncology Nursing

My entry into oncology nursing was through the mastectomy study, but the process was far from easy. I was new to the field of research and was not well grounded in any theoretical foundations. Despite very good help from Lucille Agee who collected data with me and from Harold Garfinkel, a consultant on methods, I found the experience carried many unanticipated consequences. I had to give almost continuous attention to interpersonal relationships among many different people whose actions could jeopardize the success of the study. I might note that the women who consented to participate posed fewer communication problems for us than did physicians and nurses. In 1961 it was not uncommon to hear physicians say, "Whoever heard of a nurse doing research?"

I had to make many decisions about protocols, procedures, and personnel for which I was not prepared, and I made some mistakes along the way. I often had the sense that I did not know what I was doing, and I felt at times like a lost soul in the wilderness. Like many of the pioneers in oncology nursing, I learned the trade in a context of social isolation—one reason being that nursing research was very much in its infancy, and oncology nursing was not yet born.

Yet the completion of the study brought a tremendous feeling of personal achievement. The mentorship of Anselm Strauss was a significant contributor to the successful completion of the project. Under his direction I learned much about the ways and means of analyzing these data. Between 1962 and 1965 I published six articles based on the results in medical and nursing journals. At the same time we began to publish articles from the dying patient study, and thereby my work became known to other nurses.

The publications from both studies triggered many invitations to give papers, conduct workshops, and provide consultation. The most common request was concerning nursing care for dying patients. During that time I provided consultation to the Veterans' Administration, M.D. Anderson Hospital in Houston, and Ellis Fischel State Cancer Hospital in Missouri, among others.

On the trip to Houston in 1968 I met Renilda Hilkemeyer and learned about her tireless effort to make continuing education in cancer nursing available to all nurses. At the VA Hospital in San Francisco I had my first meeting with Cicely Saunders in 1965. In 1969 at the Ellis Fischel interdisciplinary conference, I met Elizabeth Kübler-Ross, also on the program, in the hotel coffee shop as we watched a snowstorm in progress outside. Over the next 20 years I worked with these three talented women on several occasions as influential networks of oncology nurses and "death people" began to develop.

Some of my invitations pertained directly to the study of women's adjustment postmastectomy. Presentations based on these data were given at ANA conventions in 1962 and 1964 (the latter focused on the problems of the women and the nurse researchers) and at an AMA convention in 1965. Although my primary responsibilities at UCSF were research-related, I guided one or two nursing students who were interested in breast cancer in independent studies. I also made presentations from the study at several seminars on oncology nursing held in 1963 and 1964. Attending one of these seminars was Jo Craytor, and I was much impressed with her efforts to develop a combined teacher–clinician role in oncology nursing at the University of Rochester. I imagine we probably talked about the social isolation we felt as we struggled to create new roles that made many other people uncomfortable.

Between 1966 and 1970 I participated actively on the nursing education subcommittee of the Professional Education Committee of ACS, California Division. We initiated several programs for nurses with emphasis on effecting change. During that same time period I met Jean

Johnson, probably at the ANA National Research Conference in 1969. Because we were both pioneers in nursing research, our paths crossed fairly frequently through membership in the ANA Council of Nurse Researchers and attendance at research meetings.

Between 1967 and 1969 my research interests shifted to diabetes mellitus. My dissertation research was focused on the process whereby adolescents with juvenile-onset disease establish an identity as "diabetic." After graduation, I took a faculty position at UCSF and used that year to develop and offer a course called "The Threat of Death in Clinical Practice." Ironically, the course was in progress at the time of the shootings by national guardsmen at Kent State during protests by students about the Vietnam War. This experience in teaching confirmed my belief that helping nurses learn how to deal with death-related issues required experiential as well as intellectual learning opportunities.

In the midst of these many professional changes, I met Bob Benoliel in 1964, and we married on Valentine's Day in 1970. That summer we moved to the state of Washington where I joined the faculty at the University of Washington.

Putting Things Together

With this move I went from the relatively quiet life of a research faculty position into full-time faculty life, and all of the stresses and strains of performing well in three different areas—research, instruction, and community service. To add to the complexity, I agreed to become chair of one of the new departments when the School of Nursing was reorganized by Dean Madeleine Leininger. Over the next five years, I (and many other faculty) felt overextended as we struggled to work within these new structural arrangements while at the same time engaging in curriculum revisions and efforts to gain approval for a doctoral program.

At that time I was involved in many research-centered activities with national nursing organizations (ANA, ANF). Through invitation I participated in many workshops, conferences, and consultations dealing with cancer, death, and caregiving issues. I found these trips out of town a pleasant relief from the stresses and strains of everyday faculty life. They also provided me opportunities to meet with people who were involved in cancer nursing research, such as Gerry Padilla at City of Hope Medical Center and Barbara Given at Michigan State University.

In 1972 I gave a paper on the concept of care for the child with leukemia, published in *Nursing Forum* in 1974. Because of the ideas in that paper, Ruth McCorkle was stimulated to meet with me at the ACS First National Conference on Cancer Nursing in 1973 and to discuss the focus of her dissertation research. In 1975 Ruth joined the faculty at UW, and we began a period of collaboration in the broad area of psychosocial oncology, formally ending with her move to the University of Pennsylvania in 1986.

The first ACS National Conference on Cancer Nursing was important for me in yet another way. I was asked to give a paper focused on pain. Why I was asked to do so was never clear to me as pain was not my acknowledged area of expertise. But the opportunity led to my writing a paper in collaboration with Dorothy Crowley (whose expertise was in pain), an endeavor that was a highly rewarding professional experience. Published originally in the proceedings of the ACS Conference, that paper has been reprinted several times over the years. From feedback, I learned that it stimulated the thinking of a number of nurses and physicians.

During my first year at UW I initiated a new course, Death Influence in Clinical Practice, that was offered as an elective for any graduate student. Later, when Ruth and I created the Transition Services option in community health nursing, the course became a requirement for those students.

Because of my belief that students learn about the meanings of death out of experiences that bring them face-to-face with their own concerns, I gave a lot of time and energy to teaching the course. In addition to arrangements for a variety of community assignments, I made a concerted effort to be sensitive to the feelings and reactions of students. I used written dialogues to allow them opportunities to write about thoughts they could not share in class. And I made myself available for personal conferences as they wished.

I taught the course for 20 years at UW. Most of the students were nurses, but occasionally there were students from psychology, education, or medicine. Teaching it was very hard work. Each year brought together a group of people with different patterns of interaction and openness, and some groups were harder to teach than others. The process of trying to offer an intellectual challenge in combination with emotional support took a lot of energy, and I often left class rather depleted. Yet teaching the course was one of the truly rewarding experiences of my professional life. According to a number of former students, the course was a highly influential educational experience and refocused their ideas about caregiving issues in practice, as well as their personal concerns about death.

Teaching the course in the summer of 1974 was a particularly challenging experience for me. Early that summer I learned that a good friend was diagnosed with Alzheimers at the age of 52. Midway through the course my mother died following a stroke. I shared some of my experience in relation to my mother's dying in discussion in class. I think it was helpful to some students, upsetting to others. That summer I really felt down a lot.

Transitions and Collaboration

After Ruth McCorkle came to UW, we initiated a program of research through small studies focused on developing instruments for studying what we saw as major clinical concerns for cancer patients—symptom distress and enforced social dependency. Because I was well established and tenured, we agreed that it would be to Ruth's advantage to be PI on the research proposal submitted to the division of nursing (funded 1979–1981). This was the first of several research grants that got us into all of the complexities and communication difficulties that go along with work being done by people from different disciplines and with different ideas about what to do, why, and how. These studies also made possible the employment of nursing doctoral students as research assistants, many of whom learned a lot about the realities of research from watching us in operation.

Soon after Ruth arrived, we began work on a framework to guide a master's level program to prepare nurses for leadership in the creation of community-based services for advanced cancer patients and their families. We spent a lot of time bringing our ideas together into the transition services framework. I found this activity to be one of the most enjoyable of our efforts together. Over the next few years I learned a great deal about oncology nursing practice from Ruth, who had been a clinical specialist prior to her doctoral work.

We were awarded a training grant from the division of nursing to initiate the Oncology Transition Services program (1977–1980). Yet we were almost blocked from its creation by political infighting among members of the faculty. I must say that Ruth played a pivotal role in gaining support from key faculty members in our department to open up the roadblock.

When I think back on that proposal, I think we should have had our heads examined. In addition to spelling out a curriculum plan, we committed ourselves to preparing a set of videotapes for instructional purposes and to having a full-time evaluation component. Implementing the program meant recruiting students, developing courses, finding physician preceptors, making arrangements with agencies for clinical experiences, and having faculty available for the various essential tasks.

The first cohort of five students entered in 1977. I much admire that first group because they were the recipients of our trial-and-error efforts to get the program going, and they all survived. In the second year the program was facilitated by our employment of Barbara Germino, a new doctoral student, as a teaching assistant, and by Donna Moniz, a FNP who left in 1979 to enter law school. We also employed a sociologist to serve as evaluator on the project. After Fran Lewis joined the UW faculty, she participated part-time with us.

In many ways my experience with the OTS program was something of a mixed blessing. I learned a great deal from those efforts to offer a program dedicated to collegiality and collaboration in the highly competitive work arena known as academia. I was the only tenured member of the faculty group, and the others behaved toward me as an authority person more than as a colleague. Thus communication often was not open, and I learned about some problem situations after the fact. There were other tensions among the faculty relative to teaching strategies, ways of working with students, and personal concerns about making tenure.

The assignment to work with cancer patients at home created stresses and strains for the students, as did the more or less nondirective strategies used for clinical teaching. They were bothered by some family situations they saw. Some wanted explicit direction on what to do. As is often the case, there were a number of conflicts involving faculty and students. I spent a lot of time in conferences with students and/or faculty in efforts to help them work out satisfactory resolutions. There were also certain tensions and conflicts among students, and these also required attention in the interests of effective communication. Some days I gave a lot of effort and energy to being a counselor. Fortunately, I had a husband who understood the emotional energies required for this kind of professional investment.

The positive side of the OTS Program was the reward of observing the professional growth and development of nurses as able clinicians and to see many of them become leaders in hospice nursing and other forms of community-based services. I was also excited at the chance to make basic principles of ethics an integral part of the ongoing program. This step was aided by my participation in 1977 in an intensive bioethics course given by the Kennedy Institute at Georgetown University. A third reward was provided by periodic social get togethers with graduates of the program to exchange news and learn about personal and professional happenings.

At the time we started the OTS program, I was invited to serve on the National Nursing Advisory Committee of ACS. There I renewed my professional contacts with Jo Craytor and Renilda Hilkemeyer and met other oncology nurses who were leaders in administration, clinical practice, and research. Virginia Barckley, nursing consultant at ACS, was one of the admirable people I came to know through those endeavors—a lady with a marvelous sense of humor. This committee consisted of highly productive people who put pressure on ACS to provide guidelines for cancer nursing education at the master's level, provide scholarships for nurses in graduate study, and develop criteria for professorships in oncology nursing. That was an impressive network of people, and I am proud to have been one of them (Benoliel, 1989).

Another whom I admired was Vernice Ferguson who in 1977 invited me and a group of influential nurses to a meeting at the NIH National Center with the chief medical officer of NCI. The purpose was to consider ways and means of making federal funds available for cancer nursing research. I was impressed with Vernice's skills in promoting communication, thoughtful discussion, and movement toward a productive decision. Later I saw her demonstrate the same political sensitivities and skills while serving on the governing council of the American Academy of Nursing and in Sigma Theta Tau.

During these years I was invited to serve on a number of site visits for NCI. I found these to be marvelous opportunities to learn how people in different disciplines approached problems and reached solutions. This experience was very useful when I became coinvestigator on a multidisciplinary NCI contract to implement a cancer prevention course for nurse practitioners and physicians assistants and to evaluate its effectiveness (1979–1982; 1982–1984).

The period between 1975 and 1980 was flawed for me by the progressive pain of arthritis in both hips. I began to use a cane and found that much energy was required just to live on a day-by-day basis. In 1981 I had successful hip surgeries, in February and in May. In September I went to Europe with my husband on a business trip to London, Paris, and Italy. I had served visiting professorships in Israel (1972) and in Japan (1975), but Bob and I had not as yet traveled overseas together. We had a wonderful time.

Connections, Rewards, Separations

I found professional visits to other societies extremely helpful for two reasons. I began to make connections with influential nurses many of whom were interested in oncology nursing. I began to understand how culturally institutionalized values and beliefs about women influenced societal images of nursing and nurses and contributed to obstacles in nurses' efforts to improve the status of nursing. I also was impressed with how much some of these women in nursing could accomplish in their efforts to bring about change.

In the 1980s Ruth McCorkle and I continued our research with support from several federal grants. With help from NCI, we also initiated a research training program in psychosocial oncology for pre- and postdoctoral students (1984–1987) among whom were Letha Lierman, Judith Saunders, and Mel Haberman. At the same time we were awarded another training grant to extend the transition services model to the care of children with cancer as well as adults (1981–1984).

This project was even more difficult than the first because its implementation required the collaboration of faculty in two departments of the school, and schedules did not always fit well together. For a time, the two sets of faculty met in values clarification sessions with a counselor, but these efforts were not completely successful in helping us move toward more open communication. Ironically, the faculty members were not viewed as good role models by many OTS students who saw us as overextended professionally and not very collegial in our working relationships together. Yet, despite our limitations, the students came through this program successfully, and many went on to assume leadership positions in oncology nursing in the community.

My life was even more complicated by the program to create a cancer prevention course for FNPs and PAs and to evaluate both process and outcomes. When the original PI on the contract (a physician in public health) left UW to take a position elsewhere, a political fight ensued to determine who would take over that slot. It brought me into direct confrontation with another physician, relatively new on the project, who assumed he should be the new PI and who treated me and others like second-class citizens. In a private meeting, I reminded him that I was a full professor, did not expect to be treated in a condescending manner by a faculty member of lower rank, and was prepared to file a formal grievance procedure if his actions continued. Fortunately, he left the university shortly thereafter.

In the late 1970s Ruth was very active in the newly created Oncology Nursing Society. She was a leader in bringing into existence the Puget Sound Oncology Nursing Society. I participated to a lesser extent because of my commitments to other organizations and activities. However, I gave many presentations on oncology nursing at local, national, and international meetings.

In 1986 Ruth took a professorship at the University of Pennsylvania. Our research collaboration continued through the completion of the spouse bereavement study (1986–1988), and I took over the directorship of the psychosocial oncology training grant through its termination in 1987. My next research collaboration was with Letha Lierman to study the effects of support on breast self-exam practices of older women. This project (1987–1990) was a gratifying experience because the same team of competent and productive people stayed together for the full three years and had few communication problems.

After Ruth departed UW, I realized that no other faculty members were interested in assuming responsibility for the OTS program. Because I knew I would soon retire, I took steps to make certain that the OTS option for graduate study was eliminated. The faculty liked the framework that we had developed and used it for a new option on Long Term Care. In 1988 the tenth group of OTS students completed their studies and moved on to the world of practice.

In the decade of the 1980s my contributions to oncology nursing were recognized through the Distinguished Service Award given by ACS in 1984 and the Distinguished Merit Award from the International Society for Nurses in Cancer Care in 1988 in London. In 1986 I was privileged to participate in Judy Johnson's slide-tape show about pioneers in oncology nursing. I was honored to share this experience with, among others, Katherine Nelson who offered the first college course on cancer nursing back in 1947. I also was invited to teach a seminar on Research in Psychosocial Oncology in Umea, Sweden, to a multidisciplinary professional group of people who were highly motivated and productive. Later I was told that one nurse taking the course said that the experience changed her life.

At UW I was honored to be appointed the first Elizabeth Sterling Soule Professor, named to honor the founding Dean. I held the title from 1987 until I retired on January 1, 1990. Throughout the 1980s I also was active in organizations and activities related to my interest in death, dying, and bereavement, and in women's issues. But those, of course, are other stories.

In 1989 I was honored to be asked to give the keynote summary address at the ACS First National Conference on Cancer Nursing Research. This invitation allowed me to review the historical events that led to the appearance of cancer nursing research and to see clearly how the connections among influential nurses contributed to the birth of this activity. Reviewing the work of others as well as my own gave me a powerful sense of continuity about the work of oncology nurses who lived through different periods of time but shared a common vision about the care of people. I experience this same sense of continuity when I think about the contributions of my former students.

At the conference in 1989 I received a Special Recognition Award for Leadership in Cancer Nursing, along with Jean Johnson. The most exciting award for me occurred when the Jeanne Quint Benoliel Celebration Day was held at UW on May 15, 1989. Among those planning the celebration were Ruth McCorkle and former students, Lesley Degner and Barbara Germino. During the day, ten former students presented papers describing salient research and/or practice activities, followed by Ruth's summary comments about the influence of my work on nursing and nursing science. In the evening a reception and dinner were held. One of the highlights of that event was a skit in which a former colleague served as JQB and the participating students, dressed as fancy earrings, danced around singing "Wear me. Wear me. Wear me." To appreciate the symbolism of this humorous event, you need to know that I was as well known for my colorful and sometimes outrageous earrings as for my contributions to oncology nursing.

Life Goes On After Retirement

After retirement from UW, I was appointed Professor II at Rutgers in Newark to help in getting a new doctoral program off the ground. Those two years introduced me to east-coast nursing and the depressing effects of living in an inner city ghetto. They also allowed me to renew my working contacts with Ruth McCorkle through consultation at the University of Pennsylvania. But I left that position at Rutgers in 1992 because of my husband's health, and returned to my home in Washington.

Soon thereafter I was invited to join the Ethics Task Force of ONS, an activity that was both enjoyable and productive. It brought me into contact with a new generation of oncology nursing leaders, including Betty Ferrell and Elaine Glass. It resulted in a set of thoughtful papers that focused on different ethical issues relevant to oncology nursing.

In May of 1993 I was honored to receive the Distinguished Researcher Award from ONS and to be given an honorary degree, Doctor of Science, by the University of Pennsylvania for my work in the broad field of loss, death, and bereavement. On the first occasion, in Orlando, I was pleasantly surprised when a woman came up to me and said, "You won't remember me, but I was one of your students at UCLA. Because of you, I became an oncology nurse." On the second, I had the occasion to meet Hillary Rodham Clinton, another recipient of an honorary degree.

As I look back on my life, I am aware that my sister's death was influential in my learning to live one day at a time. I entered into my professional work with the same emotional investment that I used in my personal life, and I enjoyed what I did—even when the experience was painful. In 1990 I received a written commentary from a former student concerning my teaching in the death influence course: "You seem to have a deep calm and peace, and yet to be a skeptic of sorts—quick to question, challenge, and support." I think this description sums me up in a nutshell.

References

Benoliel, J. Q. *From research to scholarship: Personal and collective transitions.* (Atlanta: American Cancer Society, 1989).

Schorr, T. M., & A. Zimmerman, *Making choices, taking chances.* (St. Louis: Mosby, 1988), 15–22.

6

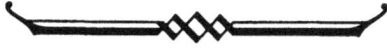

Jeannine Brant

In the summer of 1990, I returned home to Billings, Montana, from graduate school at the University of California in San Francisco (UCSF). On my first day as the new oncology clinical nurse specialist, butterflies filled my stomach. I was looking forward to my new position, and yet I couldn't help but feel a bit nervous. We stopped at the ward clerk's desk to glance at the list of patients. A young man had just been admitted with recurrent schwannoma and bilateral metastatic lung nodules. Then I heard the name, Paul Smith, a high school acquaintance. I graduated from Billings Senior High School just one year behind him and his wife, Tory. Paul had been diagnosed three years prior with a schwannoma on his right thigh. He had limb-sparing surgery with adjuvant chemotherapy at that time, and he had been doing fantastically. It was a routine chest X-ray that revealed the pulmonary metastases. I felt a sense of disbelief, but reality checked me, yes, this was really happening. I was quickly reminded that I was back in my hometown.

Although I had just finished graduate school, I had no idea that I would have to tap into that knowledge and experience bank so quickly. I had always wanted to be a CNS, and I was about to find out what that meant. I believe that my educational preparation over the past eight years allowed me to face Paul's situation and other crises that lay ahead. As I reflect back on my Montana-to-California-and-back adventure, I am grateful for the experiences and mentors that led me to this place in my oncology nursing career.

I didn't always want to be an oncology nurse. It just sort of happened. My first choice was to work in the intensive care unit. Isn't that where all of the excitement is? That was my vision as a "new grad." But I was hired in oncology nursing, taking care of cancer patients. It was mysterious to me. I had never really known anyone with cancer, and I only took care of a couple of people with cancer in nursing school. But as a new grad, any job sounds good! I was assigned a preceptor, and he showed me the ropes of oncology nursing. He even encouraged me to join the Oncology Nursing Society within the first week on the job. He kept me on my toes and quizzed me about everything I was doing as a new nurse. The questions never ended: "Why are you giving that medication? What does it do? What's your plan of care?" It was sort of a game to me, because I loved the challenge of answering the questions. I'm convinced his goal was to stump me.

I learned how to hang IVs, and I quickly learned about chemotherapy. That was all easy, but what I really struggled with was how to "care" for patients. How do I make them physically comfortable? How do I give them emotional comfort? What do I say to a husband whose wife is dying? I was young and naive and so idealistic about life. I remember the night the first patient I felt close to died. I cried for a week. I had cared for him night after night for a total of six months. I grew close to his wife and kids. I knew all about his hometown. I felt a deep loss when he died. I'm still in touch with his family ten years later. I believe we'll always have a special bond between us. In a positive sense, oncology nursing helped me to look at the world in a real light at a very young age. In the midst of joyful living, there's pain, cancer, and death.

Even though I relished my first year and a half as an oncology nurse, I had to try my hand in the ICU. I needed to go there and find out what it was I wanted there. I worked in an ICU for about a year, and I learned tons of new stuff. But it was the worst job in nursing that I have ever had! There was trauma and cardiac arrest, in a feast-or-famine tempo. The staff were extremely competitive, and I missed the teamwork of the oncology unit. I missed educating patients about their treatment regimens. I missed sitting on their beds and listening to their struggles as they faced cancer. While I was working in the ICU, patients would call from the oncology unit requesting that I come to visit. I would run over to the oncology unit on my break; it was always great to see the faces of those incredible cancer patients. After spending about six months in the ICU, I knew that I was called to another place: oncology nursing. Oncology nursing was both technically stimulating and psychosocially rewarding. It was just the right combination for me, and I never would have known that if I had been hired in the ICU initially.

I left the ICU "unharmed" and went to work in the outpatient chemotherapy area. The outpatient clinic added another positive dimension to my experience as an oncology nurse. There was almost always a sense of wellness in the clinic. In many ways, I enjoyed the clinic more than acute care. It was exciting to give patients their "last chemo" and send them on their way, hopefully forever. The outpatient nurse I worked with became a very dear mentor to me. She had been a nurse since the "beginning of time" as she would say, and she taught me how to care for patients. I was always amazed at her compassion for oncology patients. She always had time to listen to their struggles and hardships with cancer, and to their personal stories. She consistently followed up their visits with a phone call just to see how things were going. As I watched her, I began to mature in my role, to feel more comfortable in my interactions with patients. I think that caring requires both experience and maturity. In addition to clinic responsibilities, the physicians and myself would travel to rural areas in Montana to facilitate tumor boards, see patients in their home communities, and assist rural areas in establishing outpatient chemotherapy clinics. It was real frontier nursing! I continued my involvement in ONS and eventually became the charter president of the Big Sky Chapter. I found out early that if you're willing to volunteer and do a bit of work, you could be voted president or maybe something else. It was a great experience.

About a year later, my husband's job moved us to Redding, California. I was excited because graduate school was in the back of my mind. There was no possibility of a master's degree in oncology nursing living in Montana, but now I was close to the well-known phenomenal program at UCSF. I say close, but that depends on what you would call close. San Francisco was about 250 miles from Redding! I was used to driving great distances in Montana so I thought, no problem. But I really wondered, was it going to be possible? Some would say I was crazy, but I did pursue it. I called one of the professors at UCSF who was a former professor at MSU. I'll always remember what she said, "Well, it can be done, if you're committed." Committed was the key word, and I wanted to give it a shot.

I started the ball rolling by filling out the application, and submitting an American Cancer Society scholarship request. I can still remember the day I received the scholarship letter in the mail. I was awarded $16,000 for a two-year period. I jumped up and down at the mailbox and cried out, "Thank you, Lord. This is all falling into place!" The scholarship allowed me to concentrate on my studies, as I continued to work one day a week at Redding Medical Center.

The first day of graduate school arrived. I can still remember saying goodbye to my husband that first morning. I got into my car at 5:00 A.M., and drove four and a half hours to the big city. My behind was numb, and I was even a little queasy when I arrived. I was eager and excited but at the same time nervous and fearful. Could a small-town girl from Montana even find her way to UCSF? Was I really going to do this for two years? It would be 500 miles per week, and 30 weeks per school year for two years! I really wondered if I would make it. It was one day at a time at first, but pretty soon I couldn't wait to get to the city. I also developed a great car routine for that two-year period which really helped me to survive the marathon drive. I would start out by listening to a couple of talk shows on the radio. Then of course I had to make a pit stop at the only McDonalds on the highway for my morning caffeine and sometimes an Egg McMuffin. Food choices are fairly limited in northern California on Interstate 5! There's pretty much nothing out there mile after mile. Well, back in the car I'd go for the remainder of the trip. Next on the agenda was study time. Each Sunday evening before the Monday morning trip, I discussed my class notes to myself on a cassette tape. The tape grew longer each week. I popped in the tape for an hour or two on the drive and by exam time, I was ready. It was a great way to study, and I highly recommend it! The last hour of the drive was definitely the hardest. I was exhausted, and I needed toothpicks to keep my eyes open. I listened to loud music and played drums on my steering wheel. I always ran into a good traffic jam near the Bay Bridge.

I fell in love with graduate school. Being from Montana, I had never experienced such a mecca of learning. I tried to take advantage of every opportunity, and felt like a sponge, absorbing as much information as possible. I completed the AIDS minor along with the oncology nursing major, and was a research assistant for the pediatric pain study. Pain eventually became my focus of study in oncology nursing, but not really because I liked it. In fact, it was all very difficult for me to understand. I asked myself several times, "What are you doing in pain management?!" Patients' need for adequate pain management motivated me then and still does today.

I was surrounded by several mentors during graduate school. One was always near. It wasn't that they taught me about oncology nursing, but rather they taught me how to think. They taught me how to wonder, What if . . . They taught me how to be intuitive and how to accept constructive criticism. As one professor would say, "When you get your nose buried in your own work, you can't do a good job. Make sure someone reads your 'stuff'. It doesn't matter who you are, you've always overlooked something." I have followed that advice in my career more than once! My mentor during my residency program at UC Davis in Sacramento was the perfect role model. She taught me how to be an oncology CNS, helping me develop as a clinician, a consultant, and an educator. We dabbled in the research role and evaluated patients who were receiving ondansetron, an experimental antiemetic at that time.

Graduate school wasn't all learning. There was also a lot of fun. Every Tuesday night my oncology graduate class would try a new restaurant in San Francisco. Our goal was to eat our way through San Francisco in two years! We didn't even come close, but we had a lot of fun trying. I can still taste the garlic! My friends are a very big part of my oncology nursing career. We built a unique relationship through our studies and struggles through graduate school. One large 7.1 earthquake, two speeding tickets, loads of oncology nursing knowledge, and many friends later, I graduated from UCSF. I truly "left my heart in San Francisco" the day I left the city for the last time. It was a tough decision, but my husband and I decided to move back home to Billings, Montana.

I would be working as the oncology CNS at Saint Vincent Hospital and Health Center, my first CNS job.

Here I was, back in Montana, ready to begin a role for which I had been preparing for over eight years. I knew that a lot of challenges lay before me, but I had no idea that a ton of bricks would hit me so suddenly. Paul Smith, the high school runner, had metastatic cancer. My excitement and anticipation about the new job met face to face with the reality of Paul.

The plan was to start Paul on combination chemotherapy, including ifosfamide and mesna, doxorubicin, and dacarbazine. Paul had had an extremely negative experience with nausea and vomiting from his first chemotherapy experience three years prior. He had also experienced horrible side effects from the antiemetics. He really dreaded chemotherapy. I tried to convince him that the doctors and nurses would do everything possible to prevent him from getting sick. I explained that we would give the antiemetics prophylactically, and I assured him that we would continue to try a variety of antiemetic regimens to find the one that worked best. Initially, Paul was premedicated with a four-drug regimen for antiemetic control. Unfortunately, it wasn't long before he was nauseated. He was sick for the entire five-day course of chemo. He also experienced severe extrapyramidal symptoms, lethargy, and memory loss from the antiemetic therapy. The next couple of weeks weren't any better. His nausea and vomiting continued, he felt continuously drowsy, and he wasn't able to take care of his three-year-old son, Connor. The Smiths owned a French bakery, and Paul wasn't able to help Tory with any of the business tasks. Paul was just beginning to feel better when it was time to come in for a second treatment. We tried something different, but nothing seemed to be working. In the meantime, Paul lost 10 pounds and was withdrawn and depressed. I would find him in bed with the covers pulled over his head. He refused to take a shower. He couldn't eat, and he wouldn't communicate with the nursing staff.

During the third course of treatment, Paul shared that he wanted to quit chemotherapy despite the fact that the lung nodules were shrinking. He knew his prognosis was poor, but the quality of his life was the most important thing to him. Being nauseated and vomiting continuously for three months was not worth it to Paul. He wanted to be at home with Tory and Connor.

That's when I began to wonder if the new antiemetic, ondansetron, was close to FDA approval. I remembered the positive results that patients had had with this drug at UC Davis. I phoned Glaxo Pharmaceuticals about the drug, but they were uncertain about the release date. They directed me to the compassionate use program. I was hopeful that we could get the drug for Paul. Paul's physician and I discussed this with Paul, and he was willing to give the chemo one more shot with the new antiemetic. I really didn't know what I was getting into when Paul's physician and I applied to use this drug. The paperwork and legal implications were exorbitant, but I plowed onward. I remember saying to myself, "I really don't care what it takes. Paul needs and wants to try this drug. It is really his only hope to continue on with treatment. It's the only hope for remission and maybe cure." I have found in my oncology practice that ignorance is often a blessing. If I always knew what I was getting into, I probably would be very hesitant to try new things. I waded through the process, and we had the ondansetron in our hands for cycle four.

I was excited about trying the ondansetron, but wasn't too confident about the possible results. How many times do we see new drugs released which don't fully deliver on their promise? Could this really work on someone who has tried everything? I was cautiously hopeful. How could I go on in my job without hope? How do patients survive without hope? Hope is the lifeline to my soul in oncology nursing.

Day one of cycle four was here. Paul was in his bed as usual, and I knew that the covers were ready to be pulled over his head. The nurse premedicated him with the ondansetron and then started the treatment. I felt like a "father in waiting" that day! I hovered near the room, anxiously awaiting the outcome of this new drug. One hour passed, two hours passed, four hours passed, nothing. Paul was now sitting up in his bed rather than lying down. He said, "Well, I'm usually sick by now, but I'm not getting my hopes up too high." Paul remained free of nausea and vomiting. The next morning, I was ecstatic. Paul said, "Gosh, you're almost more excited than I am!" I shared with him what a truly amazing historical breakthrough this was. I was not only thrilled about his success story, but I reflected back to so many other patients who suffered intractable nausea and vomiting throughout their course of treatment. Although I knew that ondansetron would not be the "miracle" drug for everyone, I realized that the serotonin antagonists would be another option for patients, another hope in the antiemetic bucket.

Paul continued chemotherapy, and ondansetron was approved by the FDA during that time. He was in complete remission by the end of his treatment, and during his last three cycles he gained back the 10 pounds he had lost. Family and friends were able to visit Paul in the hospital. Paul and his wife would walk the halls as Connor rode the IV pole. The Paul I knew was back. He was joking with the nurses and treasuring the quality of life he had once again. I can remember when my antiemetic philosophy was "Make them sleep so they won't have to throw up." Even better, "It's best if they won't remember the negative experience of chemotherapy." And then I saw Paul and his family actually enjoying life in the midst of highly emetogenic chemotherapy.

My perceptions about chemotherapy and antiemetic therapy quickly changed.

I shared Paul's incredible success story with the local Glaxo representative. Of course he shared this with the national office, and Glaxo Pharmaceuticals asked Paul's family, his physician, and myself to participate in an educational video about ondansetron. It was called, "New Horizons: Prevention of Chemotherapy-Induced Emesis." Although reluctant at first, Paul agreed, and we were "in the movies." The video was an inspiration for patients receiving emetogenic chemotherapy, and it won a Golden Eagle film award. Paul's family and I were invited to North Carolina to receive the award, along with the other video participants. The award ceremony was a tearful yet joyful time for all of us as we reflected on the last year of Paul's treatment. The award was indeed a representation of another chance at life and a new beginning.

I grew professionally as I worked with the Smith family. I received a request shortly after filming the "New Horizons" film to speak at the Zofran™ (ondansetron) launch meeting in Atlanta, Georgia. I couldn't believe what I was hearing. I was honored and astounded by the invitation. I called my boss, my husband, my mom and dad. This was my first "hired" speaking engagement. My assignment was to prepare a 20-minute speech that would be presented in seven separate sessions to 5,000 Glaxo sales representatives. The talk was entitled, "The Role of the Oncology Nurse in Antiemetic Therapy." I think I spent weeks preparing that talk. I had my entire lecture typed out including when to push the next slide. I arrived in Atlanta and practiced over and over at the slide preview session. I remember how nervous I was as another colleague who was also presenting watched me rehearse. She didn't practice, but just reviewed her slides. I thought to myself, "She must do this a lot. I wonder if I will ever be comfortable presenting in front of an audience like this?" The next day came, and it was the real thing. Seven sessions did it! After about two or three sessions, I began to interact more with the audience, I was prompted by the slides, and I felt at ease. I was truly focused on communicating something very real to me and something very dear to my heart. It was my experiences with Paul and other patients that helped me share my knowledge that day. That talk grew into several other speaking engagements around the United States, and each one was another opportunity for me to grow in my professional role as an oncology nurse.

Paul stayed out of the hospital for almost a year. He looked great, had a full head of hair, and life was back to normal. Then, unexpectedly, Paul was admitted for a high temperature of unknown origin. I was so afraid to walk into his room that day. What would I say? Is this a recurrence of his disease? I hadn't seen Paul for a couple of months. He was orange and I immediately thought he had liver metastases. Paul saw the look on my face and said, "No, it's just the carrot juice!" I've learned that people will do many things to prevent the recurrence of cancer, even drink gallons of carrot juice daily. The source of the temperature was an infection in the Groshong® catheter. It was removed, and Paul recovered fully.

My relationship with the Smith family continued to grow. Our families spent time together, and an unspoken bond developed between us. We walked on a long journey together, and our families' common faith in God and experiences with Paul's life-threatening cancer bonded us tighter. I had my first child that year, and Paul and Connor were two of my first visitors. I was flooded with gifts from other patients as well, and it was a gentle reminder of how oncology nurses are many times a part of their patients' lives. I'm an oncology nurse day after day, but I'm also a friend many times.

Paul and Tory adopted a baby during Paul's second year in remission. They felt blessed at the opportunity to adopt a baby and become a family of four. Christmas of 1992 came, and our families united for fellowship, food, fun, and photos. We took a great picture of ourselves to send to our friends at Glaxo. Glaxo continued to send the Smiths a gift basket every Christmas in recognition of the special relationship they had. Life couldn't have been better for the Smiths. Paul's cancer was in remission for two years. I kept hoping that Paul would experience the miracle cure.

The spring of 1993 came, and so did the pain, right-sided pain. Paul entered the hospital, and I could see the fear on his face. We didn't want to admit we knew what it was. In fact, as a health care team we tried very hard not to find anything. We didn't want to. The physicians and nurses had grown to love Paul, and it hurt deeply. The tests confirmed our fears—pleural effusion and a positive liver biopsy. Cancer had won again. It sounds so defeatist, and yet sometimes I feel so overcome by this terrible disease, especially when it touches somebody I know and love. Are there ever any positive outcomes? Sometimes when the nurses on the oncology unit get discouraged, they start to list all of the success stories. It keeps us going day to day.

On April 30, 1993, Paul and his family listened to the shocking and painful news that the cancer was terminal. Their pastor just happened to walk into the room at that moment. He always happened to show up at the right time. God has great timing! The pastor was there to lend support and to simply be there. I saw Paul later that day when he was alone in his room. I found it difficult to enter the room. I always thought that oncology nurses were supposed to know what to say, but sometimes I don't know what to say. We sat in silence for quite some time, and then we began to talk. This was no ordinary talk. It was as if we had to get a lot said for fear there wouldn't be enough time to say it all. Paul shared that he did not want any more chemo. He understood his terminality and the seriousness of his disease. What he wanted more than anything was to share the time he had left at home with his family. I feel very privileged that patients share an intimate part of themselves throughout their cancer illness, including when they are dying. I have learned so many "life principles" from patients.

I often wonder what patients looked like before they were diagnosed with cancer. Sometimes I ask patients, "Do you have a picture of yourself before you had cancer? Do you have a picture of what your hair looked like?" Sometimes I get so busy educating patients about chemotherapy and side-effect management that I forget to stop and say, "Who are you?" I don't mean that in a derogatory way, but I do want to know what life was like for patients before cancer came into their lives, and I wonder how cancer has changed them.

Many patients are not afraid of death but rather the dying process. One thing I can do for them is to help lessen their fears about "actually getting" from this world to the next. I let them know that the care team will do everything possible to provide general comfort, relief from pain, and relief from dyspnea. My faith is a great stability for me as I work with cancer patients. I know I could not make it without God.

When Paul died, I had difficulty separating out who I was in the situation. Was I a nurse or was I a friend? It seemed a little awkward to be there amidst the family, in the middle of a very intimate and private time. I felt privileged to be there, and I was grateful to share tears with them. There was a real peace after Paul's death that overwhelmed me. I knew he died in comfort, surrounded by love. And I know that God had prepared a place for him, and he was living in that glorious place, free from cancer and pain. So is death all that bad? No, I like to think of it as the ultimate healing for many. It was for Paul.

I look back on the past ten years of my life, and I'm truly amazed at how I have been directed to a career in oncology nursing. Some call it fate, but I believe that my work as an oncology nurse is a true calling from God. I feel blessed by the fact that although painful at times, I enjoy my work. It feels so good to say, "I can't think of anything I'd rather be doing!"

Notes

Groshong is a registered trademark of C. R. Bard Division of Davol, Inc.

Zofran is a trademark of Glaxo Chemicals.

7

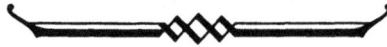

Cynthia Cantril

The old man thought he was lucky to be in a private room after being transferred out of the surgical intensive care ward at St. Louis County Hospital. He was anxiously waiting for the doctor, the chief surgical resident, to tell him about the results of his surgery. The old man was not able to understand the young Puerto Rican doctor's accent or the implications of his diagnosis. The physician arrived and told him, "You have Duke's C adenocarcinoma of the colon with possible spread to the liver. We will send you home with plenty of morphine." He only understood the words morphine and home. He was clearly confused and concerned as the doctor very quickly left the room.

As a twenty-one-year-old, new graduate nurse, I stood at the bedside and was appalled at the insensitivity of the resident and the lack of caring and support the patient must have felt. Although this incident occurred in 1972, it still seems as if it happened yesterday. It was the pivotal moment in which I decided I wanted to take care of patients with cancer. I wanted to gain the skills and knowledge to help people who had this terrible disease.

The world of cancer nursing was not new to me. I had worked each summer during high school as a candy striper on the head and neck cancer surgery unit at Barnes Hospital in St. Louis, Missouri. Perhaps that is where I began to see the need for emotional support and communication along with sophisticated treatment technology. As a naive teenager, I experienced all kinds of emotions as I delivered and read mail, washed the stainless steel tube-feeding cans, and delivered materials to the quiet and cold intensive care unit. I was only allowed into the unit when asked. I remember feeling so helpless and sad to see only swollen eyes peering out from the heavy bandages. Even then, I was drawn to those who needed to communicate so much and yet were given little time or chance to do so.

I learned important lessons as a candy striper which shaped me into the person and nurse that I am. While I could not articulate the words then, I learned about issues such as power, perceived power, and personality characteristics of the many persons who work in the health care industry. I remember the charge nurse asking me to take the staff elevator to central supply for a "stat" pick up. The elevator door opened and there stood the famous doctor who had pioneered the partial laryngectomy. Residents and nurses lived in both fear and awe of him. As I was about to step into the elevator, he glared at me and said, "Do not come into this elevator—I do not ride with candy stripers." He was smiling as the elevator door shut and I, in contrast, was humiliated and devastated! I was extremely intimidated by that doctor. As years have gone by, I often think about that situation. Since that time I have learned to believe and trust more in myself. So very often my beliefs or convictions have been challenged. Yet the times in my life that I have taken the most risk are the times that I have been most rewarded by the outcomes.

In 1973, on my twenty-second birthday, I interviewed for my first job in oncology. I met with Dr. George Hill, professor of Surgery at Washington University School of Medicine in St. Louis. He would be my first and most important mentor. I was hired on the day of my interview and became the first "nurse oncologist" for the university's department of Surgical Oncology at Barnes and Jewish Hospitals. There were no other nurses working in this role which was constantly evolving. My initial responsibilities included chemotherapy preparation and administration, clinical trial patient management, patient assessment, education and advocacy, and interdepartmental patient management. Very shortly after I was hired, Dr. Hill left to become the Visiting Professor at the University in Saigon, Vietnam. Along with an attending professor and a resident, I was left to follow and oversee the patients in our department. The secretary had rescheduled all of the chemotherapy patients to receive treatment after Dr. Hill's return. But a few days after his departure, I was called by a nurse at an outpatient internal medicine research office. She told me that one of our research protocol patients was waiting to receive his chemotherapy. When I entered the treatment room, I saw the biggest syringes that I had ever seen on the tray next to him. The nurses had prepared the chemotherapy drugs for me. I had observed Dr. Hill giving chemotherapy before, but this time I was on my own. I took a deep breath and introduced myself. The patient, in all his wisdom asked, "Is this your first time?" He winked and said, "Don't worry, I'll talk you through it." And so he did. That night my dreams were nightmares of syringes, butterfly needles, blood return into the tubing, and probably other career opportunities. The next morning I could not get to the office fast enough to check on Mr. M. You cannot imagine the relief I felt when he answered the phone with a cheerful voice and said thanks for the "great job" I did with his chemotherapy. I recognize that this episode could seem unbelievable or archaic. Yet early on, only doctors gave cancer therapy. Eventually, nurses became more involved in cancer care and all aspects of care delivery changed. For a long time, there were no other nurses at Washington University with whom I could share this experience. All too often I felt alone and unsure of my skills. I suspected there were other nurses in similar roles and slowly I found other oncology nurses at many research institutions.

I was invited to present my first lecture in November 1974. The title of my presentation was "Clinical Indication for Chemotherapy." At the time, the only widely used, commercially available drugs that were not classified as experimental included 5-Fluorouracil, cyclophosphamide and methotrexate, and nitrogen mustard. We had been using such drugs as doxorubicin, bleomycin, carmustine, lomustine, and others for research purposes only. After the seminar concluded, many nurses stayed and we discussed administration techniques, job roles and functions, and symptom management issues. I wish I could adequately express the intensity and excitement of that day. The invitation to speak that day provided a window of opportunity; I met Lisa Begg (Marino) who was working in Chicago. She told me that a few other nurses working with cancer patients had begun to seek each other out to discuss the special needs of oncology nurses. I expressed my desire to see if a special group could be formed. We planned to attend the American Cancer Society–National Cancer Institute national conference on advances in cancer management in New York later that month. Seventy-one nurses attended a special discussion session and we were filled with excitement. The conference provided us the opportunity to discuss and exchange ideas about establishing a formal communication mechanism. We discussed many possibilities for a structure including affiliation with the American Cancer Society, the American Nurses Association, or the American Society of Clinical Oncologists. I presented the advantages and disadvantages of an independent nursing specialty group formation. An attorney had told me that an independent nursing group would "be easy to form—you could write your own ticket but it (the group) would have little clout since communication with other groups would be difficult."

Needless to say, I should call that attorney today as ONS approaches 26,000 members! Looking back, I have so many memories of the development of oncology nursing and ONS. In May 1975 a nursing meeting was held at a local junior college during the meeting of the American Society of Clinical Oncologists (ASCO) and the American Association for Cancer Research (AACR). It was then that our dream came true. We decided to establish a formal oncology nursing organization. The initial four officers were Lisa Begg (Marino), president, Chicago; Connie Henke (Yarbro), treasurer, Alabama; Daryl Maass (Mathers), secretary, New York; and myself, Cindi Mantz (Cantril), vice-president, St. Louis. We really had no concept of the time, energy, amount of commitment, or expertise that would be required of us over the next months and years. We did know that our timing was right and that we were absolutely dedicated to promoting our specialty of nursing. The first officers had individual personalities and strengths that allowed us to face the many challenges that lay ahead. Frankly, I do not remember being apprehensive over the challenges—only excited.

Our employers were incredibly supportive. Without their support and belief in us, individually and collectively, I do not believe ONS could have been established. One particular incident captures the essence of our early struggles. Dr. Hill asked about an unusually high departmental phone bill. I gulped, smiled, and told him we were trying to get the ONS bylaws written. Another question arose about a significant amount of Xeroxing and mailing that was occurring during evenings and weekends at the office. Often, this strong, reserved, and gentle man would just shake his head at me. He knew I was a determined woman with a mission! While these past events may appear trivial, I am not sure that ONS could evolve today given the current health care system problems. I am so very, very appreciative of the support that all of our employers gave. Like our ONS leaders today, the first officers balanced busy work schedules and other professional and personal obligations. ONS was just beginning and no one really knew how the organization would ultimately take shape. The founders had an unshakable determination and commitment to define and promote our specialty. We took risks. Often, we were unprepared in dealing with the rapid growth of the society. For example, when the concept of local chapter formation first appeared, we had major concerns about whether or not we should approve them. If the board approved the development of chapters, how would they be structured?

Some of my memories are unpleasant. I can look back and accept that we were young and inexperienced with respect to the evolutionary challenges involved in developing and managing a new organization. Nonetheless, I think there were some who were hurt and insulted by our lack of experience or naivete. The first officers faced some insults too. Our personal budgets also were taxed with travel and other expenses associated with the organization's development. At one business meeting I was angry when a member stood up and questioned the use of her dues. She wanted to know if the officers were using the membership dues for their own personal gain. I replied that she could look at my personal checkbook to realize how much of our own personal finances had gone into the initial development of the society. It takes years of experience to realize that there are always "new waters to chart" and continual challenges to face. As I look at the ONS staff and board of directors today I feel secure about the Society's caretakers.

I do not remember really questioning myself about the personal and professional resource requirements. I believed in a dream and a promise. One promise I made to myself was to see that resources would be developed for oncology nurses. I did not want others to feel as isolated or unsure as I often did. Chemotherapy guidelines did not exist. I read drug package inserts to see if administration tips were provided. I sometimes stared at syringes of chemotherapy drugs that I had prepared, wondering what side effects would occur. Where and how I could learn more about symptom management? Every day, questions emerged for which there were no answers.

Finally, there was the wonderful feeling of being able to call another nurse. A nurse who could share both the happy and sad moments of oncology nursing. Today I hope that every nurse caring for persons with cancer knows where to find support and use the resources available. So many people have and continue to define, refine, and promote our specialty. I am grateful to have been able to participate in making a dream come true.

By the time I was 24 years old, I had worked with several hundred people; many of whom had died. Through this work, I learned an infinite number of life's lessons. One such lesson came from a patient named Bill. He was a twenty-year-old with testicular cancer. When I first met him, he had a metastatic lung lesion that responded quickly to chemotherapy. Over the years of working with Bill, we had become close. When he was admitted for chemotherapy, we often talked until late at night. His disease progressed despite all available treatment. Bill knew that I would usually write his admitting orders. We discussed special requests he had prior to admission. One day after he had completed his last experimental drug and his disease was progressing, he asked a favor. He knew his family could not bear to see him die at home. He asked that I make sure that no "heroic" measures be attempted when he was admitted for terminal care. "Please let me die with my dignity, Cindi," he pleaded. I promised I would be there for him when that time came. Every Wednesday I went to the inner city hospital to assist residents in the oncology clinic. One week, I was late getting back to the office. When I got there, I found a "stat" message that Bill was in the emergency room. The message had been taken at least an hour or two before I actually got it. I ran to the ER. Down a long hall, I saw a stretcher surrounded by interns, nurses, and residents. I prayed that the person they were surrounding was *not* Bill. When I got to the stretcher, I felt as if my heart was in my throat. I saw Bill lying naked with barely a sheet over him. I felt intense emotions of sadness and anger. I also felt that I had betrayed Bill. I saw the tracheostomy tube, ventilator, subclavian line, and various other tubes and equipment. When I reached the head of the stretcher, I saw his face and our eyes met. His eyes expressed anger and anguish;

mine filled with tears. How could I have let him down? How could I have made a promise that I could not keep? That night in the intensive care unit, I kept a vigil with his family. I silently prayed that he would not die. Then I realized that my prayer was truly selfish. I had no right to ask that Bill endure more suffering. He, not I, had extensive metastatic disease. He, not I, was emaciated and in almost constant pain. The lesson was clear—I was feeling guilty that I had not been able to fulfill my promise. I was unable, for my own selfish reasons, to say good-bye. Later that night, Bill became extremely restless. He communicated to all of us, his family and others around him, that it was time to say a final good-bye. He had private moments with his family. He expressed gratitude to me, which I did not feel I deserved. A short time later, he unhooked himself from the respirator and died.

Over 20 years later, I remember the inconceivable sense of sadness, failure, and loss I felt as I left the hospital after his death. I did not return to work for many days. I was emotionally exhausted and sad. I rejected the support friends and colleagues offered. I wondered if I was capable to continue in oncology nursing. A few days later, I did return to the hospital, a much wiser person. I am thankful for knowing and caring for Bill.

Of the innumerable lessons that I have learned over the years, my experience with Bill and his family remains one of my most profound. I learned that all too often we caregivers confuse our roles and "agendas." We have the potential to mix our own personal life goals with those of the people we care for. I learned that patients and families need, and have the right, to control what happens to them. I also learned that I should never make a promise that I potentially could not keep. This experience continues to show me all sorts of things about living and dying. Despite the obstacles we put in his way, Bill was finally able to die with dignity. He taught me that there can be peace after so much pain. I miss him still.

Each day oncology nurses say initial hellos and final good-byes within a matter of minutes. We are blessed with the opportunity to care for others and share some of the most precious of life's moments. Every oncology nurse frequently hears, "Is your job depressing?" Each of us has our own special way of responding to the question. For me, there is no greater gift than being part of such a special time and place in nursing. I know the world is a better place because of our contributions to the quality of life of those affected by cancer.

Many people have served as mentors and role models to me. My mother has been a very significant role model in my life. I am the youngest of six children. My father died when I was a few months old. Mother was faced with raising six children alone. My older siblings tell me that one day some men came to our house after my father's death to "counsel" Mom. They told her she would have to sell the house.

Women in those days did not have credit and they questioned her ability to make the payments. She was told that arrangements were made to separate the children and place us into foster homes. They also told her she did not have the earning capacity to provide for us. I suspect my mother threw them out! We were never split up and we continued to live in our home in a small rural town in northern Illinois. During the week we were cared for by other families and mom would commute to Chicago to work. She remarried when I was six and was able to fulfill her lifelong goal to become a nurse. She entered a licensed vocational nursing program when she was 54 years old. She is now 84, and until a few months ago, worked full time on the night shift at a nursing home. My stepfather died from vascular disease when I was sixteen. Our family resources were not very good. But I was determined to become a nurse and entered nursing school right after high school graduation. By working in a nursing home on weekends and during the summer, I was able to pay for tuition and expenses. My mother has always been a cheerleader for my career. I wonder how my mom endured all the losses she has experienced. Because of her, I learned a great deal about loss, strength, conviction, and perseverance.

In 1978 I married and moved to a small rural town south of St. Louis. I began working in an entirely different type of environment—an eighty-bed osteopathic hospital. Again I developed a job and role that was new to health care in that area. There I gained great respect for the doctors and nurses who in one day would deliver babies, set fractures, assist at and perform surgeries, stabilize trauma victims, and many other tasks required in a rural hospital. I learned that folks living in rural areas are often isolated and as a result are very self-reliant. Just some of the challenges I found there included teaching colostomy irrigation techniques to a person who had only an outhouse, coordinating clinical trials in a rural area, providing outreach education, administering chemotherapy in the emergency room, teaching symptom management, and teaching a nurse's assistant program at the local community college. One once-in-a-lifetime experience was when I organized a colo-rectal screening program. I can't forget being eight months pregnant, standing in Wal-Mart during the Christmas shopping rush, and passing out hemocult testing kits. Try to imagine explaining to shoppers how to prepare for and perform the test. The test kits were returned to my office at the hospital for me to develop!

In 1979 I was recruited to a developing cancer center in Cape Girardeau, Missouri, 110 miles south of St. Louis. As the coordinator of oncology services, I was responsible for the development and implementation of the inpatient and outpatient medical and surgical oncology services. It was another dream come true to be able to work with the entire cancer care spectrum. All of my past experiences in cancer care could come together. The staff and I created a comprehensive community-based cancer care program. We implemented "I Can Cope," "Make Today Count," and hospice programs. We provided social service, nutrition, counseling, and rehabilitation programs in both inpatient and outpatient areas. The overall program was highly successful.

Shortly after I was recruited to Cape Girardeau, the director of nursing was terminated because of a threatened nurses' strike. Up until that time, I had not experienced the level of anxiety that results from change happening too quickly. Luckily, the oncology staff was receptive to change and we were able to continue expanding our cancer program. I worked with some of the most caring and committed nurses I have ever met. But once again, my convictions were challenged as I faced a volatile situation. I found that a powerful oncologist was, in my opinion, practicing in a questionable manner. He asked nurses to have a permit signed *after* a procedure had been done. He refused to involve his patients in teaching and support programs. He was often rude and unsupportive to staff, patients, and families. I decided, after careful consideration, to deal with the situation. I went through all the appropriate channels with administration, the hospital board of directors, and the medical staff. The state Board of Healing Arts became involved, and to sum it up, a real mess was created. I knew I was facing formidable odds but I also knew I could not just "sit by and watch."

Memories of those days are bittersweet. I was recruited to create a comprehensive cancer care program and I still feel very good about the final outcome. Yet I believe I was too aggressive in my timing of dealing with the problem physician. A few years later, one of the medical oncologists called me to say that the problem physician had totally "lost it" and had barricaded himself in his department threatening suicide. Years later, he died alone, as he had alienated all those around him. From this experience I know how important it is to consider all the possible ramifications of "taking a stand." I was fully aware that I was involved in a power and influence scenario.

I knew that I might lose my position as a result of my challenge of the "status quo." Moreover, I knew that the director of nursing was not capable of understanding the significance of my stand. In fact, she came in one day during her vacation, terminated me, and left the hospital. I immediately called the chief executive officer to tell him what had happened and he stated that she could not terminate me and that I was *not* "to clean out my desk." The situation went from bad to worse. The story spread throughout the hospital and the primary medical oncologist and internal medicine specialists threatened to boycott the hospital if I was let go. I stayed on for many more months but was truly unhappy. My personal life was crumbling with a divorce and I had to make some difficult choices. Ultimately, after realizing I was in a "no win" situation,

I left the hospital and returned to St. Louis with my two-year-old son. I still would do the same thing if faced with the same experience today. Admittedly, I would have approached the situation with more caution— one of the great things about getting older!

Back in St. Louis I took a new role in "joint practice" with a medical oncologist who was beginning a new practice. I worked part time for him and also worked as a consultant for a large community hospital. In the office I mixed and administered chemotherapy, counseled patients and families, and established our practice in the cancer care community. For the hospital, I taught chemotherapy classes and set up psychosocial support services for the staff and patients. In addition, I was working on my graduate degree part time, working on committees in ONS, and juggling my new role as a single parent. After all the years of having my whole world seemingly revolve around oncology nursing, I was ready and open for a more satisfying personal life.

I met a remarkable man who understood my commitment to my career. He was also a single parent and we shared the ups and downs of the responsibilities involved. The only obstacle was that he lived in San Francisco and had a very busy radiation oncology practice there. We decided to get married and I had to leave my job. I went to the hospital's director of nursing who was incredibly supportive. As I described a six-month time line for my move, she interrupted me and she said, "This is an important time for you—life is short and you need to go to San Francisco sooner." She helped me complete all of my responsibilities and prepare for a new person to take my place. Her sensitivity was so special. Later I learned that her husband had died a few years before. She helped me reprioritize my goals from strictly my career, to a new marriage. In my experience, that type of support has been rare from nurse administrators.

In November 1983 I entered a whole new world as a wife and mother to four children. My husband's former wife had died of melanoma when she was only 42 years old. My stepchildren were ages 9, 15, and 18. Eventually I wanted to become more involved in nursing and took a position as the oncology nurse specialist at a hospital in San Francisco, ironically, the same hospital where my husband was the chief of radiation oncology. I was accepted with mixed reactions from the hospital staff. The hospital had never really had a successful clinical nurse specialist role and I felt under the scrutiny of many people. One prominent medical oncologist asked me during my first week, "Do you really know anything about oncology or did you get this job because of your husband?" At that time, only doctors were administering the chemotherapy (déjà vu). I asked why the nurses did not administer therapy and one nurse said, "We don't want to." She went on to say that if the doctors gave the chemotherapy, the nurses did not have to worry about it. I wondered how that rationale evolved! Over time, the nurses consented to a chemotherapy certification program and began to administer the chemotherapy. Over the next year I served as the nurse specialist, acting nurse manager, occasionally as fill-in for staff, and helped with outpatient HIV treatments. My supervisors changed five times and there were three different vice-presidents for nursing.

The oncology nursing community of San Francisco was wonderfully supportive and the local ONS chapter was very active. I met Pamela (P.J.) Haylock who became a close friend and professional colleague. She was acutely aware of the issues I faced and I am forever grateful for her continual support. She helped me work through a major career transition as I decided to move away from acute care. I realized that I could stay at the bedside for the rest of my career and not make the impact I wanted to make. I wanted to work more actively in education, prevention, and detection. P.J. suggested that I look into the field of public health and I was accepted into the master's program of Public Health at the University of California at Berkeley. Following graduate school, P.J. and I set up a cancer care consulting partnership.

In 1992 my husband experienced significant vascular problems and underwent a bilateral aortic femoral bypass procedure. He decided to retire early and we moved to the San Juan Islands off the coast of Washington state. My experiences were again helpful to a rural community when I was elected to the Orcas Island Medical Building Association board of directors. I was reminded of the special needs of rural dwellers and of the challenges of maintaining quality health care services and access to care in rural areas. I learned about the issues of blending allopathic and naturopathic medicine practices. I also had the time to commit to a special passion—cancer survivorship. I served on the board of directors for the National Coalition for Cancer Survivorship (NCCS) and chaired the 1993 NCCS Assembly in Seattle.

Currently we live near Bozeman, Montana. I chair the state steering committee on breast and cervical cancer detection for the Department of Health. I also work with the Montana State University School of Nursing in grant writing and research. I am a member of the ONS Archives Committee and look forward to becoming chair of the committee in 1995.

Reflecting on my career, I am thankful that I chose nursing, most especially oncology nursing. I am reading stories and autobiographies of nurses of long ago. They describe the many rewards of nursing that still seem real today. Frontier nurses speak of taking risks, and facing challenges, rough travel, unknown and strange diseases, and low pay. But they also speak of the intangible rewards and the satisfaction of working as a nurse. So, despite continuous changes in roles, finances, and standards, perhaps the fundamental reasons I chose the profession of nursing remain the same.

Oncology nursing has provided me with an infinite number of lessons and relationships. I must say that there are some days I wonder how long I will stay in oncology nursing. As quickly as the question enters my mind, the answer appears. I will remain as long as I feel I can contribute and make a difference in the lives of persons affected by cancer.

8

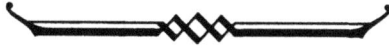

Sandy Creamer

In the very beginning, I wanted to be a nurse because I liked the "costumes" worn by the students at a nearby hospital. They could be seen walking back and forth from the hospital to the residence with white caps, white uniforms, and navy blue capes. I didn't know what they actually did, but it seemed important and honorable.

Nurses have always looked like stars to me, even as I get older. In the dictionary, a star is defined as a twinkling point of light, a celestial object, self-contained and self-luminous. A star is a superior performer. That's what I wanted to be.

I entered a diploma nursing school and started to investigate what it really was about. During "nurse's training," I was eager and excited. I loved all phases of it and could not choose my favorite field. As part of the educational/social experience, we had shows, skits, and role-playing. It was a joyful experience.

I worked in pediatrics and in the nursery at first, followed by many years of med/surg "floating" (where did that word come from?). I floated everywhere including critical care areas, not always liking it as my stomach was filled with knots, for fear I could not rise to the occasion. I was indeed looking for my special niche.

It was after many years of marriage and three children that I found my spot. A colleague informed me about the planned opening of a small oncology clinic. The position was merely one day a week. I decided to go for it and I would continue my three evenings of "floating" also. Oncology appealed to me as it was a brand new road that not many had traveled. I got the job, perhaps because few applied, due to the scariness of cancer.

Early on, I studied drugs and medical terminology such as "adenocarcinoma" because it was so unfamiliar to me. Nursing school had brushed over cancer as a fatal, gloomy disease. In fact, the word *oncology* didn't exist, at least not in my life. As the months passed, I grew to love it more and more. It had challenge, compassion, and caring. It felt joyful. The patients brought such meaning to my life. Ongoing relationships with patients and families created a dimension I had always longed for, but I thought it was forbidden territory. In nursing school we were taught never to get involved emotionally with our patients. In fact during one of my student evaluations, I was told that I laughed and smiled too much, and not to "get so involved." I was told to act more professionally. So years later, when my patients hug me and tears well up in our eyes, it seems like a whole new ballgame. On the job, I started learning the meaning of "therapeutic use of self." Intertwining my own special qualities, sharing myself and being a risk-taker worked for me. My work felt joyful. It was and is a source of pleasure.

In the past, maybe nursing instructors wanted to prevent burnout, or unacceptable attachments, or they were just plain picky. No matter what, joy is essential in nursing, and in oncology nursing we walk alongside of our patients, helping them, supporting them. It's a compassionate pathway, which is ever so close and intimate to the patient and family. It resembles parallel lines, one track for the patient and one for us. This is an acceptable, desirable relationship, not possessing, merely "taking the journey." I was well on my way.

The oncology department grew. I kept studying and learning. Karla, a mentor of mine, along with Dr. Evjy and Dr. Gan, inspired me to coauthor a patient education book as well as numerous other projects. My mentors shared their knowledge daily as they were pioneers in our community. Those admirable people, and my love of the specialty, were instrumental in my goal-setting. In 1980 I stated that I would return to college and by 1990 I would have a master's degree and become a clinical specialist, just like Karla. Well, I did it and it wasn't easy, but I felt joyful. Amidst the studying and exams, and throughout the subsequent years in oncology, I have attempted to bring pleasure and meaning to patients and staff alike. Joy has a place in cancer care. Finding ways to incorporate joy has been a priority. Joy is the fuel for the body. It is not always present to patients, but helping them identify and use their coping skills and once again find meaning in their lives often contains a sense of enjoyment.

Little did I realize when I entered oncology nursing 18 years ago, that I would bring to my practice those theatrical genes from my relative, Mary Pickford. (Honestly, she's my mother's cousin once removed.)

One of my diversified roles has been producer/director of the annual Cancer Christmas Story/Bethlehem Star Search. It takes place in early December and is a celebration of survivors and living. It is a drama, it is a mystery, it is a comedy, it is nonsense, but most of all, it is wonderful. It is loaded with joy. The oncology team shelves uniforms, needles, and chemotherapy for one spectacular evening, for "the show must go on."

From October 1, auditions and recruitment take place. Secret rehearsals are scheduled and costumes are created as we prepare for our annual surprise cabaret. The performers include oncology nurses, doctors, volunteers, pharmacists, social workers, and patients. On occasion, some local amateur entertainers have participated. This gala event takes place in a small auditorium at our hospital, Saint's Memorial Medical Center in Lowell, Massachusetts. Patients, families, and friends are invited.

This affair evolved from the concept "therapeutic use of self." We were risk-takers, and over the years it has become a team-building and lifegiving experience.

Joy to the World

More than 16 years ago, when Sister Anne and I started our weekly support group, we were greenhorns. We were nervous, excited, and eager to make it work. Sister Anne is a social worker, but my previous experience with support groups was fairly limited, except for Weight Watchers. Nevertheless, we believed group support was beneficial for patients, families, and staff. I was new at oncology nursing, but it felt different from my med/surg practice. It seemed to offer a lot of room for individuality and creativity with many opportunities. I realized that whatever qualities I possessed could be brought to oncology with therapeutic value.

Soon I invited a part-time oncology nurse, Rhea, to participate. We attended a facilitator's training session at the Boston ACS office and were on our way. Some group sessions were dynamic, some were not, but all were supportive. When December rolled around and much of the world was celebrating, we decided on the spur of the moment to have a cancer Christmas party. It was simple. We signed up for the food. Helen brought deviled eggs, Bob brought Twinkies (because he couldn't bake), others brought chips and dip. Sister Anne brought tea sandwiches, and Rhea and I brought punch and dessert. There was an instant celebration. Just before leaving home, I called Rhea and told her to bring a flared skirt and boots. I brought pompoms, batons, and my similar attire. Under pressure I quickly composed a victory cheer for cancer patients. I borrowed my husband's band music tape, John Philip Sousa's greatest hits, plus a tape player. Sister Anne located a large, worn Santa suit. The excitement was mounting. Group started, and after a brief sharing, the party began. We ate and exchanged pleasantries about the excellent deviled eggs and how good the Twinkies tasted. After a while, I motioned to Bob (the Twinky man) to follow me to the anteroom along with Rhea. Bob was undergoing treatment for advanced brain cancer, but was soon to be a star in our first production. Rhea, Bob and myself assembled and quickly practiced our skit. We laughed like children as

Bob (now bald) donned the Santa suit. He looked silly. He was a Harvard graduate, a business professor, and never in his life had acted so spontaneously as on that night. After an introduction by Sister Anne, we turned on the tape and marched into the room, attempting to twirl my daughter's batons—Santa Bob and his two chubby cheerleaders. We looked hilarious, and the crowd roared. We laughed heartily until tears appeared. We shared intimacy, vulnerability, and fun.

Joy Has a Place in Cancer Care!

That was the beginning. Every year since, the oncology department plans a Christmas party. All patients and families are invited. A potluck supper is organized. Usually a volunteer and Lorraine, our secretary, take charge of the food list. We advertise in the clinic and the inpatient unit with a colorful invitation. Eventually we outgrew the support group room. Now we book the hospital's auditorium, complete with stage, microphone, and an old piano. I recruited my talented friend Barbara to be our musical director. We include a sing-along with lyrics and accompaniment for group participation. In addition, I attempt to create a few skits with a musical comedy flair. Our Santas have varied from patients to doctors, each bringing a sense of hope and love to all. We share gifts that are donated from well-known businesses, and favors made by several oncology nurses.

This holiday gala has gained notoriety in the hospital and in the community. The director of the local cancer program asked to videotape it. An amateur theater company and a local choral group have performed. Students from the Boston Conservatory of Music and from the Tewksbury High School band have joined the fun. A hospital pharmacist asked to be involved as well as social workers, visiting nurses, the IV therapist, the chaplain, more oncology nurses, and the volunteer department. The doctors became enthusiastic. Dr. Gan was the official photographer, Dr. Evjy, a Santa, and Dr. Anamur does anything I ask from playing the organ to acting. As producer/director, I delegate jobs to all and devise a formal program of events just like in real theater. Initially I choose a theme. The themes have varied and have included the 50s, the Olympics, Broadway, and Country/Western, to name a few. We start discussions and brainstorming approximately six weeks before the show. Each year we receive phone calls from patients and families inquiring about this special evening as December approaches. The clinic staff invite people on their discharge instructions. Many cancer survivors participate year after year. Several new patients undergoing active treatment attend, maybe in an attempt to hold on to hope and positive reinforcement. Patients disfigured with radical head and neck surgery have danced and sung on stage with confidence and self-esteem. Richard, with cancer of the mouth and dysphagia, dressed in western attire and performed in a cowboy skit. He also prepared a delicious casserole for his food contribution.

Another memory is of Mary. She was a teacher, a wife, and a cancer patient. It was six months after her lung cancer diagnosis that she mentioned how radiation had affected her singing. She enjoyed music as a hobby but was dismayed about her altered voice. It was Mary's idea to try to sing "O Holy Night" in front of everyone and I prodded her on. She brought her own arrangement, gave it to the pianist, and beckoned me to introduce her. That night Mary wanted to sing for us, even though her voice might crack. Her song was angelic and moving. She did it. She got through it with minimal problems. We cheered with a standing ovation and misty eyes. She gave us a wonderful gift of voice and courage.

Kick lines are always a hit, so when Angie, while receiving chemotherapy, told me that she previously was a dance instructor, the wheels started turning. I asked her to be the choreographer for our next Christmas show. She was 68 and had metastatic cancer of the liver. She didn't know if she would have enough energy to do it. Realizing I was asking a bit much, I reassured her. I told her not to worry, that if she wanted to quietly show me the steps or describe them, I'd jot them down and teach the others. So we collaborated every week for about 15 minutes, usually while waiting for her lab work. We decided on two different dances. Our costumes were black top hats, black skirts, and red blouses. We borrowed canes from the physical therapy department. We practiced in the clinic hallway after hours. We wanted to make Angie proud. We were the "Onc-ettes." Undoubtedly the hit of the evening was "New York, New York." Angie felt well enough to lead us on stage. She beamed. Her husband sat in the audience in awe. Like most of our acts, this was a surprise for all. I can't explain my feelings. I felt the way I do when I watch the Jerry Lewis telethon, or when I witness heroism, courage, and joy. In my opinion, heroes are those people who, in the face of adversity, stand up and dance.

The years have come and gone. Our oncology department has witnessed more than five hospital administrations, an onslaught of HMO rules and regulations, tough insurance mandates, and a variety of Joint Commission woes. We have lived through several nursing vice-presidents, enormous employee restructuring, layoffs, the merger of two hospitals, and the five relocations of the oncology department. We have assisted many to achieve remissions and cures, and supported others through death. Extraordinary people have walked into our lives and many have gone, including our close friend and oncologist, Dr. Gan. We are eternally grateful to him and to all those who have taught us well.

Our most recent venture was the grand opening in July 1994 of a state-of-the-art oncology center. As a cofounder of the oncology practice, I felt fortunate to participate in this event so many years later as oncology/hematology coordinator of all services. Our oncology team of 30 people is dedicated, experienced, and competent. They are joyful. The journey so far has been difficult, meaningful, and exciting. Our environment has undergone much transition. There are many days when we "just hang in there." Through it all we continue our annual Christmas cabaret. It is a refuge from sadness for patients and staff alike. It brings fun and excitement and is contagious. The atmosphere represents love. We mingle, we listen, we affirm, we enjoy, we hug, we smile, we celebrate humanity. Joy to the world.

9

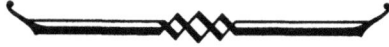

Karen Hassey Dow

I wanted to be a labor and delivery nurse. The year was 1975 and I was a new graduate vying for one of three labor and delivery nursing positions at a large teaching hospital in Washington, D.C.

"Sorry, but we only offer those positions to nurses with *experience*," the nurse recruiter informed me. "How about our gyn-oncology unit? You don't need experience to work there."

Yes, probably because the nurses don't stay very long there either, I thought quickly. Well, I enjoyed working on the surgical units when I was a student, and I did have some experience taking care of patients having cancer surgery. Oh, why not? And besides, I needed THE FIRST JOB as an RN. Thus began my professional career and journey as an oncology nurse. Looking back I wish I could say that my career was carefully plotted and planned. It wasn't. But, like most things in life, the lasting experiences are usually unexpected and the most enduring lessons often come serendipitously.

Twenty years ago we didn't have preceptors. Most often, we were left to fend for ourselves. Basically, new grads had two weeks of inservice orientation to the general hospital routines, procedures, and benefits. After that we were pretty much thrown into the general chaos of the units. In looking back, since this culture shock was the norm, we didn't think it was so unusual. There was always an endless stream of new nurses starting new jobs with little or no experience. The gyn unit had its share of complicated cancer surgeries. I was so young and naive, and it seemed that so many young women with advanced cancer were having radical pelvic exenterations. It was really hard not to identify with them. While other patients were in and out in a week, these patients stayed for a short lifetime. They were so sick and their surgeries were so extensive and mutilating. Many of my fellow new grads shied away from taking care of these patients. They were too frightened or too scared to take care of them. The residents and interns weren't much better. Bored with this rotation and wanting to get into the excitement of labor and delivery, many really didn't care much for oncology patients. I doubt that the oncology patients much cared for the residents either.

Our knowledge of cancer treatment was very rudimentary. Clinical nurses had very little information on proper mixing and handling of chemotherapy agents. We knew that caution had to be exercised, and unfortunately, that was about the extent of the knowledge on my unit. "Be extra careful with this drug. Make sure you don't put too much pressure in the bottle when you draw up the med and make sure you don't squirt it all over the place," warned my assistant head nurse. The drug was doxorubicin. Radiation safety information was a little bit better, but not much. My first experience with radiation therapy was with a patient who had endometrial cancer. "Make sure you don't walk too close inside this circle," warned my assistant head nurse. She was great about warning me about land mines to watch out for on the unit.

"What do you mean?" I eagerly wanted to know.

"Well, see this circle marked off with masking tape on the floor?" she pointed. "You have to stay outside the circle as much as possible because of the *radiation*," she whispered. "Make sure you get in and out as quickly as possible and don't talk too much to the patient." Unfortunately, those were the days when we focused more on learning about cancer treatment and less on what was happening with our patients. We were still concentrating on learning the technical, even though there were so many physical care needs to attend to.

Such was my first year's experience in both nursing and oncology. Patients with cervical cancer, endometrial cancer, breast cancer, and other cancers came and went. Beyond their physical needs, we nurses were facing patients' and families' anxieties over disfiguring surgery, the pain of advanced cancer, and endless return visits for numerous complications. Patients' needs were overwhelming to a very young nursing staff. We were long on shortages of all kinds, and short on long talks and reflections about our practice. No wonder the recruiter said we didn't need any experience. We got it all and much more in the first year. Today it is nice to know that prior experience is usually required for working on oncology units. We have come a long way. It is also wonderful to see preceptorships and clinical internships for new grads to help them through the first year's work. It is tough. It is wonderful to know that new grads have a supportive preceptor to ease many of their burdens and concerns. Thankfully, the road today is a bit smoother.

By the end of my first year in practice, I was preparing to leave the D.C. area. I was getting married and moving to Boston. The hardest part about leaving was that I had gained a lot of clinical experience on my unit and I felt comfortable and proficient in my nursing care. I would miss the patients whose lives I got to know beyond the surgery and chemo and radiation. And I would miss the other nurses on the unit.

We had developed a strong bond and camaraderie. Once again my assistant head nurse warned me, "Don't change jobs too fast and too quickly." "Okay, I won't, but why not?" I asked. "Well, it will look like you can't keep a steady job. Besides, it doesn't look good on your resume." Well, I didn't have a resume so that didn't bother me one bit, but I told her that I would heed her warning about switching jobs too much or too often.

Before I left the hospital, another of many serendipitous moments arose. A new nurse by the name of Kathy had just started working on my unit. She was different from the other nurses because she had prior nursing experience and wanted to specialize in gyn-oncology. Kathy had also just moved from Boston. Even though I was already planning to interview at a very famous teaching hospital, I casually asked her advice as to where to look for a job in Boston. She told me that she had just come from a little-known hospital, but they had just started using primary nursing, and she had loved working there.

"Which hospital is that?" I inquired.

"Beth Israel," was her reply.

Because of this casual conversation, I went to Beth Israel to check it out, was hired the first day there, and began my long career and association with Beth Israel Hospital in Boston.

The BI. Looking back, I heeded part of my favorite assistant head nurse's warning. I didn't leave this hospital in search of another job, but I did have many positions at the BI over the past 17 years. I have had appointments as a clinical nurse on the gyn-oncology unit, a nurse clinician in radiation therapy, nurse manager, clinical specialist, and nurse researcher. Each time I was ready to pursue another course in my career, there was a position that was ready-made or available for me to enter. That was another wonderful experience in working at the BI. Whenever I was ready to make another professional move or advancement, this change was always welcomed at the hospital.

At any rate, returning to 1976: In many respects the BI wasn't all that different from other Boston area teaching hospitals. Even though the hospital was just beginning its primary nursing practice system, it too suffered from terrible staffing ratios, low patient satisfaction, and high nursing turnover in the mid-1970s. This time, the nurse recruiter brightened when she heard that I had experience in gyn-oncology and was looking for a position on that unit. The head nurse hired me on the spot. What a difference a year makes, I thought. Those were great and really exciting days. Most nurses were excited about the prospects of instituting primary nursing. Anything was better than what we had experienced with the disjointed team approach. And that is what was exhilarating about implementing a new care delivery model. When you are on the bottom rung just about anything looks good and change is exceedingly welcomed. When you have a big stake in keeping the status quo, anything new is exceedingly threatening.

Continuity of care by maintaining your own primary patients, 24-hour accountability, and collaboration with physicians and other care providers were buzzwords that actually became reality. Administrators placed the emphasis on the goal of patient care and the petty territorial issues were gradually stripped away. Patients' faces became attached to their names, and primary nurses placed their names over their patients' headboards to denote their accountability. Nursing care plans and integrated documentation soon were the norm. We owed so much to Joyce Clifford, my VP for nursing, and her vision of what nursing could be. But we owe so much more to the clinical nurses who took that vision and made it a lasting reality.

I think that we are fortunate as oncology nurses because we have almost a built-in guarantee of continuity of care. We see our patients for such a long time over the long course of their disease or recovery. But with the added structure of a professional practice model that I experienced at the BI, we could really soar in our patient–nurse relationships. Like other nurses, I have literally taken care of several hundreds of patients over the course of 20 years. It is true that patients teach us so much more than we have to offer them. And while I cannot remember all of my primary patients' names, several stand out as really memorable to me.

One of my first primary patients was an exceedingly large woman named Hazel. Admitted with DUB (dysfunctional uterine bleeding), we later learned that Hazel had advanced endometrial cancer. Cancer prevention was still a very theoretical notion in both the public and the professional eye. I remember explaining to Hazel what the surgery and post-op course would be like, how we would take care of her after surgery, and I reassured her that she would have pain but we would give as much relief as possible. Hazel wasn't much interested in the surgical procedure or what I had to say about it. Hazel worried that her voice would drop a few octaves after the hysterectomy and wondered whether she would "still be a woman." Patient education is important, but here was my patient telling me that her emotional response was her major concern. I learned a lot from Hazel. Just when we think we have prepared our patients adequately, they refocus our attention to what is really important. Well, Hazel got through her surgery, her voice did not drop, she did not have much pain (she rarely complained), and I sent her home. She was scheduled to receive several weeks of external radiation therapy. I had very little information about outpatient radiation therapy. I knew very little about its side effects and what it meant to patients. Besides, the radiation was done in the outpatient department, and surely someone would be taking care of her, I reasoned. As I later learned, radiation was a very difficult course. Hazel needed six weeks of daily radiation treatment. She lived in the city and transportation back and forth from the hospital was a huge problem. She had trouble with her bowels and couldn't eat many of her favorite foods. She became tired and had little energy for even managing her household chores. Hazel had no family to rely on; she also had little support in getting through her treatment. Yes, the technologists giving her treatments every day were very capable, but they were also very busy treating patients and she had few outside resources to lean on. All this she told me when she returned to my unit to have her radiation implant procedure. I learned a lot about radiation therapy from Hazel and in looking back, she was one of the reasons why I became so interested in this treatment modality. Surely we could do better to improve patients' care.

Over the next few months, Hazel became weaker and more debilitated and I knew that her battle with cancer was drawing to a close. We both knew that she was dying and when the time came, Hazel came back to my unit to die. I remember the other nurses calling to tell me that Hazel was admitted probably for her terminal admission. They thought it best that I come in early on the day shift to say good-bye. But I instinctively knew that Hazel would wait until my evening shift before she died. And that is exactly what happened. When I came in that evening, her condition continued to deteriorate. She died later that evening. It is a peculiar thing about our relationship with our primary patients—we can sometimes sense when death is imminent. It seemed that my primary patients were not admitted on the days that I didn't work or was on vacation. Most of my patients seemed to wait until I cared for them before they died.

Jenny was another primary patient. She came from a large, loving, extended family who were always bringing in food and drink that Jenny couldn't tolerate, but they brought it in anyway. She would get diarrhea. But they felt that Jenny needed to eat a lot. They equated her losing weight with her dying, so if they kept her weight up, Jenny wouldn't die. This was something that I didn't stop. Jenny knew that she was sick, they knew that she was sick, and so what if they kept on bringing in food that she couldn't eat. Jenny complained a lot. Her family didn't really listen to her complaints but gave it right back to her. She needed a private room because there was always a lot of commotion going on in there and whenever she had other roommates, they couldn't take the noise. Jenny had cervical cancer. She had pap smears, but too infrequently and with too little follow-up. She only came to the hospital seeking care when the bleeding interfered with her life. Like Hazel, she had advanced disease. Like Hazel, Jenny had surgery and lots of radiation therapy. She too had many side effects and made darn sure that everyone knew how she felt. It wasn't difficult to learn from Jenny about her disease. Jenny later died of her disease. Her family couldn't bear to be in her room in the end. It was too painful for them. I was at her side when she died.

It was tough going seeing so many patients whose disease had run its course. It seemed that many of our patients died around the holidays. It didn't matter whether patients were old or young. It didn't matter whether they had radical surgery or extra-radical surgery like an exenteration. It was still tough. Primary nursing has its share of joys because we take care of our patients for a long time. It has its share of sorrow when patients that we had cared for come back to die.

Nurses on our oncology unit, just like many others around the country, developed a strong and special camaraderie with one another. I know that people who are not nurses would think us morbid, but we learned to find humor in the most ridiculous situations. And when we had comic relief we relished it. This was yet another joy in oncology nursing practice. We could laugh, cry, and giggle over the seemingly endless routines of inpatient hospital nursing. What little recognition there was in those days, we gave heartily to each other. One particular nurse on my unit was full of humor and had a big heart. She was like Lucy Ricardo—always getting into some kind of scrape and laughing at herself. She became one of my best friends and still is to this day. Her name is Judi Hirshfield-Bartek. She had such a long name, so we just called her Judi H.B. We were primary and associate nurses for most of each other's patients. We also loved to do pre-op teaching. Hard as it is to imagine today, patients were admitted the night before surgery just for pre-op procedures. At 9:30 each evening, we held pre-operative teaching classes in our solarium. We dragged out our teaching bags loaded with IV tubing, foley catheters, and other paraphernalia. We called patients into the solarium and gave them instructions on what to expect, what it might feel like, what pain meds they would get, and when we would get them up from bed. Judi and I were quite a team and to this day we still have many lasting professional associations and collaborations, and a special friendship with each other. She has been a true and honest friend—one who tells you what you need to hear not what you want to hear; one who helps you through the ups and downs of everyday practice. One wonderful aspect of oncology nursing is that we make friends, often for life.

By 1978 I was one of the senior experienced nurses on my unit. Already I was precepting new grads and helping to smooth their transition to the unit. I was eager for more formal education. Fortunately, Boston University was providing special oncology programs for nurses, funded by a grant from the National Cancer Institute. Its purpose was to provide a week-long educational and support program for nurses in practice. I applied and was accepted to the program and I loved every minute of it. I learned a lot more about oncology nursing and had ample time to reflect on where I was heading in this specialty. I remember many of the nurses who were teaching the program peppered their didactic presentations with many personal experiences and hardships. After taking the program, I was ready to expand my practice. Once again, serendipity stepped in. A new oncology nursing position was created in the outpatient hematology-oncology unit to meet the demands of the larger numbers of patients being treated. The nurse coordinator was Barbara Farley. She was experienced, bright, and had a vision for oncology practice. I wanted to work with her. The decision for the position came down to two individuals: Debbie, another nurse, and me. Debbie was chosen. I was deflated. Yet, it turned out to be O.K. because another one opened just a few months later. This time the position was in the little-known field of radiation oncology. This was a major turning point in my life. It is hard to believe today, but there were few nurses lining up for this position. Radiation therapy? Who wanted to work in radiation therapy? Besides, exactly where *was* radiation therapy? No matter, I wanted to work in radiation therapy. And I was hired for the position.

There was little in the way of nursing practice in radiation oncology in those days. It was not difficult to make major advances since they were needed and welcomed in every part of this practice setting. Symptom management and how it differed from or was similar to chemotherapy, enormous skin care problems, transportation issues, pain management, and social and family concerns were major areas in need of attention. Developing relationships with the radiation oncologists, radiation therapists, physicists, and administrative staff was very different from developing relationships on inpatient units where there were a *lot* of nurses. In radiation oncology, we were fortunate to have one or two nurses. And the work was new, stimulating, and satisfying. I feel that forging new roles and charting new paths have been hallmarks of oncology nurses. Whenever a new technology or a new way of delivering old treatment methods was being developed, nurses have stepped in and brought a richness and diversity to that practice. I feel very fortunate to have been one of those individuals in radiation oncology.

Back to the 1970s. The use of breast-conserving surgery and radiation therapy for breast cancer was in its infancy. I recall many a red-faced surgeon trouncing through our department (often for the first time) to rant and rave that we were killing their patients. We most often thought that the object of the sentence was *business,* not patients. There were other surgeons who were skeptical at first, but eventually were great supporters of breast-conserving surgery. At any rate, women desiring a choice in the matter, whether it was to preserve their breasts or have a mastectomy, sought out our department. A new day dawned in breast cancer care. Alternatives and choice became new cancer care buzzwords, and Massachusetts became the first state in the nation to mandate that information on alternative breast cancer procedures be given to women. I enjoyed the challenges in my role and the diversity of my responsibilities. I loved talking to patients and their families about alternatives to mastectomy. I presented and even wrote about the topic in the *American Journal of Nursing*. Since we had so many new patients receiving radiation therapy for breast cancer, I began to focus more on breast cancer care. I helped start programs to teach the nurses on the unit about the implants and how they differed from the gyn implants. We discussed the procedures with women and their families and saw them coming to our unit more and more. So within my emerging subspecialty of radiation oncology, I delved deeper into the care of women with breast cancer.

In 1979 I heard about a new group of nurses who were meeting on a yearly basis to talk about their practice, the Oncology Nursing Society. This was the first time I had heard anything about them. I vowed that I would attend the 1980 meeting. That year the annual Congress was held in San Diego at the Sheraton Harbor Island Hotel. All 500 attendees could actually attend meetings and sleep at the same hotel. Convention centers, multiple hotel listings, and endless "dress for success" wardrobes were still things of the future. During one very memorable abstract session, as we sat in shorts smelling of suntan lotion, a petite and vivacious woman stepped up to the podium. She then proceeded to describe her practice and how she collaborated with a clinical psychologist and radiation oncologist in providing emotional support and educational programs for their patients. I sat there enraptured. I had dreamed of starting such a program and now someone was telling us of such a reality. Her name was Laura Hilderley. She was in a radiation oncology practice in Providence, Rhode Island. I raced up to talk to her after her presentation and invited myself to visit her. She laughed and agreed. Later that month, I spent a day with Laura and the other nurses and radiation oncologists that she worked with and who obviously had a great deal of respect for Laura and her vision for oncology nursing. Much more, her patients and their families loved her. The feeling, I am sure, was mutual.

Here was another turning point in my life. This chance meeting in 1980 became the first of countless encounters, discussions, and collaborations with Laura around radiation oncology practice that has spanned the last 15 years. I sought out Laura's advice about day-to-day care, about skin care practices, mouth care routines, and relationship issues. Laura understood the difficulties in practicing in a struggling subspecialty where much of oncology care was focused on chemotherapy. Laura understood what it meant to practice in a unit that was so far away from the general patient care areas, a unit few people knew even existed. She knew what it meant to have patients understand the differences between radiation therapy and radiology. She was there in so many critical ways to help me grow both personally and professionally. And she helped nurture and develop a new generation of radiation oncology nurses as well.

I remember she called me one late fall afternoon in 1981. The unit was in its usual uproar, I still hadn't had my lunch, and I wished that no one knew my name. I was two months pregnant and was feeling the rush of hormones.

"How would you like to present a topic on symptom control in radiation therapy?" she asked.

"Sure," I gulped. "When is the presentation?"

"At the next Congress in Saint Louis," she casually replied. My heart sank, my knees buckled, and after I picked myself up off the floor, I told Laura that I would love to participate. Sure, this would be a great opportunity, but I hadn't the slightest notion of what it was to entail. All I knew was that I had to have some slides! I ran down to our audiovisual department and had a crash course in slide-making. Our usual low-key AV staff obliged a near-crazy pregnant nurse. Of course computer-generated slides and software programs were at least eight years away from the clinical setting. For the moment, we actually had to type out our information on an antiquated machine called a typewriter. Forget about point size and typeface; we were dealing with the basics. The AV personnel actually took a picture of the typed information and then produced the slides in blue diazo. When we really wanted to get fancy and impress our audience with sophisticated slides, we switched to a black background instead of the blue diazo and then colored in the different lines with different magic markers. Great! Now I had slides and learned how to load them onto a carousel. Turn the left bottom of the slide to the right top and you're all set!

By the time the ONS Congress in St. Louis arrived, I was seven months pregnant but I had my slides! This was my first major presentation to a national audience (actually, it was one of my first presentations ever). My parents who lived in St. Louis were also coming to hear me speak. I had all the usual presentation jitters—GI upset, dry mouth, and heart palpitations. And even though I have done over 100 presentations to many different audiences over the past 15 years, I still get those presentation jitters. My presentation was a success, meaning that I could advance my slides and talk about them at the same time, and I launched into a new aspect of my professional life, professional speaking. Thank you, Laura, for giving me that chance.

Much more important, Laura and I have remained special and close friends, so close that we decided to collaborate on a book about radiation oncology nursing practice. We had talked about needing such a book for many years. As we talked more and more about it, the book became a near reality in 1985. We both loved reading Bonnie Johnson's and Jody Gross's practical tips in their *Handbook of Oncology Nursing*. We sought their advice on editors and later selected their editor. The nursing book editor liked our proposal and drew up a contract which we promptly signed. Seven years, three publishing houses, and six editors later, our book was finally published by Michael Brown of W. B. Saunders in Philadelphia in 1992. It was a labor of love. Nearly all of our original contributors stayed with us throughout the project. There were marriages, births, divorces, and other living experiences that occurred among us and the contributors throughout the course of writing and editing the book. Our next nursing book will be about writing nursing books!

At any rate, Laura and I truly became strong friends during this period of writing and editing. When one was up the other was down and vice versa. When one couldn't edit another manuscript, call another contributor, or obtain those endless permissions, the other one stepped forward. That is so characteristic of oncology nurses; we do things one step at a time (but most often have more than one thing going at a time!). We got to know about one another's family, friends, home life, and hobbies. That was a more personal and valuable an experience for me than book editing.

On the subject of writing, I found that writing helped to clarify my thoughts. Actually, I got into writing as I did with so many other aspects of my professional life, through opportunity and challenge. The year was 1981. I was leading a round-table session on skin care in radiation therapy. Even though it still holds a lot of attention at round-table sessions at Congress today, skin care in radiation therapy was a novel topic at the time. I was amazed by the diverse skin care practices out there, some of which were wonderful and some of which needed to go the way of lemon glycerine swabs. I remember that our discussion also focused on a paper on skin care during radiation treatment that was published in one of the general audience nursing journals. The paper was full of inaccuracies and promoted myths about radiation. "This couldn't have been written by a nurse practicing in radiation," I thought. I skimmed the author's credits. It was not. What's more, the paper received some writing award for innovative practice. Well, then and there I was determined to set my pen to paper and write based on the literature, my knowledge, and experiences with radiation therapy and skin care. That is just what I did, I literally set my nicely sharpened Ticonderoga pencils to yellow legal pad paper. I had no word processor to help me organize my thoughts. But I wrote my paper and I edited it as much as I could and I was satisfied that it reflected the realities of practice. I was really excited as I gingerly placed my original and three manuscript copies in the mailbox to Sue Baird, then editor of the *Oncology Nursing Forum*.

I waited and sweated it out for the next eight weeks. I was so excited to receive a letter that started out with, "Congratulations, your paper is accepted," from Sue. To this day, in my files, I still have that acceptance letter from over a decade ago. This first foray into professional writing was another memorable landmark in my professional life. I took to writing and enjoyed it immensely. Sue Baird gave me the opportunity to join the editorial board of *ONF*. I was elated. Here again we have a rich heritage. We have a long tradition of nurse editors like Sue and editorial board members who took the time to carefully read and critique my paper. They were honest in their critique and supportive in their commentary. This has had a lasting impression on me. They gave me a chance at writing and when it was my turn to review and edit other people's work, I try to keep that supportive and honest tone in my reviews.

On another memorable afternoon in 1985, I got a call from Sue Baird. Now in my department, getting a call from Sue Baird was no small event. "How would you like to move up to an associate editor's position on the *Forum*, Karen?" she offered. This time, I had no rush of pregnant hormones, just excitement at feeling the blood drain from my head.

"Well, sure, Sue, but are you sure that I am up to the task?" I had been on the *ONF* editorial board for just over a year. I loved reviewing the manuscripts and took great care in my reviews to provide careful, directed, and constructive feedback. Having been on the other side of sending in manuscripts, I tried to keep the prospective author's tender feelings in mind. Moreover, I became somewhat of a resident critic of the ads appearing in *ONF*. I loved to read and critique these ads for content and merit.

"We need an editor for the 'People and Events' column and I think you could manage it," she informed me. By this time, I had two years of experience in writing and editing our hospital nursing newsletter, *Report on Professional Nursing at Boston's Beth Israel Hospital*, better known as *Report*. The work was challenging and I was eager to sharpen my skills. Besides, I wanted to learn more about editing from Sue. She told me that our first editorial board meeting would be in New Hampshire at a lodge. The drive up from Boston took over two hours. The sun had set by 5 P.M. and it was dark by the time I found the winding dirt road path to the inn. We were still a few years away from meeting at our all-time favorite Greentree Marriott in Pittsburgh. This meeting was a delight. The innkeepers at the bed and breakfast stoked up the hearth fire and served incredible home-cooked meals all day long. They brought out fresh-baked chocolate chip cookies every day for mid-afternoon snack. This was home cooking at its best. We were truly spoiled. I was assigned a room with Micki Goodman. It was hard to imagine that I was rooming with the *famous* Micki Goodman who wrote so many of the early chemotherapy protocols. I remember that Sue Baird, Sue Dudas, Micki, Bonnie Johnson, Marilyn Frank-Stromborg, and Michelle Donehower were at that first editorial board meeting that I attended. Sue even arranged for us to go on a tour of the Dartmouth Printing Press, the publisher of *ONF*. We walked through the printing press and smelled the inkjets as the offset printing press rolled on. It was all great fun.

At this meeting, the initial conception for the *ONS News* was discussed. I was assigned by Sue to write up some ideas about what the newsletter would contain, types of columns, features, and so forth. I had already done this type of work at my own hospital. These initial ideas were set and prepared for presentation to the ONS Board of Directors. *ONS News* was launched two years later. Little did I know then that I would soon be named editor of *ONS News* in 1988 and turn over the helm to Brenda Nevidjon a year later.

By this time I was actively pursuing my writing endeavors. I can't say that I was like a reporter with a pen and paper handy all the time. But I did keep in the back of my mind a running list of what I would like to write about. Sometimes the topic was caused by my frustration, such as the first paper I wrote on skin care. On other occasions I tried to turn what I had presented into a manuscript. And yet on other occasions, I just wrote. This is the advice that I have for others: write early and write often.

Returning to the practice setting, the year was 1981. There were only two nurses in my radiation oncology practice and despite my hospital's growing renown in primary nursing practice and the professional practice model, I felt stymied in my attempt to bring more nurses to our unit. At the time, DRGs were beginning to make the scene. So was HCFA. I brought to the attention of my nursing director the increasing complexity of care in our unit. We had more women receiving radiation therapy for breast cancer who were crying out for more emotional support; we had more patients receiving radiation for head and neck cancer twice a day and we had no place to accommodate them, much less give them food and drink; and we had more patients requiring assistance with transportation, social needs, and the like. We needed more nurses. Again, I was challenged to put my pen to paper and write down all these changes in practice that occurred and why we needed to increase our FTEs. Anna, my nursing director, assured me that we could do something about it. We put together a proposal for additional FTEs in nursing based on the increased complexities of treatment, and the fact that our patients needed more care. We reasoned that nursing could generate revenue by attaching a cost to the additional nursing care that would support the additional FTEs. The third-party payers agreed to the exception and thus a system of nursing visit charges was implemented in our radiation oncology unit. The year was 1982.

So we got additional nursing staff and our care and patient satisfaction improved. We transferred to a collaborative model of one primary nurse, one radiation oncologist, and one resident team. We saw patients at the time of their diagnosis, followed them during treatment, and saw them together during follow-up. Our numbers swelled and more breast cancer patients came to our department. One day we learned that the local television station was going to highlight primary radiation therapy. The public affairs department found its way to our unit and was literally aghast at the way it looked—tired and worn out. What's more, we had an empty fish tank in the patient waiting room that sorely needed to be replaced. Patients were getting depressed thinking about those poor dead fish that had once lived in the tank.

"Can't you *do* something about the way this place looks, Karen?" begged one administrator. "It just doesn't look great for the media."

Oh sure, just for you, we'll spiff this place up in a few seconds, I thought. Did he just come down with the last rain? If we ever had enough money to make this unit a comfortable place, it certainly wouldn't be for the media, it would be for patients. Thus began another trek into a new aspect of oncology nursing care: designing an entirely new department organized around patients and nursing care. This was the 1980s and we were upscaling, not downsizing. Our buzzwords were growth and spend, growth and spend. We took a fresh look around and indeed saw a department that needed a face-lift. We were fortunate because not only did we get the face-lift, we were given an entirely new home. I was fortunate to work with wonderful radiation oncologists who knew that a unit organized around patient care needs and traffic patterns would be a well-designed unit. They encouraged me to voice my opinions and concerns and what I didn't like about the old department to the architects and planners of our new department. First of all, patients did not like the idea of being in a dark, dank unit without any windows. Could we do something about that? We were given skylights in the patient waiting area and a beautiful garden with miniature trees and flowering shrubs to enjoy all year round. Great! Now, inpatients were so sick and needed a quiet, private area. Could we do something about that? The architects devised a separate inpatient waiting area with private sections close to the nursing station. Terrific! Patients and their families needed to feel as comfortable as possible. We asked for racks and bookshelves for patient education pamphlets, and an area where coffee and tea and crackers could be made available. Larger johnnies and terry cloth robes were ordered just for our unit so that patients did not have to feel undressed in the waiting area. These are not the stuff of major motion pictures, but these small gestures with the patients' comfort in mind made such a difference in people's attitudes. The environment certainly spoke of comfort, rest, and reassurance. Since then, I became very well acquainted with hospital architects. I helped to develop the initial plans for two other radiation oncology units, one in Massachusetts and one in New York.

By 1986 I was ready for a change in practice and a change in my life. Despite the wonderful support that we receive from one another, I needed a change. The balance between the personal and professional life is a delicate one, and I started to see my life through my professional self more and my personal self less. I needed a reversal and a change of perspective. In 1986 I had a four-year-old daughter, Lauren, who demanded more, not less attention. This was a child who had cut her teeth on Sesame Street, Peter Rabbit and Aunt Jemima Pudding Duck books, and my presentations. I remember when she was an infant she loved to hear me talk to her. She was not one of those quiet children content to sit in front of a white wall. So I would get out the text of one of my upcoming presentations, make her my audience, and read to her. She would chortle and gurgle and throw up. As she grew older, she demanded more of my attention. So despite my enjoyment of my work, it was time to move on in other aspects of my professional life. I remember Joyce Clifford saying to me that it is sometimes better to leave a position when you still love it rather than when you hate it. Those words had a great impact on me and motivated me to move on.

I had also experienced the death of my father of leukemia and it was a terrible ordeal. Now I was on the other side and waited expectantly for oncology nurses to comfort me. Shortly after his death, I remember attending an ACS conference on cancer nursing. The speaker at the podium was talking about mouth care, and thoughts about my dad's struggles with managing symptoms came crashing around me. I got up and left the presentation in tears. I knew I had had enough for a while. It was too hard to bear. I needed a rest.

Writing once again came to the rescue. The editor of *Report* was moving on to another project at the hospital. Joyce Clifford offered me the new position. I accepted. It gave me the time away from patients and families to rethink, recollect, and recover. Writing and editing are great ways to develop creatively. I was in charge of the monthly meetings. I worked with clinical nurses, specialists, and managers. We thought about our practice and got so involved in writing about the day-to-day practice of day-to-day nursing. This was a great way to get grounded in the realities of practice once again. And even though I missed patients after a fashion, I was glad that I had the break in care.

I didn't take a break from oncology nursing practice for very long. In 1987 the graduate program in nursing at the MGH Institute for Health Professions was expanding. Debbie Mayer was leaving her teaching position at the Institute to work full time in the Biological Response Modifiers program at Mass General. Sylvia Paige, the coordinator of the oncology tract, gave me a call. "Would you be interested in teaching graduate students about oncology?" she asked. While I loved precepting graduate students in the clinical setting, I had never really considered a formal teaching position. Here was my opportunity to give it a try. Here again was another turning point in my professional life. I came to enjoy teaching about oncology nursing and the position was the shot in the arm that I needed. Plus, I got to work with some great nurses like Judy Spross, Debbie Mayer, and Sylvia Paige. Before this time I had only read about their work in nursing journals; now I had an opportunity to work with them. I have grown to value their friendships, their expertise, and their humor immensely. We laughed a lot at the seemingly endless political struggles that go on in practice, the kinds that need "chin straps" to keep our jaws together from amazement. They also knew how to relish special moments, one of which was high tea at the Ritz or the Four Seasons. We all loved the special attention to detail in high teas, so we planned to mark our end-of-semester work with high teas.

In 1988 I was moved to write a paper about pregnancy after breast cancer. I wanted to focus on a message of hope and life after breast cancer. The inspiration for this paper came from my experiences of two of my special, primary patients, Marcia and Barbara. I learned a great deal about going through adversity and getting to the other side from them. Both women were young, full of life, and both had breast cancer. They wanted desperately to have children. So, I went back to the literature and looked up all I could on breast cancer and pregnancy. To my surprise, most of the articles were published in the surgical oncology literature starting as far back as 1937. I researched the topic and found that women were no more likely to have recurrence after subsequent pregnancy than other women who had no subsequent pregnancy. I shared these thought with our radiation oncologists. We then set about talking with younger patients about their concerns and indeed found that many patients had these thoughts, but did not always voice their concerns. We tried to bring to the foreground what their background thinking had been. Barbara and Marcia eventually became mothers and I relied on them immensely to talk more about their experiences with other young women.

The fall of 1988 was my last year on the *ONF* editorial board. One evening at dinner at the infamous Greentree Marriott, I sat next to Peggy Lamb. We exchanged pleasantries, and I asked what she was doing. "I'm at BC," she replied. My eyes widened. "What on earth are you doing there?" "I'm in the doctoral program," she smiled. My eyes popped out even more. "You ARE?" "Yes, and I love it!" I was amazed. Judy Spross and I had attended Boston College's first open house for the doctoral program and were less than impressed. We were looking for a doctoral program focused on clinical, and we had decided that this program wasn't for us. Well, never say never. In the fall of 1989, I found myself in the second entering class of doctoral students. And in the fall of 1992, Judy Spross was on the student rolls herself.

Once again, here was another chance discussion with a fellow oncology nurse that changed my course. Peggy Lamb is one of the funniest, most talented, and most generous women that I have ever met. She was a great encouragement. She very much enjoyed being in the doctoral program, had a great mentor in Dr. Callista Roy, and was learning about an entirely new and exciting area of nursing—research. She gave me an entirely new and different perspective on doctoral studies at Boston College, and I wanted to pursue it even more.

One of the things that I have agonized with was how to blend family with professional life. There seem to be so many opportunities in oncology nursing. The trick is not to take advantage of them all. One of the lessons that I have learned is that despite how well we take care of our patients, there is always another skilled oncology nurse who can care for them, but no one, not anyone, can take care of our families and children any better than we can. We alone are uniquely qualified to do that job. So by 1989 I was working on a part-time basis to have more flexibility in my family schedule. Pursuing doctoral studies would require a change in my work and family schedule, and I knew that I needed as much love and support from my family to make it through the program intact. The decision to pursue a doctoral course was a family decision. My husband Norman and my daughter Lauren were cautiously support- ive. One of my jobs had to go and that was teaching. I had to keep my family first in my life and my work second, and doctoral studies would be my work for the next three years.

I was delighted that Boston College accepted me and extremely delighted that I received scholarship money. I found doctoral studies wonderful in every way. This was my opportunity to enjoy scholarly debate and writing and to grow in my research endeavors. I was the only oncology nurse specialist in my class, and the first thing that we students had to do that first day was to acknowledge that we were experts in some area of practice, and then to get on with the business of learning a broader perspective. The next two years were full of classes and SPSS-X and statistics. I had a wonderful mentor in Dr. Callista Roy and an equally supportive and talented doctoral committee in Dr. Victoria Mock and Dr. Jay R. Harris.

In the summer of 1989 I received a telephone call from Jennifer Bucholtz. She informed me that the *ONF* Editorial Board wanted to nominate me for the Schering Clinical Lectureship. I was shocked, delighted, and of course extremely honored to be nominated by my friends and colleagues, and this lectureship was very special to me. I thought back to the other recipients and how I was moved by their presentations—Judy Spross on pain, Debi McCaffrey on the elderly, Roberta Strohl on radiation, and Mary Cunningham on creativity in nursing. They were tough acts to follow.

This clinical lectureship was certainly another major turning point in my career. I don't know exactly how to articulate it, but it's a bit like being crowned Miss America. You go through months and months of thinking about what you want to say and how you want to say it. The paper on cancer survivorship was one of the most difficult ones that I have ever done. I knew that I wanted the topic to cut across treatment modalities, cancer types, gender, and roles to focus on the issue of surviving and living with cancer. I read as much as I could on the topic of survivorship from different perspectives. How did people survive other traumatic or life-threatening events? Were there any aspects that were similar to cancer patients? I think it helps to see cancer patients less as being different and more as being similar to other survivors. I read and re-read all the previous Schering papers and tried to glean new insights into clinical practice. Next I took anti-diarrhea medication and set myself to writing my thoughts. It was helpful just to sit at my computer and let the thoughts work through my fingers on the keyboard. I sent my first draft off to Judy Spross and Judi Hirshfield-Bartek to read. They were great friends, but more important, great critics. At first, Judi asked me, "What's your point here?" Judy Spross remarked, "I think you are onto something, but I don't yet know what it is." So I kept writing and rewriting until I knew I had it right.

The next step was to think about how I wanted to portray this presentation in a very large room with lots of people just finishing their big lunch. Here my husband helped me tremendously. He said, "Why do you nurses always have to have things look so *clinical?* Why not add a touch of beauty as you tell your story?" And with that, we set about thinking of survivorship as seasons using Fitzhugh Mullan's prototype and literally took different shots of the changing seasons. And that is how that lecture was organized. The year after the lectureship, I was not prepared to "go on the circuit." I traveled to lots of new cities and towns, both large and small, across the country. I had the opportunity to meet so many expert oncology nurses sharing their experiences in practice. I think we need to give special recognition to the numerous oncology nurses out there who give 100 percent each day and still find time to put together educational programs. Here truly are the unsung heroines and heroes who constantly get after others to write down their objectives, send in their CVs, make sure they have the right slides, and so forth and so on. They carefully plan programs to benefit clinical nurses and don't always receive recognition for the work they do.

On one memorable trip to Chicago in the fall of 1990, Susan Leigh and I were on a panel about cancer survivorship. It was late on a Friday afternoon and we were both traveling to St. Louis: she was going on to another talk and I was going on to visit my family. We got to O'Hare airport only to find that swirling high winds had closed the airport down. We figured that we would have to hunker down for the night at the airport. It turned out to be one of the most enjoyable evenings that I have ever spent. Suzie is a fighter, a tireless worker for cancer survivors, and a sheer delight to talk to. We sat for hours on the TWA gate floor talking about our lives, our hopes, our aspirations, and our families. Our work intertwined in the discussion, but always our families and our lives came first. I think that is an extremely valuable lesson that we have all learned from our patients, not to sweat the big stuff and take each day as it comes. To enjoy our families and the very mundane pleasures of day-to-day living. This is what it is all about.

In April of 1992, the day that I arrived home from defending my dissertation, a package was waiting for me. In it was an invitation to join a newly formed commission, the Breast Cancer Commission. There would be 17 members and I would be the only nurse on this panel. Debbie Mayer had nominated me the previous fall. She had thought it would be a long shot but was so committed to nominating a nurse for one position. Well, there it was. I spent the next 18 months traveling mostly to Washington for hearings. The commission heard testimony from nearly 200 scientists, advocates, activists, and clinicians from all across the country who brought their passion, knowledge, research, and hopes about eradicating and curing breast cancer. This was another major turning point in my life. To think that I represented the views not only of oncology nurses, but of all nurses was extremely weighty. To think that I could influence in a very great way the course of thinking and research about breast cancer was incredible. To see how politics, breast cancer, and policy were intertwined was another major eye opener. After thousands of pages of transcript were distilled down to approximately 20 pages of a report, we presented the report of our findings to Hillary Clinton at the White House in October 1993. But I think the most important things that I received were so many beautifully handwritten notes from nurses across the country who talked about how breast cancer was affecting their practice and their patients. I received notes from nurses who developed innovative teaching and support programs for breast cancer survivors, from nurses who wrote about insurance issues and concerns, and from other nurses deeply concerned about managing symptoms. These are the everyday work of nurses.

In building a legacy from the voices of oncology nurses, mine is but one voice, one of the building blocks of the legacy. I know that for every lecture that I have presented, there were dozens of nurses quietly working in the background of program planning. For every paper that I wrote, there were those nurses who spent hours reading and re-reading the manuscript to help me better present the information. For every subject that I wrote about or spoke about, there were hundreds of my patients who richly taught me about the topic. For every application that I have ever made for a new job or a new educational program, there were those mentors who spent careful hours writing out thoughtful letters of support. And for everything that I have accomplished in nursing, I know that my family and faith in God have been the driving force behind my work. This is what our legacy is, to receive much from those who have laid the groundwork before us and to hold out our hand to help the next nurse in line. That is what makes our link in nursing strong and that is how we will continue to weather many a stormy day in the future.

I know that our work proceeds from a base of family and friends who love us and support us and are honest with us in our work. Looking back to the beginning of my journey, I realize that I have really not carefully planned out my career even though I have had one wonderful ride. I never even set out to be an oncology nurse, although I would never trade my work for any other specialty. I never planned on writing or editing papers (English wasn't even my native tongue), but I have grown immensely from the discipline. Today, I also know that God's hand was in all of the seemingly serendipitous turning points in my life. God has given me a measure of faith and I have a humble and a grateful heart for what God has done for me. This is the bedrock of my faith and one that helps me to work each day and to comfort those in need of comfort, and to help those in need who cannot do for themselves.

I feel that I have at least 25 more years of work in oncology nursing ahead of me. I do not know where the paths will lead but I do know that I will be taken care of. When God closes one door, He will open another and will continuously look after me. I can trust that each day He will give me no more than I can handle, and I thank God for all the blessings that He gives me each day.

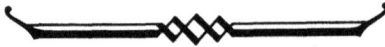

10

Coni Ellis

My first memories of wanting to become a nurse are tied to my one and only hospitalization as a child. Ill with what sounded like a fatal disease, "pharyngitis," I spent three days in a military hospital where I was treated in a really special way as the only child on a women's ward. I thought the nurses were the greatest, going from patient to patient taking care of whatever they needed. I remember playing nurse to my dolls with my room being a hospital and receiving a nurse's kit for Christmas.

In high school I was in the Future Nurses Club and worked as a nurse's aide at the base hospital and loved it. I also enjoyed writing for the school newspaper and teaching Sunday school. I felt in nursing I could do all three, care for people, write, and teach. Little did I know . . .

I originally was accepted to attend a three-year diploma program in Alabama but as fate would have it my air force dad was transferred from Mississippi to New York in my senior year and said I couldn't stay behind. As I was writing to New York schools, his base was closed and we were transferred to San Antonio, Texas. I was lucky to be accepted by Incarnate Word College.

Now as I look back on my 25 years in nursing I see six critical decisions that have had major impact on my career. Graduating with a B.S.N. from Incarnate Word College, San Antonio, Texas, in December 1968 was number one. When my best friend Margi Ciatto and I decided to leave Santa Rosa Medical Center, where we did our clinical rotation, and move to Houston, Texas, was number two. Margi had worked at St. Joseph Hospital (also owned and operated by the Incarnate Word nuns) as a nurses' aide while in high school and strongly recommended we start our careers there. We started as floaters at the 850-bed general hospital, going from one unit to the other. Once we passed the boards in May of 1969, I chose to be permanent on the oncology floor while she picked OB/GYN.

It was on 5 South, the oncology unit, where I was first mentored by a "well-seasoned nurse." Lola Smith, 15 years my senior, was a "young nurse at heart." Filled with boundless energy she opened the world of oncology nursing to me. The memory of one particular patient we cared for stays with me even today. Mr. H. was a 75-year-old gentleman with cancer of the throat, who had had a radical neck dissection with laryngectomy. One week was very distressing for Mr. H. and we couldn't seem to please him. He became very angry with me and even threw a full urinal at Lola. She just took it in her stride and began to teach me, although I'm not too sure how conscious I was of it at the time, that we need to allow patients to express their feelings. Anyway, I decided to make a special effort to answer his call light whenever it came on. He usually called because he needed to be suctioned, which I would do and he would frown and signal that he was O.K. This continued for a week or so. I felt that he needed more from me but I didn't know how to give it. Then one day he put on his light and when I came in he was smiling and had written this note: "I hear you're leaving next week." I responded, "Yes, I'm going to have a baby." He wrote, "Name him after me?" Up to that moment I think I thought I had been meeting all of his needs but realized I had focused on the technical skills and not those that would recognize his humanness.

Our unit had cancer patients who received surgery and chemotherapy as their major treatment modalities. We worked with Dr. John Stehlin, who was one of the first physicians to give intra-arterial chemotherapy to patients with liver cancer. The first patient I cared for was a young man named Chuck from Arkansas. He was close to my age, recently married, and had a son. I became very attached to him and invited him to join me and my fiancé for Thanksgiving dinner that year since his family was still at home. I made sure I got assigned to care for him whenever I was on duty. When it came time to discharge him, I was depressed for days worrying that he wouldn't get the care he needed at home. Lola helped me to see the difference between meeting the psychosocial needs of patients and my own needs, and that there were boundaries that needed to be maintained.

As a new nurse caring for cancer patients I was both threatened and energized by the variety of patients we cared for and the treatments and procedures that needed to be done. The surgical patients who initially frightened me later became my favorites, those with head and neck cancers, who at that time had radical laryngectomies. Trach care, with Lola as my teacher, became as routine as providing mouth care for a patient. Along with another new grad I became interested in developing continuity in trach care; we didn't have standards of care and quality assurance monitoring in those days. We instituted simple things like changing the suction catheters, solutions, and bottles every eight hours as opposed to the previous practice of once every 24 hours, or "whenever." Our primary goal was to heighten awareness of aseptic technique.

Now when I care for these patients we have a multiple set-up that includes suction catheters, gloves, containers, and saline—a far cry from what we had.

IV therapy was a procedure that seemed to separate the "new" nurse from the "real" nurse. Initially, when I knew the surgical residents were available, I had difficulty starting IVs (with the old syringe needles). Once I became learned, this skill was second nature to me. Later in my teaching career I would teach a basic IV therapy course and even later would present a class to orientees. I always tried to instill in the "new" nurses to act confidently with their patients, showing their care and compassion, and that this in turn would help their patients to have confidence in them as they gained their competence.

Chemotherapy, now that was new to me. We hadn't been exposed to it in nursing school, other than in lectures. While floating on the medical units I had learned to mix and deliver IV chemo. That was the only route we used and the only pumps were sigma motor pumps for intra-arterial infusions. My buddy, Pat Bucheck, and I compiled our school notes and would have discussions during our breaks. We experimented with an intra-arterial pump trying to figure out how the drug went in versus the saline. There were no drug company representatives or nursing inservice instructors to enlighten us so we would share our notes with the rest of the staff.

My only exposure to radiation therapy was caring for patients with intercavitary XRT-tandoms and ovoids. Time, distance, and shielding weren't as stressed as they are now. If you had a dosimeter badge you were given "the impression" that you were safe. When I later took care of those patients in the late 1980s and 1990s the technology was similar but the safety concerns were much better addressed with lead-lined doors and selectron rooms.

Margi, my best friend, and I lived together and after work would compare notes about our day. One night she asked me if I'd ever put down an NG tube and had immediate returns. I said no. The next day was an experience I wouldn't soon forget. I not only got immediate returns upon NGT placement, but the patient coded. It was my first CPR experience after taking a CPR class the week before. Luckily, the patient survived.

Whenever I think of the early days of my career I remember another patient. Mr. Z. was a Jewish gentleman from New York who loved to tease me. When he wasn't teasing me, he and his wife were introducing me to different foods from Alfredi's Deli. I never did develop a taste for lox but to this day I enjoy bagels and cream cheese and matzo ball soup.

During his course of treatment Mr. Z.'s scrotum became very edematous and painful. He made me feel like I was taking good care of him when he noticed a schedule change one day and demanded, quite loudly down the hall, "Only Ellis takes care of my————!!" I hadn't realized that through all his joking he truly appreciated the respectful way I provided his care.

While evolving from a new grad to feeling comfortable as a new registered nurse, I also became new wife, daughter-in-law, and sister-in-law. Adapting to these roles was made easier as my husband was and remains a great soul mate. He could sense when patients weren't doing well and would be especially understanding. I've been fortunate never to have felt overwhelmed by maintaining a home and a job or graduate school, as we naturally share the housework and childcare, sensing when one needs relief from one job or the other. Alan has also been my editor, critiquing my papers, thesis, and now manuscripts.

Pregnancy with my first child ended my working on 5 South. A month after I left, Cindy was born on July 14, 1970. I really enjoyed being home with my daughter but looked forward to returning to work. However, this was not to be because six months later I became pregnant with my second child. Teffa was born in October 1971. Life in a two-bedroom apartment and two little ones in diapers wasn't as fun as it could be, but with the lack of funds, TV and reading were my only two distractions. Again, Margi recognized the "danger"—she saw me watching the "soaps" and knew my brain was turning to mush. First she bought me a few craft kits, which I completed in record time. She realized I needed more stimulation. It was time to go back to work!

St. Joseph Hospital had been affiliating with Houston Community College (HCC) for a nursing assistant program and had decided they would have their own program. They now had a nursing education department with four instructors. While I was interviewing at HCC, Margi was discussing me with the director of nurses at St. Joseph's and I was simultaneously hired for the same job by both places. My third critical decision came in February 1972 when I began a two-year stint teaching nursing assistants. I developed the program from the ground up. Initially it was a four-week course. I was unable to check off all the students in two weeks so the clinical was expanded and the course grew to six weeks. I would teach one course, have a two-week break, and then start another one.

During one of those two-week breaks, I had the most traumatic event of my life as a parent. One Saturday afternoon Margi and I were out shopping. My husband was at home with the girls. Teffa, 22 months old, adventured out on our two-story balcony and fell through the railing to the pea gravel below. Margi and I would have never known it had happened except that we had stopped by her dad's and he said Alan had called and that they were down the street at Spring Branch Hospital. We arrived as my black-and-blue bruised little darling came out of X-ray where they had determined she had four skull fractures and a broken leg.

That began a 2-week vigil for me at her bedside 24 hours a day, allowing for only minimal breaks from her sight. She was a real trooper and showed me how a sense of humor can help get you through times like these. Laced up in bilateral leg traction, wearing my sunglasses and my size eight pink sequinned slippers, she would swing her little fanny in the air and play peek-a-boo. When I look at the pictures we took, it still makes my heart ache to see her bruised face and big smiles. But it was her little giggles and playfulness that reassured me she was going to be O.K.

Besides being her mommy I was her nurse and did whatever task needed to be done, from the first night of around-the-clock neurovital signs to changing her diapers. I learned the value of having loving parents and supportive friends. Margi was there when I needed a "nurse" to relieve me, so I could break away and be with my husband and Cindy at home. Flowers, cards, and calls made the days pass faster. I encourage families today to tape them on the walls and when holiday time comes to decorate with them for the season. These simple distractions can make their stay a little more bearable.

Once the two weeks were up I was worried about having to leave Teffa alone in the hospital when my mom informed me she had taken time off from work and if I could show her what to do, she would do it. What a relief!

Teffa went from traction to a hip spica cast (nipples to toes in plaster) for three months. We automatically assumed I'd have to give up my job and stay at home with her when once again the manager of their day-care center came through. She told us if we could take care of her at home they could care for her there. So for three months we would bring her in with her tilt board her dad had built and her wagon and she was happy as a lark to be there with her friends. Six months later Teffa was fully recovered and had relearned to walk, swim, and pedal her trike.

Upon my return, it was decided we needed to present the nursing assistant courses back to back to increase the number of support staff for our hospital. The women attracted to this course were from lower socioeconomic backgrounds and had had no formal education after high school. As their teacher I had the pleasure to see them grow in their communication and interpersonal relationship skills as well as in the technical nursing skills they needed to care for patients. Although no longer a "caregiver to patients," I felt I was in a very powerful place for imparting my philosophy of care to others.

There were numerous frustrations during the two years I taught the nursing assistant course. The first was the physical size and location of the classroom—two blocks away from the nursing education department. I learned to troubleshoot every possible audio-visual equipment problem over the phone. But teaching 20 students handwashing with one sink and bedmaking with one bed was too much. Finally, after negotiating with St. Thomas University School of Nursing, the class moved to their skills lab.

Another frustration was the expectation of trying to develop a caring individual when the students selected often didn't have the basic qualities or attributes you would want in a nursing assistant. Once my peers who did the screening realized I couldn't rehabilitate someone in six weeks they developed better interviewing skills and this wasn't quite the problem it was in the beginning. I was relieved because I felt we were taking tuition money from those who didn't have it to spare and then watching them fail.

The challenge in managing these 15–20 students came when they went into the clinical area on five to eight different units in two different buildings. I was helped by my previous experience as a floater: I had worked with many of the nursing assistants and, along with their head nurses, selected them to be "buddies" for my students. I recently returned to St. Joseph's as part of my enterostomal therapy nurse clinical experience and was pleased to see so many of "my graduates" still there. Three of the buddies, Ms. Dixon, Ms. Osby, and Ms. Richards (all are in their 60s) are still delivering the quality nursing care they modeled for those students 20 years ago.

Once our nursing staff was supported by enough nursing assistants, my role changed. For the next two years I developed and taught a four-week ward clerk course mixed with "Adventures in Attitudes." The students were usually employees moving from the nursing assistant role or another position within the hospital. As I began a two-year assignment teaching this course, I felt myself moving away from the bedside. Teaching medical terminology, receptionist duties, and transcription of orders, although fundamental to providing quality care, was not as fulfilling as the nursing assistant course. However, I still received the gratification of seeing someone learn and implement a new role with success, which is one of the primary reasons I enjoy being a teacher.

My lack of bedside contact was brought home to me very distinctly by a former student of mine. During an inservice on the application of patient restraints, Rachel Barch kept sending me nonverbal messages of, "Oh, yeah, right!" After the inservice she told me how "unrealistic" I was. I hadn't mentioned the difficulty one might have trying to restrain the patient *prior* to putting on the restraints. From that day on, I made sure either to *have* the clinical experience I needed to "be real" or have someone who did teach through me.

After teaching nonlicensed nursing personnel for four years, in 1976 I taught my first peer-to-peer class. As the secretary for the Texas Nurses Association District 9, I was involved with our attempts to change the nurse practice act and was a supporter of mandatory continuing education for relicensure. The first class was on this very subject which was not well received by the RNs at St. Joseph's, or the rest of the state's nurses, since it wasn't until 1993 that this became law.

During this time I had enrolled in graduate school and was struggling with how much of an adult learner I wanted to be. Pregnancy with my third child, Alan, put school on the back burner.

My childbirth experience at Northwest Memorial Hospital was uneventful except that two of the RNs caring for me turned out to be former nursing assistant students of mine. As they each shared with me how I had influenced their choice of nursing for a career, it was indeed a doubly proud moment for me, seeing them providing care as registered nurses, and having a healthy baby.

While I had been off from work for a total of 22 months with my first two children, I was only off for three months with my last. Returning to work with a two-month-old son was distressing for me. Besides the guilt of delegating his care to others, I had the guilt of wanting to return to work. When my private sitter cancelled and we were able to make childcare arrangements at the day-care center that had cared for the girls earlier, I felt better. Although it was several miles out of my way to work, it was worth it to know who was caring for Alan.

Upon my return to work, Alan began having a series of ear infections. After undergoing five myringotomies and an adenoidectomy, the physician decided he was allergic to milk. Once milk was withdrawn from his diet at age two he did well. His father also started taking him to work with him so he wasn't exposed to the sick kids. Hence, he developed an incredible bond with his dad.

For the next two years my teaching focus now became general orientation and CPR. This perhaps was the least stimulating part of my career yet it *was* challenging to act positive and upbeat about the same material over and over again. Recognizing the potential for burnout in inservice education, Doris Yordonoff (who was my boss for 15 years) encouraged me when I wanted to develop a variety of courses over the years. Doris also encouraged us to participate in our professional organization (ANA, TNA) and took an active role herself in these activities. In 1976, the U.S. Bicentennial year, I was responsible for designing and implementing a huge three-sided poster that depicted the history of nursing in Houston for the Texas Nurses Association convention. The convention was held in San Antonio, and I visited my school of nursing for the first time since graduation. I was pleased to see some of my college instructors so they could see that I "turned out O.K."

Doris was one of four nurses at St. Joseph Hospital with a master's of science in nursing. She encouraged all of us in the nursing education department to attend graduate school and made sure we were able to get off on time to attend classes. She would make arrangements for us to teach from 3 to 11 P.M. to enable us to attend day classes.

Decision number four occurred in 1981–1983 when Mae Jean Carr, a fellow instructor, and I enrolled in graduate school, carpooling together to Texas Woman's University twice a week for two years. We were great supports for one another as I hated tests and she hated papers. It was great sharing Xerox costs and other resources too.

Graduate school was a very energizing time for me. I love to teach as much as I love to learn. A lot of what I had learned "by the seat of my pants" was validated in the education role classes I attended. Our classes were very small so we received a lot of attention. We actually presented the content, which was a different student role for me. With encouragement (and pressure) from my children I made the As and Bs I didn't necessarily make as an undergrad and was honored by becoming a charter member of the Eta Phi chapter of Sigma Theta Tau.

Through the years I had really missed patient care, especially caring for patients with cancer. They always seemed to be grateful for everything we did for them. In a profession as stressful as nursing, it's energizing to be appreciated. Therefore, I selected the oncology unit in Hermann Hospital for my medical/surgical clinical experience in grad school. Although there wasn't much hands-on nursing to do I was nervous about getting back in the clinical area. Once I met a few patients I was glad I had made the choice. I especially loved one elderly woman's spirit. She shared with me that she was frustrated and tired with all of the different levels of folks coming in and asking her the same questions. So when an intern came in at 3 A.M. to do a history and physical she not only kicked him out but told the chief resident when they made rounds that morning. From that point on I was careful to record as much about a patient as I could from their chart and to do my assessments as efficiently as possible and not travel the same ground for the tenth time. I find I can be just as thorough without the redundancy.

Doris was also futuristic in her staff development strategies. Seeing that the institution could no longer afford to send nursing staff carte blanche to continuing education programs, she made it one of our priorities to present three or four conferences a year highlighted by nationally known nurse leaders and speakers. This is when I learned the fine art of program development from the ground up, from objectives to budgets to negotiating with speakers.

Unfortunately, Doris didn't see how the changes that were occurring in health care (including the implementation of DRGs) would impact the hospital in general and the nursing education department in particular. From 1985 to 1987 the hospital downsized from 830 to 350 beds and eliminated ten directors, including Doris. The nursing education department was dissolved. These two years were very stressful for me trying to complete my thesis and not knowing whether or not my job would be cut. In the end I was one of the two "spared." Always a med/surg or backup to OB/GYN, I now found myself assigned to the psychiatric hospital. My immediate supervisor was my former peer (ICU/CCU) instructor and nurses who were "clinical coordinators" were now in the role of instructors. My assignment was to conduct orientation while orienting to psych on the side.

Philosophical differences came to a head when the plan for delivery of nursing care was changed to "modular" nursing: one RN, assisted by an LVN or nursing assistant, caring for 12 patients. I've always felt that as a part of nursing I had to support the administrators in their decisions and now found myself in a dilemma. I knew I couldn't provide the quality of patient care I would want to deliver with those ratios and no support systems. So how could I continue to promote this plan?

During this time I was attending an American Heart Association CPR corporate update when I ran into one of my graduate school buddies, Cheryl Wirth. She told me that if I was still unhappy with my job they had an opening at M.D. Anderson for a clinical instructor for the general surgery units/clinic. I went home that night and discussed it with my husband and family. I decided to give it a shot. There's nothing like interviewing for a job when you already have one. Two weeks after I received my master's, I applied and was accepted (decision number five).

In June 1987 I began working at the mecca for an oncology nurse, M.D. Anderson Cancer Center. My two-month clinical orientation focused on the gynecological and general surgery units. The radical nature of the surgical procedures, wound care, and medical equipment was overwhelming to me. I was afraid I had been away from the bedside too long. To supplement my orientation, I worked one Sunday a month the first year and then increased my time to two double shifts a week.

When I first started working extra on 4LP (General Surgery), I was nervous as a cat about being evaluated as an "instructor," carrying a full load, and developing the skills to care for such a variety of surgical patients. I shouldn't have worried as the staff recognized where my real skills were, in meeting the psychosocial needs of patients. Therefore, my assignments usually included patients and families whose predominant needs were for psychosocial or spiritual support. Since I knew how to provide this care I became more relaxed as I learned the technical aspects of patient care. With a nurse/patient ratio of one to four on the 3–11 shift, I had the time and the resources to help my patients and their families.

To charge myself up I used to start walking rounds with a song or chant such as "Boom Chug a Lugga" as we proceeded from patient to patient. Most of the staff are younger (by 20 years) than myself, so I have to explain how these little things help me "get through the night."

They soon looked forward to finding out what Coni was going to start the shift with tonight.

I love a good joke and enjoy infusing humor in my teaching. It usually spills over into my caregiving. Post-op patients are uncomfortable with their NGT tubes. When I'm doing my assessment I usually reaffirm this discomfort, explain bowel sounds, and if they are three to four days post-op I tell them to dream about beans or I show them a cartoon of a fellow blowing out the bottom of his bed with his "first post-op gas." This usually gives them a laugh and distracts them for a moment. One patient was nine days post-op with no bowel sounds and frustrated by being asked over and over again, "Have you passed gas?" I made a sign for her; on one side it said "no" and on the other it said "yes, hallelujah!" and told her to use it whenever a nurse or doctor asked her. She thought it was great. The next evening I came in, gave her a quizzical look, and she flashed me the "yes, hallelujah!" side and her family clapped. The patient and her family knew I was concerned yet this served as a distraction from her discomfort. I have used this approach successfully several other times.

In meeting patients and their families for the first time, I like to put them at ease and reassure them that I'm there for them. I remember one night when it almost backfired. I innocently asked the woman sitting next to a much older man, "How's your dad?" She replied, "He's not my father." I returned with, "So, how's your sugar daddy?" Both of them burst into laughter. (I learned to ask, "What is the relationship here" after that!)

My most frustrating night caring for a patient taught me humility. I was having a particularly busy night when this patient was received from PACU after a colon resection. In my initial assessment of the patient I found him to be in a lot of pain. His orders specified setting up a PCA pump with morphine. Before it arrived he became more agitated and impatient with me. Within 15 minutes of his arrival, we had the PCA pump and as I attempted to connect it to his IV line the port connector on his line fell off and blood started squirting everywhere. His wife was trying to reassure him that I was doing everything I could to fix the situation when he decided I should leave as he didn't think I knew what I was doing. I left and per his request called a nurse on the IV team. Together we got his PCA pump going and before the end of the shift had his pain under control. I still felt awful. Two nights later I came in for the 3–11 shift and wondered if I should request not to be assigned to him. Instead I kept my mouth shut and was assigned to him. I went in and introduced myself and proceeded with my head-to-toe assessment, sharing with him and his wife my findings and answering their questions. He looked at his wife and let out a sigh, saying, "Honey, isn't it wonderful to have a nurse who knows what she's doing? I feel like I can relax and rest now." The wife winked at me and I realized that he had been in so much pain the first night that he had no recollection of me at all. Instead of going on my merry way, I commented jokingly, "Gee, that's not the way you felt the other night," and related my frustration in trying to control his pain two nights before. What a mistake! He was embarrassed and most apologetic the rest of the night. I now use this as an example of what not to do and point out the importance of focusing on the patient not oneself.

On a lighter note, another night I received a report on Mr. R. regarding his pain level; the nurse reported seven on a zero to ten scale. In my initial assessment I didn't find the patient to be showing any signs of being in pain and he denied any when questioned. Then I reviewed his PCA record and saw that he had no continuous rate, had not been administered any doses all day, but had rated his pain level at seven or eight all day. It was reassessment time, so I asked him what the number meant and he replied, "You know how you rate a woman?" I said, "Yes, like ten means pretty fine." He replied, "Yeah, I'm feeling pretty fine!" This is a great example of the need to periodically verify with patients what we mean with different assessment tools.

Pain management is a great concern of mine. I feel oncology nurses play an even greater role as patient advocates in this arena. Most of our physicians either do a good job in this arena or call in the pain management team. However, we have new residents here for a few months who haven't covered for oncology patients or are not aware of cancer pain syndromes. One such person was introduced to me one night as "the doctor who didn't believe in pain medicine." I said, "O.K., I guess you don't believe in sleeping the nights you're on call?" He responded with, "What do you mean?" and I replied, "Well, you're not going to get much sleep when I'm here, because I will call you until my patients are comfortable." He collapsed in a chair and said, "O.K., what do you need?" I told him and from that day on he was reasonable with his responses to our pain requests.

In my first five years at Anderson I also had to cover the gynecology units as we were always short one instructor. I oriented around 200 nurses. It was frustrating for me but I could see myself over time evolving from the nurse who cared for and taught about cancer patients, to an oncology nurse.

I was already certified by the American Nurses Association as a clinician in medical/surgical nursing so in 1989 I took the big step and sat for the oncology nurse certification and passed. Then I felt truly as if I'd joined the ranks of oncology nurses. In 1994, I obtained my enterostomal therapy nurse certification. Both groups are made up of people who are stimulating to work with as they are never satisfied with the status quo. I feel the "action's there", whether at work or when I attend the annual Oncology Nurses Society Congress or the Wound

Ostomy Continence Nurse Society convention. In 1993 I was especially fortunate, because of my background of caring for patients with breast cancer, to be selected by Burrough's Welcome to present in their "Purple Breast" program at ONS in Orlando. After this experience I continued my interest in breast cancer patients with several presentations, posters, and manuscripts.

This interest evolved into real concern for our patients at M.D. Anderson as they went from three- to five-day hospitalizations to the short-stay mastectomy of less than 36 hours. Along with our general surgery CNS, Cathy Burke, clinic nurse manager Cindy Zabka, and clinic assistant nurse manager Karen McCarver, we developed a class for post-op teaching to meet patients' educational care needs. Because we were concerned with whether their psychosocial needs were being met, we designed a research project. It is in its infancy so it is too early to report on the results.

Participation in professional nursing organizations is important to me. For the first two-thirds of my career, when I didn't have a real focus, I supported the American Nurses Association and the Texas Nurses Association. This later third of my career has centered on being an active member of my local Houston chapter of the Oncology Nursing Society. As a board member for six years I've assisted with the newsletter, served as the ONS–Oncology Nursing Foundation liaison, and helped plan and present OCN review courses twice a year. Our chapter has some very fine leaders and we've seen it grow in membership from 100 to almost 200, with 30–40 regularly attending the meetings. I try to influence new orientees, especially the new graduates, to join a professional organization, and supply them with the necessary paperwork to make it easier for them. Unfortunately I'm not 100 percent effective, but I won't give up!

Our department has two nationally known nurse leaders at its helm: Betty Cody as the administrative chair and Debbie Volker as our director of nursing. We stay on the cutting edge of what is happening in nursing education because of their leadership.

From the very beginning as an instructor, I have also participated in house-wide inservices, CPR, continuing education, and outreach programs, focusing on the psychosocial issues of oncology patients, pain management, and spiritual care. This evolved into my being the psychosocial module coordinator for the Houston Area Critical Care Collaborative program which was presented the Thelma Schorr Award for innovations in staff development.

Right now we seem to be in a constant state of change which is predicted to be our "reality." Both Betty and Debbie are very supportive of our presenting at national nursing conferences. It's been through their role modeling that I started sending in abstracts which have resulted in numerous poster, round-table, and formal presentations.

In the last seven years I've also been mentored by three other outstanding individuals: Dorothy (Dot) Smith, who still encourages me to write for publications. Along with our nurse counselor Mickey Bumbaugh and our psych CNS Mary Hughes, Dot and I wrote a pocket book for nurses entitled, "Promoting Health–Preventing Problems, A Psychosocial Guide." After it was published, Shirley Morrison, a former instructor and now nurse manager, nominated me for the Oncology Nursing Foundation's Mara Mogensen Flaherty Lecture for my efforts in the psychosocial arena. This year, the Houston ONS Chapter nominated me for the Quality of Life Lectureship.

Dot has a special way about her that makes you believe in yourself. She is also a positive role model for recognizing the need for reenergizing yourself. I especially enjoyed having Dot as my director as she did what I needed at this point of my career—she provided me with the resources and encouragement I needed to do the job, got out of my way, let me do it, and jerked my chain when I needed it. Dot also has a most pleasing personality which I really miss now that she's gone to Louisiana. I try to be as cheerful as she was but don't always make it.

My number two mentor was Clara Usrey. As our outreach coordinator, Clara was responsible for meeting the oncology nursing education needs of those nurses outside the institution. One of the most successful programs she developed was our Mobile Van Education project, called, after its benefactors, "Polo on the Prairie." This program makes eight trips a year to present a total of 16 all-day oncology programs to nurses in hospitals with fewer than 100 beds that don't have access to continuing education. Clara encouraged me to learn three of the major topics so I could go on these trips. Enter Beverly Hampton, my enterostomal therapy mentor. Taking me under her wing she taught me the ostomy, wound, and skin care content, as I already knew the pain management and death and dying content. Four years later I've traveled all over Texas presenting this content and having a great time besides. Clara, who has since retired, always made sure you learned about the countryside you were passing through from the piney woods of east Texas to the desert in west Texas. Now, the outreach coordinator, Georgia White, and I have to rely on chamber of commerce information.

While I enjoyed teaching this content, I didn't *feel* like an expert. To do this I needed to take our enterostomal nurse education program, which was decision number six. After two years I was sent to the program and graduated in November 1993. I feel that a new world is opening up before me now. My job has changed to outreach/ET academic instructor. In this position I continue to keep my clinical skills up to date as I participate in patient care and plan/present CE programs on a variety of subjects. As the outreach instructor, I facilitate the clinical/education experiences for our nurse visitors who come from all over Texas, the United States, and other countries. They come for one day to two months to a year to learn about cancer care at M.D. Anderson. This year they have come from Japan, Thailand, Australia, and Nigeria. It is a real challenge to assess their learning needs and then match them up with educational and clinical experiences. We also custom make courses and take them wherever requested. Every spring in Outreach we sponsor a Student Oncology Day to which we invite nursing students from Texas and southern Louisiana. During this day, they hear a variety of lectures on oncology and have clinical skills labs where they can do some hands-on learning. Our goal has been to encourage them to consider oncology nursing as a career. We have had a good response as several students each year either enroll in our professional nursing student extern program or come as new grads to our nurse intern program.

We also have a two-week oncology program we cosponsor with the Nurse Oncology Education Program of Texas which focuses on nursing faculty. Our goal with this group is to facilitate them in integrating more oncology into their nursing curriculums and to encourage them to seek oncology clinical experiences. As the academic coordinator for the schools of nursing with which we have clinical affiliations, I can tell you it is working. We have more requests for undergraduate clinical experiences than we can meet. Now I'm seeing an increase in the number of graduate nurses seeking their clinicals here in all three roles: CNS, education, and administration.

As the ET (enterostomal therapy) instructor I help with the management and presentation of the program as well as facilitate the clinical aspects. Beverly keeps me busy as she is always thinking up new programs for us to develop and present. I'm also learning to be a photographer as it is essential to our role as educators to have current clinical pictures of the wound and ostomy problems we deal with which enhance our teaching. This portion of my role also lends itself to product evaluation and clinical research, which we hope to do in the near future.

Dot and Beverly have always taught me the responsibility to share what I know through manuscripts or professional presentations. This fall we'll be very busy with the preparation of a TV program on wounds, two wound programs for vendors, classes on ostomy and wound care for North Harris County Community College, two manuscripts on wound care, plus our regular responsibilities.

I have set a goal for myself to present at least one national conference per year and have met this goal by being selected for either a poster, round table, or presentation. It's a lot of fun to travel around the country, network with other nurses, and be looked to as an oncology nurse.

As 1994 began, working overtime as a staff nurse was deleted and we entered the managed care arena. It has become even more important for me to supplement my income, as my husband has become disabled. Reenter Cheryl Wirth into my life (my old grad school bud and former instructor mate at MDA). Cheryl is the continuing education coordinator for North Harris County Community College. I am now one of her adjunct faculty members and teach short courses in wounds and ostomy care, spiritual care, and yes, hospital nursing assistants.

Nursing to me is a vocation, not an occupation. I feel that I have received more than I ever gave. I encourage all the new employees I encounter to take time to care for themselves, reenergizing themselves on a regular basis and supporting one another. If they feel they "can't do the job another day" I encourage them to try a different clinical area, go back to school for an advanced degree, or try a different RN clinical role. I stress to them how special they are as caregivers and how important it is for them to keep their special qualities. Over the years several nurses have taken this advice and remain in nursing in a different "place" and continue to love their work.

I've stressed this to my three children also, to pick an occupation or job that they will really love to do for they'll be doing it the majority of their lives. I think they see me modeling this behavior; therefore, I'm confident that they will. Guess what, my daughter Cindy wants to be a nurse!

11

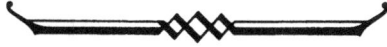

Betty Ferrell

Beginning

I grew up in a very loving but poor family in a small community in Oklahoma. At the age of 17, I went away to college with barely $100 in the bank and by the grace of the financial aid office at the community college I would attend! As a freshman I was a speech major because I was going to school on a debate scholarship and working as a secretary in the speech and debate department. By the end of that first year, I knew without a doubt that I did not want to pursue the goals of my fellow students in this department, to study law, communication, or other related disciplines. What I could not identify at the time, but later knew, was that I was really searching for a profession that provided greater meaning. I thought of nursing primarily because I was sur-rounded by several nursing majors in my freshman dormitory. Thus my decision to become a nursing major at that time was more of an issue of, "Why not?" than a true understanding or dedication to the profession.

As a sophomore without a job or scholarship in the speech depart-ment, I was desperate for employment. I applied for a job at a local hospital, quite convinced that they would welcome me with open arms. After all, I had declared a major in nursing only a few months before. However, the hospital felt that the only position I was qualified for was that of a housekeeper. Thus I began my career in nursing cleaning toilets in the early hours, afternoons, and weekends! This job was undoubtedly my real nursing education. During that year I was able to enter every area of the hospital including the emergency room, patient rooms, and nurses' lounge (a real source of education). I was also able to observe interactions between nurses and patients and between patients and family members. I often had conversations with patients that began with, "I haven't told my doctor this, but . . ." I learned a lot as an observer during that year which undoubtedly has influenced my role as a nurse.

As a junior in the nursing major, I was accepted into a nurse extern program for the summer of my junior/senior year and extending until my graduation. I attended a hospital orientation at a major hospital in the area during the peak time of a nursing shortage. After a two-week orientation, the nurse externs were assigned to units. I remember getting my assignment on a piece of paper that said, "Oncology." I did not even know what the word meant, but I was so glad to have a job that I smiled and proceeded to go to the unit to meet the head nurse, trying at best to hide my ignorance and to quickly find out what "oncology" really meant. I worked on the 3–11 shift at what was the height of team nursing. This meant that for the entire oncology unit, there was one RN, myself, one other nurse extern, and two nurses' aides assigned to the team. Thus, in a few months, I graduated from being a housekeeper to being a team leader in caring for 20 oncology patients.

I remember clearly the first patient that I cared for on the oncology wing. It was in the evening of one of my first days, and a patient rang the call bell to ask for pain medicine. I entered the room to find an elderly man who was in severe bone pain from widely metastatic disease. As I entered the room and the patient turned to see me, I realized that even this movement was provoking extreme pain. I remember the look in his eyes as he asked if I could please get his pain medicine and "help" him. My heart was racing; it was a revelation: "He's the patient in pain—I'm the nurse—I'm going to relieve pain and suffering!" I went to the Kardex to look up his pain medicine. I saw the order on the Kardex for the dose of medication that I was sure must be an error. Still at this stage of having my medication cards securely in my lab coat pocket, I reached for the cards only to find that the dose prescribed for this man was ten times more than that on my medication card. I felt in that moment that my life was passing before me! If I gave this dose of medicine, this patient might die and surely my nursing career would end before it began. On the other hand, I also remembered this man's face and his need for pain relief. I remember giving the dose of pain medicine and praying that the patient would not quit breathing. My prayer was not for his own safety, but clearly for my own career! Of course, what I learned in the subsequent hours was that the pain medicine only barely relieved his pain.

A year later, upon graduation, I looked for a position. The hospital that I had selected to work in did not have positions open in oncology at that time. I accepted a position for a day-shift job as I also was a newlywed. I was assigned to work on the postpartum unit. The excitement, fulfillment, and commitment to nursing that I had learned in the past year in caring for cancer patients came to an abrupt halt. Those six weeks on postpartum felt like a void. One day, while going to lunch, the nurse supervisor for oncology, Pat Tolsin, saw me and remembered having seen me at an oncology nursing function and my being an extern on the oncology unit. She asked me what on earth I was doing working on postpartum, to which I informed her that I certainly did not know. The supervisor informed me that she in fact did have a position opening on oncology and thus "rescued me" back into the place I belonged—in oncology.

I worked for three years as an inpatient staff nurse in oncology. During that time, I became very interested in the family members of the patients and particularly intrigued with what happened after the patients were discharged from the hospital. Even then, in the "pre-DRG" era, I was very intrigued as to how patients and families were managing this devastating illness at home. I left the hospital environment to begin working in home care. Over the next several years I worked in a number of roles from staff nurse to director of nursing and administrator in home care and hospice. In a way, my career since that time could be described as, "the rest is history!" Since those days, I have focused all of my work clinically on my research on patients and families at home with the primary focus on pain as a clinical problem.

The Next Ten Years

Challenges

In my career as an oncology nurse, I have faced many challenges and controversies, most which seem to stem from raising questions or taking a different perspective. I have felt many times like a small voice in the wilderness trying to get attention for problems that I feel have been ignored. I recall a patient who was an inspiration for me early in my career while still an inpatient nurse. This was at a period of my professional life when I was very consumed with the ideas of increasing patient compliance, teaching patients to follow the regimen, and assuming that the best care for all patients was to be "good patients" so that they would live long lives and be successful with cancer treatment. However, I met a patient who defied all that I knew. He was a patient who decided to live life, including the experience of cancer, on his own terms. He was the kind of patient you would find in the stairwell smoking marijuana or hosting a party in his room despite isolation precautions. He was the patient who preferred margaritas and nachos to Ensure® and created havoc amongst the staff. I learned many things from this patient about the nurse-patient relationship, but what I most learned was that he was an individual who lived life on his own terms and who made a choice about the quality of his life. Shortly before he died, he presented me with a T-shirt that someone had given to him that he felt expressed his philosophy and perhaps one that I could learn from. The T-shirt reads, "No guts, no glory." I have thought about that patient and shirt in the ten years that followed.

My greatest challenges are in taking stands on issues that are controversial. I think within us all is a tendency to believe that we are doing a good job, that all is well, and that our patients are comfortable and supported. I recall that when I began my work on pain management, I was greeted by many colleagues who thought the ideas were ridiculous and assumed that pain was managed well at home. As I began my pain research, I became aware of the fact that, because of advances in treatment, we had been able to improve pain management but in the process had made other aspects of the quality of life much worse.

I remember doing the first home visit on a patient who went home with an epidural catheter. I observed a patient who was in an absolute crisis. She had not slept, was not eating, and had lain immobilized for fear of dislodging her epidural catheter. Her children, to whom she had gone home so she could be close to them, were terrified because they had been warned "not to touch their mother" for fear that they would interfere with the pump or tube. I witnessed a husband who was very stressed from this caregiving at home. I asked this woman about her pain, and I remember feeling nauseous when I heard her reply. She told me that she had no *pain*. But as I stood at her bedside, I realized that while we had succeeded in reducing her pain, we had made every other aspect of her life worse for both her and her family. It was then that I began my research into the quality of life as an outcome of pain. Working with colleagues, such as Marie Whedon, I have attempted to advocate for scrutiny in advances in pain management technology. This has not often been an easy message to share. I am very concerned about the safety of new drugs and innovations in pain management. I remain committed to being careful as we advance in pain management that we do not create harms or complications in the process.

More recently, my interest has been in issues of ethics related to pain management. The advances that we make in pain management through efforts such as the Agency for Health Care Policy and Research (AHCPR) pain guidelines are very important. However, I often feel that our textbook approach to pain management and the advances in the science of pain management overlook the *art* of caring for those who are suffering and the human experience of pain. I believe that advocating for issues such as this are important, yet one definitely pays a price for taking such stands.

The second challenge for me has been to bridge the two aspects of my role, being a clinician and a researcher. The more I have devoted my energy to research, the less of my time has been focused on clinical care. I have benefited from focusing all of my research on clinical issues, but struggle to find ways to be personally involved in direct contact with patients. I have felt pulled between the roles of researcher and clinician. I believe very much in the need for research-based practice. I believe in the importance of research to the Oncology Nursing Society, the nursing profession, and to the care of patients with cancer. However, I have always struggled with the need to keep research clinically focused and relevant to the daily care of patients and their families. The time that I served as a member and subsequently chair of the ONS Research Committee was very challenging as I worked toward implementing research within ONS in a way that would promote both the advancement of research and the benefit to clinicians. We are so lucky within ONS to have the most dedicated and excellent nurse researchers. My research colleagues within ONS have truly served as a source of inspiration for me.

Frustrations

There are two issues which continue to irritate me and probably also keep me motivated to go on. The first is the continued perspective of oncology in many professional and political arenas as one of only aggressive treatment and cure. I believe that the importance of concepts such as hospice care, palliation, and supportive care have moved forward tremendously in the past decade. However, I still experience situations in which the need for supportive care, symptom management, and recognition of cancer as a terminal illness are neglected. Many oncology nurses have worked in settings where it is almost unthinkable to utter the word *pain* for fear that such a discussion might imply that not all patients in that setting would be cured of the disease of cancer. I believe that the social stigma of death and the institutional value of cure still impede tremendously the care of those patients who will not be cured of cancer but in fact will die from it.

The second frustration that I face daily is in advocating for the role of nursing within the field of oncology. Nurses have made tremendous strides in all levels of cancer care. Efforts by individual nurses and by the Oncology Nursing Society have undoubtedly altered the course of care for persons with cancer. At times, I become incensed to find situations where nursing is absent. I see educational programs, committees, and organizations in which nursing has been clearly ignored. It feels as if for every two steps forward, we take one back. Despite this, I think we are making tremendous progress.

Successes and Celebrations

The greatest cause for celebration in my professional life has been to know that what we do as oncology nurses makes a difference. It is sometimes difficult in my area of pain management not to become overwhelmed with the reality of how frequently we fail to provide adequate relief from pain and other symptoms. However, I have had many causes to celebrate in seeing patients whose pain has been relieved and whose quality of life has been improved as a result. Being an oncology nurse means being able to celebrate the victories achieved one at a time. Seeing one patient able to get out of bed, go to church one more time, or be made comfortable enough to hold a grandchild is enough reinforcement to outlast many frustrations. I can honestly say that most of my successes and celebrations as an oncology nurse are directly linked to my involvement with ONS. The Oncology Nursing Society has provided me with colleagues, friends, and "soul mates," and has undoubtedly made me proud to be a nurse and most important an oncology nurse. As I list my mentors, friends, and heros, I realize that I have known most of them through my association with ONS. During moments of feeling alone, I have also felt very connected to a nationwide network of people who may be distant geographically but who I know I can count on for support.

Mentors

My earliest mentors in nursing were those I met through the local American Cancer Society in Oklahoma. Nurses such as Gay Jones and Zelma Reid served not only as examples of professional commitment, but also as invaluable role models of individuals who balanced both professional and family commitments. Two other people who served as mentors for me were Jean Haught and Johnita Rolling. Jean Haught was the nurse educator who worked in the hospital and conducted my orientation as a nurse extern. She is the person who handed me that slip of paper assigning me to oncology. She also became my best friend over the next ten years. Jean was killed in a tragic accident in 1988. What I most remember about her was her dedication to issues of patient care, her friendship, and what I have thought of since as her "passion" for nursing. The second early mentor was my sister, Johnita. She was two years older than me and was the first member of my entire extended family to attend college. Although we were very different, I have later thought of how she influenced my choices, particularly my interest in education. Johnita was killed during the second year of my nursing career. In many ways these two individuals have inspired me, and I feel that I keep a part of them within me. The "spunk" of these two people is probably what empowers me to fight some of the battles that I endure.

My Family

My family has undoubtedly been my greatest strength. I am fortunate to come from a wonderful family and to have married into a wonderful family. My family has not always understood my focus on education, but has definitely supported and believed in me. An early childhood experience that I think has influenced me was one that I did not recognize at the time. During my adolescent years, my mother worked as a nurses' aid in a children's convalescent hospital. She cared for children who were comatose, had severe birth defects, and were both physically and mentally severely disabled. She worked the 3–11 shift at this convalescent home. I would sneak in to visit her in the evening on many occasions, and discuss my current adolescent crisis. This was clearly at the stage of my life when I was convinced I never wanted to pursue any health career and definitely would never be a nurse. I can remember standing in a corner, hiding (as I was not supposed to be there), and quietly observing her interactions. I watched her care for physically and mentally incapacitated children in a way that no one else did. She would talk to children who everyone else said could never hear; she would lovingly treat these children with tremendous dignity. She created the images that I have of what it means to be a caring nurse.

My husband's support has been *the strength* in all that I have accomplished. He is my most honest critic and most ardent supporter. He has been nothing but supportive throughout our 17 years together. We have experienced many things. The greatest influence of my career is undoubtedly my husband who is the most compassionate of spouses, fathers, and physicians. My daughter Annie is the light of my life. I went into labor with Annie one night after class in graduate school. She attended her first class when she was one week old (Nursing Theory in my master's program). From ages two to six, I left home once or twice a week to attend my doctoral classes in Texas. Until age six, Annie believed that all mothers left the state once a week. Annie has taken all of this in stride and expresses that she must hold honorary membership in the Oncology Nursing Society after having attended six congresses and two fall institutes! Annie's humor and love are my greatest supports in my work.

The Balancing Act

When you love your work, it becomes even more difficult to balance the demands of professional and personal life. I have many interests outside of work including arts, theater, travel, reading, and most important, time with my family. In the first years of my nursing life I lost my best friend

Jean, my sister Johnita, and my son Andy who died at nine weeks of age in the neonatal ICU. The loss of these three people taught me that what matters most is relationships. Whether it is the relationship of family, friends, or colleagues, I value relationships with people more than anything else and feel that relationships are probably the balance to my life.

I often hear a saying, "No one ever looks back and says 'I wish I had worked more.'" I disagree with that sentiment. I believe that as women and particularly as mothers, we often sacrifice professional goals because of unrealistic expectations of being perfect mothers and wives. While I thoroughly agree with the ideas of balancing one's life and respecting the need for both physical and mental health, I also believe that it is not a sin to love one's work nor to be committed to one's profession. Although there is a great need for us to respect the diversity within our profession, the greatest need is to respect the choices that each of us makes with regard to work, education, family commitments, and other life choices. While I have observed some people frown when they see someone holding a baby at the back of a session at an ONS Congress, I always smile. I consider it a privilege when someone brings their baby to a session, and see it as a symbol of hope for us as we try to balance our personal and professional lives in ways that may be scrutinized publicly and yet personally rewarding.

What keeps me in oncology nursing is that through my profession I have found an ability to find tremendous meaning in my work. I value greatly my association with the Oncology Nursing Society and my many ONS friends.

Note

Ensure is a registered trademark of Mead Johnson Company.

12

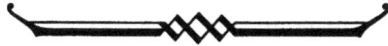

Rosemary Ford

Last May, after accepting the position of outpatient nurse manager, I organized a retreat for the nursing staff. I asked each member to bring a picture of themselves at or around the time of graduation from nursing school, and to share why they decided to go into nursing and their goals at graduation. I was amazed and a bit envious of those who knew they had the calling at an early age. This was definitely not my experience.

My father was a career army officer, retiring as a colonel when I was 12. My mother was a nursery school teacher during World War II, then a homemaker until my father's death in 1978, when she became secretary for the parish church. I am the oldest of three. My brother Greg is 2 years younger, and my baby sister Carol 11 years younger. My sister is also a nurse and my mother continually states that she is amazed that we are nurses, acknowledging that we received no direction in this area when we were young. My mother always thought I would have a good head for "business" (never elaborated) and had the notion that I would never have considered nursing because I was averse to the sight of blood. I have yet to figure out what she bases this on. My sister is one of those enigmas mentioned above who knew since the time she was a candy striper that she would be a nurse. She says her decision had nothing to do with following in my footsteps, and I believe her as, thinking about it now, it seems to me we both decided to enter nursing independently in the same year (she at 10 and me at 21)!

I was a recluse as a teenager, never participating in class and rarely talking to anyone aside from my best friend Anne. I attended a Catholic all-girls school in the heart of Berkeley from 1963 to 1967. This was confusing to say the least as the free speech movement raged a few blocks from my school and the nuns declared that the devil lived on Telegraph Avenue. The nuns lavished their attention on those girls who excelled scholastically. The myth was that if they worked very hard they could enter into the most esteemed group of women (aside from those in the convent of course)—nurses. I never was a good fit with that school, never applied myself (as teachers are wont to say), and so was left with the notion that nursing was a field beyond my abilities.

After graduation I entered a junior college where I felt revived by the discussions, the debates, the focus on current events, and yes, it was great to be in classes with boys. The highlight of these two years was my English 101 instructor, Sheila Wander. She expected us to think. Her approach and style were completely opposite from the rote memorization and compliance which characterized my high-school years. Of the 35 who started in her class, only 7 of us finished. No one received an A; I received one of the two Bs and I consider this grade the highlight of my first four years of college. Ms. Wander invited me to enroll in a study group the following semester and this acknowledgment enabled me to push out of the low self-esteem I had developed in high school.

Another experience during this time which I probably should have paid attention to but didn't, was how excited I was about my physiology class. Most of the other students were in a three-year diploma program for nursing. This class was an easy A but somehow I never put it together that maybe I should pursue this interest. Instead, I followed what was the most obvious influence on me at the time, and decided to major in either English or sociology. Because it was 1969 and because I had to declare a major to transfer to San Jose State, it seemed most relevant to choose sociology to try and figure out what was happening in those chaotic years.

My first real encounter with a nurse was with my dorm roommate Jill who was a nursing student. I was in awe of her dedication to arise at 5 A.M. to make it to her "clinicals," and was happy to roll over knowing my first lecture started at 10 A.M.

I continued to enjoy my classes and was peripherally involved in the war protests. In my last semester I was shocked to learn that I was about to graduate and was not very employable. A few months later I found a job as a receptionist at an association for government employees which was affiliated with a large labor union. The politics were far to the left and the field representatives were constantly holding heady philosophical discussions which I found exciting and seemed like a continuation of my sociology classes. In a year I had advanced from receptionist to secretary to office manager, but knew that I was not satisfied with and really not that good at clerical work. The women's rights movement was in full momentum at this time. I was trying to figure out what to do next with my life and made a conscious exercise of looking for women role models. Social work was an obvious area to consider because of my degree, but my attention and admiration quickly was drawn to the public health nurses. These nurses were the most cohesive group in the union, used the union for their own needs, were articulate, involved, vocal advocates for their patients, worked independently, seemed to be having fun, and were relatively well paid. They seemed to be involved in important work as I watched them fighting for funds for a juvenile diabetic teaching program or organizing their clientele of elderly ladies with blue and pink hair to crowd the county council meetings to argue against cutting funds for visits to the elderly.

I was dating one of the field reps at the time (whom I later married), and Julie Grisham (then Venkus), the public health nurses' representative to the union, was a friend of his. Julie and I became (and still are) friends and she was very supportive of my decision to go to nursing school. It did not take long to make the decision, and once made it felt right. I enrolled in night school for the prerequisites and two years after my initial graduation, I found myself back at San Jose State majoring in nursing and getting up at 5 A.M. A few of the public health nurses had warned me that nursing school was an obstacle course to go through, but that it would be worth it. It was helpful to keep that in mind. Nursing school was a love/hate experience for me. At 23 I was one of the oldest in the class, and found it amazing that the nursing department seemed to function in isolation from the rest of the campus. I enjoyed participating in the classes as I had before and I think I was identified as a thorn in the side of a few of the faculty. I remember one meeting where I was called into a room as the only student with several faculty members and was asked to define the term *Third World*!

For the most part I have learned to appreciate (in hindsight) much of the curriculum that was covered. I still feel that the program had too little actual clinical experience and am thankful that my last semester clinical instructor allowed me to spend an extra day a week at Stanford's intermediate ICU when she was present with another class. Because of the emphasis on ICU skills that I had encountered in school, and the tight job market in public health, I had turned my attention to intensive care nursing.

At graduation a few of us tried to get the consensus of the class not to wear caps—after all, male nurses didn't! However, there were no males in my class and tradition won. A few of us did not comply anyway. I overheard some of the spectators comment on how embarrassed those of us without caps must be to have forgotten them. So much for symbolic protest!

After graduation I moved to Seattle where my husband had been accepted to graduate school. In 1976 nursing was experiencing one of our periodic job shortages. I applied to every hospital in the city which would give me an application, but the only one willing to interview me was the county hospital. I explained to the nurse who interviewed me that I was interested in intensive care and she said that the burn unit was a good step into intensive care.

I think I have been lucky at the various turning points in my life and this is certainly one where I feel I was at the right place at the right time. I was the last nurse hired in the burn unit for almost a year. Because of that and being a new grad, I was able to gradually take on responsibilities as I was ready and not be thrown in over my head as I saw happen to others later. My preceptor, Lori Macko, was a wonderful nurse and great role model. (I have talked to many nurses about the trend for new grads to exhibit a bit of hero worship for their initial preceptors, but even from this distance in time I still hold Lori in awe.) She was able to handle emergent situations while at the same time making sure I was learning what I needed. She was protective and supportive without smothering. In my first year of burn nursing I gained the skills and experience I had complained about not receiving in school. I still consider some of the nurses on that unit the best I have ever encountered. I saw with amazement that they valued and used care plans, often staying after a shift to update them. In nursing school, care plans had been the equivalent of a referenced term paper without any indication of how they could be utilized on an actual unit. I really enjoyed the work. The debriding was definitely the most stressful part of care. However, the more skilled we became, the more efficient we were and the less pain the patients experienced. The patients were on the unit for long periods of time so it was easy to get to know them and their families. There was a sense of satisfaction in becoming expert in a specialty and knowing this made a difference in patients' experiences. The unit was a blend of an intensive and nonintensive care unit. It was nice to get the break from ICU and not have to float off the unit.

My second year on the burn unit was an education on different issues. There was a chasm between the staff nurses and the nurse managers. I observed those nurses who I admired being criticized in staff meetings for incidents which had occurred when they had been in charge. I knew from firsthand experience that some of the criticism was unfounded, but even if it had been, the method used to reprimand was inappropriate. The staff schedule was another major issue. Nurses worked seven-day stretches, split between either days/evenings or days/nights, had two days off, and then were on again for another seven. Eventually the schedule allowed for four days off in a row. However, we were routinely asked to work one of those days.

Another issue was that the surgeons required that all intensive care patients be "open for rounds" twice a week. This meant that we had to wash and debride all these patients by late morning, and have them covered with large gauze "burn dressings" soaked with saline until the surgeons came around to see them. After that we could apply the cream to the burns. These days were horrible as the patients were in increased pain without the cream, and lost their body heat into the sopping wet dressings no matter how high we turned up the heat shields. Several nurses attempted to change this policy. The patients were washed twice a day, and the nurses' position was that the physicians should come into the "tank" rooms and see the patients during these times. The nurses were told this was not convenient. Morale deteriorated quickly. At the beginning of the summer of 1978 there were about 42 nurses working this unit, and by the end of August there were about 24.

I had an incident occur which led me also to look for work elsewhere. I was caring for an elderly woman and did not feel the medical team was giving her the attention she needed. The assistant nurse managers agreed with me in private but did not support me when I approached the medical team with my concerns. I was also reprimanded at this time for breaking the rules on evening shift regarding visiting hours. I had allowed the wife of a severely burned patient to stay an extra hour because the patient had seemed more alert that evening. The patient was in a private ICU room, the shift was quiet, the patient was probably going to die (he did), and in my assessment what he needed most was her. I was extremely frustrated, missed the nurses who had recently quit, and decided to do something constructive with my anger—join the exodus and apply somewhere else.

One of the nurses who had recently left had accepted a position at the Fred Hutchinson Cancer Research Center and she had encouraged me to apply as well. I told her I had no interest in cancer nursing but she said something vague about it being research and enticed me with the fact that the nurses worked five days on and five days off. This sounded too good to be true, but I thought it was worth checking out. At the end of a shift I walked the six blocks to "the Hutch." Despite a shaky start with the director of personnel ("We only hire RNs." "I am an RN." "We only hire RNs with ICU experience." "I have ICU experience." "We don't have any openings." "I'd like an application in case you do."), I filled it out and then forgot about it. A couple of months later I received a call that there was an opening and asking if I was still interested. I was so enmeshed again with issues on the burn unit that I considered calling and saying I was not interested. My husband reminded me of my constant stress and strongly urged me at least to interview.

Peggy Hutchison, the evening shift coordinator, interviewed me and by the end of the interview I thought I had found the best of all nursing units. There were so many similarities with burn care and they seemed to appreciate their nurses! The patients were on the unit about the same length of time, it was a mix of ICU and acute care, and even the patient care in terms of central lines, blood product administration, infection/sepsis complications, and age of the patient population (mix of adult and pediatrics) was the same. In addition, there were *no* visiting hours; families were encouraged to stay overnight, and the five on/five off schedule was real. Peggy offered me the position. I feel I was lucky because I accepted the last evening shift position available for years. I gave notice at the burn unit and started at "the Hutch" in December 1978.

I was precepted by Judy Campbell who had been with Dr. Thomas's transplant team almost since the beginning. I saw the physicians listen to her assessments and suggestions with respect. Rounds were an interdisciplinary event (not an oral exam for medical students) with nurses expected to participate and acknowledged as having unique information that the team needed. I was given a couple of articles, probably the entire literature on BMT at the time, which I scanned. Having only a cursory background knowledge of leukemia I did not have much of a foundation on which to place bone marrow transplants. During the first couple of months this did not bother me as I was trying to learn the specifics of the tasks needed to care for these patients, the charting system, and the unit's culture. Intensive care was a skill which was valued highly and not all the nurses had the strong background I did. I was at home with a ventilator and Swan-Ganz® set-ups and once intubated these patients were certainly more stable than many of the burn patients I had cared for.

My first evening shift started out with an assignment of two boys around the age of ten. One had just had a lung biopsy but was very stable on an oxygen mask. His mother was extremely anxious and kept asking me if he was going to be intubated. I look at him and he looked fine, was ambulating and acting like a normal kid so I said not to worry. Eight hours later he was intubated, on 100 percent oxygen, and 15 of PEEP. His biopsy had shown him to be infected with histoplasmosis. He survived on the ventilator another seven weeks before finally dying of the infection. I remained as one of his primary nurses. I apologized to his mother several times and learned a lesson regarding how quickly the acuity of these patients could change. I also learned to respect parents' intuitions.

During this time I was disturbed by comments from other nurses regarding the improbability of Jeff's getting off the respirator. In the burn unit, most patients who were intubated were then weaned off when their respiratory tracks healed from either the initial smoke inhalation or subsequent pneumonias. How could everyone be so pessimistic? I soon learned that in fact 20 percent of our patients died of pneumonia—usually CMV. This resulted in usually two ventilators on the unit at a given time. It seemed to be an especially cruel virus as the peak incidence was around day 60 after transplant when the patients were usually well engrafted and discharged. The shortness of breath was usually sudden, occurring over a matter of hours. The patients were always taken to surgery for lung biopsies to rule out the slight possibility that the organism was something other than CMV and therefore treatable. Usually the patient's respiratory status had deteriorated so much that they were unable to tolerate extubation post surgery. This pneumonia was one of the main reasons patients were kept in Seattle for 100 days post transplant. The main reason was to adequately support these patients through the period of acute graft versus host disease, as well as to perform the initial assessments for the possibility of chronic graft versus host disease.

I would like to depart from my story for a moment to describe the usual care and therapies we had for these patients in 1980. All the patients had single lumen Hickman® catheters. Dr. Robert Hickman had been a pediatric nephrologist consulting on our patients in the mid-1970s and was often called on to attempt to start some type of venous access in our end-stage leukemic patients. He often resorted to arterio-venous shunts for which he had to cut down to the actual vessels to access. He thought there had to be a better way and invented the tunneled right atrial catheter. Dr. Hickman placed all the catheters in a small room on the transplant unit in the evenings. He trained us to be his surgical assistants. In the early 1980s he modified the catheter to have two lumens to help meet the growing number of IV infusions administered to patients. He was enjoyable to work with and had a wonderful ability to establish a quick rapport with patients. In subsequent years he moved into a real OR, and finally retired about five years ago.

All of our patients were on hyperalimentation, although it was often turned off to run other infusions in the single lumen catheters. Patients were on prophylactic antibiotics when their ANCs dropped below 500. Amphotericin-B was widely used. A major focus of care on the unit was the laminar air flow (LAF) rooms, sterile units inserted into a private patient room which divided the room into two sections with a heavy plastic curtain. One wall is covered with filters which constantly filter the air; all supplies and food must be sterile. The plastic curtain has "access gloves" and a stethoscope inserted into the middle for short patient assessments. Patients stayed in LAF for 50 days. Methotrexate was the only graft versus host disease prophylaxis.

During this time we performed one of the first unrelated donor transplants on a girl who had a very common HLA type but did not match anyone in her family. One of our lab techs matched her and consented to be the donor. We kept the patient in LAF for 100 days. She sailed through the transplant, had no sign of graft versus host disease but unfortunately did relapse.

At 6P.M. every night, half of the hallway lights would be turned off which seemed to be the signal that it was now truly the evening shift. We ran 20 beds with six nurses and one charge nurse. My usual assignment was either an ICU room or three LAF rooms.

During this time I had no appreciation of where marrow transplantation or Fred Hutchinson fit into the larger scope of medicine. I had no historical sense of how unique this unit was. I knew the list of patients waiting for admission into the program was usually around 170 and we gave priority to patients according to the recruitment needs of our protocols. My focus was on my primary patients and the friendships I had established with the nurses.

I did have a glimpse of how marrow transplant was considered by others in 1979. I had a primary patient who had survived just about every complication on the list. She had arrived from Florida along with her husband, three daughters, two sisters, one brother, and both parents. They were a very gregarious group and the seven-month saga of her time in Seattle often seemed like a Tennessee Williams play. She was transplanted from her HLA-identical sister and subsequently endured and survived acute graft versus host disease (her physician told her she would not survive and she was insulted), CMV infection (not pneumonia), and herpes zoster. She wanted to go home and the physicians finally agreed if a nurse accompanied her. My five days off fit the schedule and so I agreed to go. I met the oncologist who had referred her who was very interested in her transplant course. However, while I was in his office, one of the partners in the practice came by and said "Oh, you're from Seattle? No one believes any of that data." Then he laughed and walked away. I was shocked and defensive. The transplant research team was a very dedicated group who from what I observed had high standards for respecting patients and individuals as well as high standards for research. As the years went by and I became more involved in the workings of the clinical division this belief was confirmed. In 1990 when Dr. Thomas was awarded the Nobel Prize, that physician in Florida crossed my mind and I had the last laugh.

Another primary patient I cared for during this time also made an impact on how I viewed nursing. John was a hematology fellow who had diagnosed himself with CML. I always tried to get into his LAF room when "Jeopardy" was on. He rarely missed a question and I'm sure qualified for millions of dollars on all those evenings I listened to his responses. He developed the worst grade of gut graft versus host disease. He was taken to surgery at one point to attempt a bowel resection but the surgeon said his bowels looked like cobwebs. One evening he told me that he had made a terrible mistake deciding to go on to transplant when he did. In hindsight I think he was right. To me, patients with CML had the hardest decisions to make since they might live normal lives for years before entering into a blast crisis. In John's case, I have my own "if only" because if he had waited another couple of years he would have been given cyclosporine for GVHD prophylaxis, and definitely would not have died as he did. After John died, I helped his wife and parents pack up his belongings at their apartment and they thanked me for the care I had given John. My initial reaction was to be embarrassed since he had died and I felt a sense of failure. But then I realized the advantage we nurses have over medicine whose focus is on cure. We make a difference in our patient's daily experiences—whether they will live through this night or for another 50 years. We can, and should, revel in the part we play when patients are cured, but we can define our successes in increments and feel immediate satisfaction in the short term. John's family's thanks had been genuine and touched a sense of accomplishment in me for the job I had done. This focus on making a difference for a patient today has helped me cope with working with this population of young patients many of whom will not survive.

In May 1988 my husband and I separated and I dealt with that stress by focusing even more on work. In June of that year we had an epidemic of CMV pneumonias with eight patients on ventilators. We stopped admitting patients since all of our staff were needed for the patients on ventilators. I volunteered to work most of my scheduled days off. Working as much as I did during those months allowed me to put my own problems in perspective compared to the tragedy I was witnessing.

During that summer a new protocol was introduced using a drug called cyclosporine to prevent graft versus host disease. It had been utilized in the dog lab and seemed very promising. It was only available IM or PO as it had not been purified enough for IV use at that time. Five patients were enrolled in this protocol and we immediately began to see problems with renal failure. Apparently this was not expected to be a major problem from the dog studies. The physicians were reluctant to reduce or hold doses in fear of graft versus host disease developing out of control. The patients were put on dialysis but all five patients died of toxicity. The study was stopped. A couple of years later the physicians announced that they were going to start another protocol utilizing a slightly lower dose of IV cyclosporine. There was quite a stir among the nurses as many of us had lost primary patients in the first trial. There were ongoing ethical discussions regarding the use of this drug, the nurses' commitment to research, and informed consent for the patients. In the long run, cyclosporine proved itself to be (almost) the wonder drug as originally advertised. I think the toxic dose and the therapeutic dose are about 1 mg apart. We have mastered the art of administering and titrating these doses. There is a story remembered by one of our staff of one of the researchers coming by the patient's room to find out why the patient had not been swallowing the cyclosporine doses since the serum assays were so low. After talking to the nurse it was discovered that the patient had been taking all the doses with cola and that the carbonation was interfering!

I know that patients' lives have been saved because of this drug. But

I also remember my patient Debbie whose brothers were going stir crazy watching her slowly die of renal failure. They had heard me say my roof needed patching and went out to my house while I cared for their sister and surprised me with new roof tiles. I moved out of that house ten years ago but still remember Debbie when I drive by. Data obtained from the experience of patients like Debbie and John paved the way for today's current success with marrow transplant. Many patients and families identify their participation in experimental treatments with pride and know they have helped future patients.

By 1981 I was very content with my niche on the evening shift and began working as charge nurse. There were changes occurring in the nursing management but I considered that day-shift business. One evening when I arrived at work I was pulled aside by the evening shift supervisor who asked me to consider the position of education coordinator which Judy Campbell was vacating because she was about to have her baby. I was surprised, honored to be asked, and very undecided. I spent the weekend making long lists of the pros and cons. I finally decided to accept on a trial basis with the promise that I could return to the evening shift if I wanted. The deciding factor for me was to be working again with Peggy Hutchison who had just left the evening shift supervisor position to accept the director of nursing position. My responsibilities were orientation of new nurses and continuing education of the nursing staff. My focus was on orientation as the unit was short five positions. Peggy and I decided that the best way to proceed was to hire one nurse per week for five weeks. In hindsight this idea seems to border on insanity, as having five orientees each at a different point in orientation with no formal orientation program was chaotic. At the end of the orientations, as I was evaluating the nurse I considered to be the strongest of the five, she thanked me and then informed me that she was resigning as she wanted to be a real oncology nurse and not just care for patients during this short phase of their total therapeutic experience!

This interaction left a lasting impression with me. This was the first of several insinuations that I perceived from oncology nurses in the early 1980s, that intensive care nurses (and therefore marrow transplant nurses) were more focused on high-tech procedures than on the holistic care of the patient. This attitude troubled me. Marrow transplant nurses are obviously oncology nurses as most of our patients have been diagnosed with cancer. It was true, however, that our focus was different from oncology units in several ways. All of our patients were entered on research protocols; all were hoping to be cured of their disease regardless of the odds; and most (especially in those days) were young. Although we gave chemotherapy, the doses were required to be high enough to be marrow-ablative and so the side effects we dealt with (indeed it was these side effects that mandated most of the care on a transplant unit) were different from those encountered in the lower doses given on oncology units. In fact we encountered diseases unique to these patients including graft versus host disease (where donor T-lymphocytes attack the patient) and venoclusive disease (liver failure which develops after total body irradiation). And yes, patients did return to their referring physicians after the acute phase of marrow transplant was over. I hope that none of us projects an elitism toward other specialties or subspecialties within nursing. Stripped of all the specialized equipment or skills, I believe and hope we all have the same basic goal—to make a difference because of our expertise for this patient's level of wellness.

I could not tell my story without describing Joleen Kelleher. Joleen started on the night shift as supervisor in the early 1980s while attending graduate school. In 1983 she replaced Peggy (who had been accepted into medical school) as the director of nursing and we worked very closely as I also wore the hat of assistant director of nursing. Joleen is a natural leader. She gives support while at the same time holding people accountable. She often asked, "Whose problem is this?" Answering this put many issues in perspective for me. If the problem is mine then I should act; if it is someone else's then they need my feedback so they can address it (and I need to get out of the way). Another Joleenism went something like, "Deal with problems now (you know, those that you know you need to address based on how much you are grousing about it internally), or you can decide to deal with them later. Just remember that if you put them off, next time the problems will be bigger and more complex." Joleen is very intuitive and encouraged nurses to blend their own intuitions with their technical skills.

This was especially true in "critical incidents" in patient care, where nurses' premonitions are often the first clues that a patient may need closer attention. Joleen expected first-line supervisors to be responsible for their staff's issues. She emphasized goal-setting and expected follow-through on those goals. In paging through some old nursing retreat minutes recently, I found a notation Joleen had written in the margin: "Take chances on people." Many times I saw Joleen take chances on staff even though it took much of her time and energy. I watched her give feedback often timed at a point in that person's life when they were ready to hear it. Joleen's belief was that staff could make positive changes if they were in a environment where they were both supported and held accountable. Joleen decided to resign her position last year. I miss her humor and wisdom, but feel grateful to continue working upon the foundation she put into place at this center.

Throughout the 1980s our nursing unit was inundated with phone calls and visitors from across the country. Use of the Hickman catheter was exploding and Bob referred nursing care questions to us. I usually answered around ten phone calls per week. As acceptance of marrow transplant as a treatment option grew, we also received numerous phone calls and visitors. Although we felt it our responsibility to share our expertise, I can remember weeks where I shook the hands of a visiting nurse group for the final time and then turned around to face my desk which had been untouched for a week. We averaged around 30 visitors per year in the mid-1980s. We eventually learned to ask for specific goals before a group arrived. This would help to focus them and to avoid the dreaded request for "everything."

In 1983 Joleen took over a project initiated by Peggy and nurses from the three other institutions performing marrow transplant in Seattle, the VA, the University of Washington, and Swedish Medical Center, to hold a nursing symposium on marrow transplant. The initial purpose was to hold a forum to acknowledge and update Seattle marrow transplant nurses on the latest therapies and results, and we decided to also invite other nurses in the country who might be interested. The response from across the country soon overshadowed our focus on our Seattle staffs. We were frankly overwhelmed by the response and the networking that occurred spontaneously. Marrow transplant nurses began to meet as "focus groups" at ONS Congresses. Since most of us belonged to ONS, it was logical to try and meet our educational and networking needs within this established and respected group. These Congresses were frustrating, however, since marrow transplant was changing so rapidly and the topics were often too specific to be of interest to a more general oncology nursing audience. Our focus group meetings were over-crowded and the most time we had for marrow transplant specific education was usually in a four-hour pre-Congress workshop for which we had to pay extra.

I remember what I consider our worst experience (even worse than being scheduled at the same time as the tours of the *Queen Mary* in Los Angeles) in Denver in 1987. We were given an area in which to meet that would have comfortably held 30 people and we had over 100 attendees. People were stealing chairs from other focus groups and slamming them down in our area. The meeting room was dark and cavernous with echoing acoustics. We tried to conduct a meeting and were asked to hold our noise level down by the smaller groups around us. The desperation was palpable in some of those who were attending in order to find out what others were doing to handle these complicated patients.

My clearest memory of this meeting, however, was Debbie Mayer sitting down in the midst of what was close to bedlam and listening to the concerns and anger firsthand. There were many "why" questions being thrown at her and I was very impressed by how she tried to listen to the actual messages. At the end of the meeting, I passed around a mailing list and agreed to be an ad hoc editor of the "Bone Marrow Transplant Nursing News" which I would mail out of the Hutch. Seth Eisenberg, one of our staff nurses (who has been and still is a great asset in many of my projects over the years) agreed to act as coeditor. His humor and dedication ensured that the newsletter was both readable and on schedule. We continued to publish this, mailing to over 400 nurses, until the BMT special interest group (SIG) was established two years later.

We in marrow transplant knew that we could easily fill two or three days with our own subject matter and did not feel our needs were being met. On the other hand, it did not make sense for ONS, which had thousands of nurses attending a congress, to give a disproportionate amount of time to what was seen as a subspecialty of a few hundred nurses each year. Debates raged about whether we were a subspecialty or our own specialty. Since most transplant units were a combination of oncology and marrow transplant it seemed that we were indeed a subspecialty, if a giant one.

In the fall of 1987 I received a call from Cheryl Lane, vice-president of ONS, asking me to be a member of a task force on the formation of special interest groups within ONS. I was surprised to be asked and pleased that ONS was taking a serious look at special interests within the membership. The task force met in October and I was impressed with the seriousness with which those present addressed this task. I knew there were strong opinions within ONS leadership that the special interest groups (SIGs) would fragment the membership. Those in favor of the SIGs, however, countered that it was the membership that was identifying the need for subspecialties and ONS needed to listen. The task force recommended to the board that the SIGs be formalized within the structure of ONS, and that a SIG standing committee be formed to establish the SIG criteria, and define how the SIGs would function within the structure of ONS. This was approved.

The SIG committee was formed in May of 1988 and I was flabbergasted to be asked to be chair by Debbie Mayer. I did have the passing thought that maybe ONS thought I should put my "money" (time and energy?) where my mouth was. I accepted and was quickly educated about the myriad issues identified by each of these subgroups. I was blessed with a wonderful mix of nurses on the committee. From my myopic point of view, I did not know who to appoint to this pioneer committee. My goal was to have as broad a representation of the different types of special interests as possible: disease specific (AIDS, GYN), population (peds, geriatric), treatment modality (radiation, immunotherapy), roles (CNS, educators), symptom management (pain), or setting (home care, office nurses). Luckily, Cheryl Lane agreed to be a member of the committee and was very helpful in suggesting other members.

She provided historical continuity to the continuing SIG development process. Joanne Hayes was my board contact and she offered a steady stream of sound advice and support when I needed it. The committee spent most of the first year hashing out the fine details of the SIG policy and procedure manual. In 1990 the first "focus groups" were approved as the SIGs of ONS.

In the middle of my tenure as chair, I adopted my son David. This new set of priorities, along with my real job and the committee, was a balancing act I had not really appreciated when observing other mothers over the years. When my committee chair term was over I must admit I breathed a sigh of relief and focused my attention more on my family and the changes at the Hutch.

In 1992 I attended the ONS Congress in San Diego. In flipping through the proceedings I experienced a great surge of pride and completion as the names of those whose first tenuous phone calls asking about how to find others with their special interest jumped out at me as presenters of instructional sessions.

In 1991 my focus at work changed. The education duties were split off when we were able to justify a nursing educator position, and I focused on standards of practice. This included the responsibility for nursing policies at the Hutch, and coordination of policies with Swedish Medical Center (which had opened transplant beds in 1980 to accomodate our increasing demand to perform more transplants within our program, and by 1985 had expanded to double the number of beds as the Hutch), as well as chairing the standard practice committee. This committee is responsible for research protocol review for clinical implications and writing interdisciplinary practice guidelines upon which the research protocols are conducted.

In 1993 the nurse manager of the outpatient clinic resigned. I agreed to fill in as I was already involved in many major practice changes about to take place. It didn't take me long to realize that I was really enjoying being closer to direct patient care issues than I had been, and in May I was appointed to the position on a permanent basis. This past year has been a whirlwind of change. The outpatient nursing staff has proven over and over their resiliency and skills. We started caring for autologous patients entirely on an outpatient basis in July 1993. This year a major focus will be on assessing and supporting the family caregivers as they are now on the frontlines in assessing and administering many therapies. One of the lessons I have learned as the manager is that if I can figure out systems to put nurses in contact with patients, problems seem to smooth out. I found that as the clinic population grew, dividing the patients into small teams with consistent nurses and physicians immediately improved patient satisfaction.

This has been an interesting opportunity to pause and reflect on my nursing career. I am pleased that those qualities I was attracted to in the public health nurses of 1972 and which led me to nursing, are still what I consider nursing's greatest strengths. Nursing is most effective when nurses are focused on their patients—paying attention to what they are telling us and what our intuition is saying about them. I heard a short news clip in which President Clinton said in an address to the ANA that nurses must represent the majority of Americans in the health care discussions as they have no formal organization as some of the subsets do. I am optimistic that nursing will come out stronger on the other side of health care reform.

Notes

Hickman is a registered trademark of C. R. Bard Division of Davol, Inc.

Swan-Ganz is a registered trademark of Pharmaseal Division of Baxter Healthcare Corp.

13

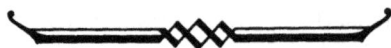

Juanita Garrison

For 15 years, I worked as an obstetrical nurse, never dreaming that I would choose another specialty, especially oncology! My experience with oncology was as a nursing student in the late 1950s and early 1960. As I remember, there were large wards of patients (very few private and semiprivate rooms). Some of the patients were diagnosed with cancer—the "Big C." I remember the foul-smelling odors from colostomies as stool leaked onto the ABD pads and handmade Montgomery straps. When the colostomy was irrigated, a round green flower pot was placed beneath it but the stool often had a way of overshooting the pot, landing on the cloth gown of the nurse and the patient's bed sheet, if not the floor. I remember the uncontrolled heart-wrenching cries of pain. Pain control was definitely inadequate! Health professionals and patients alike feared addiction, so pain medications were strictly regulated in smaller standard dosages and longer time intervals than today's guidelines. I remember the awful physical disfigurements as a result of cancer surgery or from unresectable disease, especially head and neck cancer patients. I remember the terrible radiation "burns," often requiring a cradle to keep the clothes off the skin. And I remember the deaths, especially the children, and the teenagers who were about the same age as me.

In looking back on the choice of my first specialty, I think it was the pain, the deaths, and the gloom and doom attitude that surrounded the cancer patients that made me, as a nineteen-year-old graduate, choose what is usually referred to as the "happy service"—obstetrics. Then in 1970, the death of my beloved father was to change my life as I never dreamed. A long-time smoker, my father quit the habit in 1962 after experiencing a heart attack. He used to keep peppermint puff balls in his shirt pocket in place of cigarettes. But the damage had been done and in October 1970 he was diagnosed with oat cell carcinoma of the lung, metastatic to the liver and bones. He accepted the only treatment offered—palliative radiation to his hip for pain control. The day before he passed away, he begged for more radiation treatment. Because he feared addiction, offers of morphine injections subcutaneously were refused until the night prior to his death. Late that night he agreed to take a half dose. Later, he slipped into a deep sleep and was transferred from our home to the hospital. Relatives felt it would make it easier on my mother to live there alone afterwards. He died the next morning, December 13, 1970. I felt helpless, inadequate, and angry at myself for not knowing what to do to make his two months of pain-filled life pain free.

I continued to work in OB, but the spark was missing. Then in 1975 I decided to change jobs. I accepted a position as an apheresis nurse with the division of hematology and oncology. Little did I know what I was in for! Since apheresis was not an everyday occurrence and I could only read so much before becoming bored, I sought out other duties. My medical chief taught me about protocols. For days on end I sat at a desk doing Southeastern Cancer Study Group flowsheets on patients' records that were past due. A medical dictionary and a laboratory value manual sat beside me, becoming well worn and tattered from use. Along with this recording job, I was introduced to patients who were candidates for protocols. It didn't take long to learn how to evaluate the patients for studies, develop methods of "control" over what physicians should or should not do according to cooperative group rules and regulations, and set up protocol recordkeeping. As I learned from these activities, I saw a need to learn about the diseases and the treatments. Patients asked questions, and as duly taught in nursing, I referred them to the physicians. But one day, my medical mentor and supervisor told me that I should answer the patients' questions. So off I went in 1976 to my first cooperative meeting. It was only for an overnight in Florida, but it turned me from being a nurse to being an oncology nurse. There I met nurses from different parts of the country. The cooperative group nursing leaders were nurses who were active in forming the Oncology Nursing Society and who became presidents, board members, or chairs through the years. It was in this meeting that a then-shy oncology nurse began to see oncology patients in a truly different light and to recognize potential educational strategies for patients and their families. This learning process remains ongoing. If I could have one wish, it would be to go back to 1970 and apply today's cancer education, medical, nursing, and hospice support, and pain management to my father's care. Unfortunately, I can't go back. But each year brings new knowledge to our profession and perhaps it's enough that patients today and in the future receive the benefits of those who helped us to achieve what we know today.

Although I was becoming very busy, I continued to seek out other things to do and learn. (I've often said that perhaps I should have stopped while I was ahead!) But later in 1976, as I was wandering the halls of the clinic and watching a physician do a venipuncture for chemotherapy, he looked up and asked, "Do you want to learn"? I accepted the invitation. Soon after that came learning how to do histories and physicals. I was placed in classes, informally, with medical students and fellows, given oral quizzes in front of the medical staff, and attended every seminar, tumor board, or other medical presentations within our hospital that had anything to do with cancer. I learned to count diffs on peripheral smears, work in the laboratories doing research projects, and evaluate the research findings. Then my physician mentor/boss decided I would start teaching professionals and the lay population. Doing this with the house staff, fellows, and nurses on an informal basis within our own hospital was one thing—doing a national presentation was something else! I balked—but it did no good. He volunteered me anyway. Again, Florida proved to be another turning point. It was here that I gave a presentation to the cooperative group's nursing plenary session on two brand new investigative drugs—Chips and Carboplatin. This was done with knocking knees and sweaty palms, but I pulled it off! Now I was doing apheresis, protocols, histories and physicals, and educational programs. Eight hours began to turn into 16 and sometimes 24 hours! The day I worked 36 straight hours, I decided something had to go. Apheresis went to the clinical lab. I still had a full day. But what an education I was getting. I loved it!

Over the years, help has come not only from my medical employers but from the hematology and oncology staff, staff nurses, medical techs, and house staff. In addition, I have learned from others outside my institution—nurses, pharmacists, physicians, members of the cooperative groups, staff and volunteers of the American Cancer Society, and members and leaders within the Oncology Nursing Society. They have all played an important part in my professional growth throughout the last 19 years.

There is a special group of people who have given me an education beyond my colleagues and beyond the textbooks, videos, or other forms of media. That group is the patients. These patients have taught me, among many things, about treatment side effects, how their personal lifestyles affect their decisions and recovery, what should be taught to patients and their families, and how health care professionals should interact with them. In addition, they have taught me the true meaning of humility, courage, trust, strength, and caring. They have helped me to shape my personal as well as my professional growth. There are so many special patients, each unique, that it would be difficult to single out only a certain one.

In the early years of my career, there was a special patient who tugged at the heart strings of our entire oncology team. The patient was a young student in her second year of medical school. She was diagnosed with carcinoid. Symptoms had been present for several months, but like most typical young people who are leading active, busy lives, she attributed the symptoms to one thing or another. It was another colleague in her class who encouraged her to seek medical attention. Neither dreamed it would be serious. Although she underwent chemotherapy, it was to no avail. Her death came quickly early one morning just as we started to make rounds. None of us were prepared. When her family arrived, the physician and I took them into a private area to talk to them. It was heartbreaking. Tears flowed from the family, the physician, and me. The memory of her still causes tears, not only for her but for others whose names and faces crowd my thoughts. That day there was no gaiety among the medical students throughout the hospital. Her death touched everyone. This young woman's death came on the tail end of several deaths that week, most of them expected. When she died I began to wonder if working in this specialty was worth it. A long talk from the physician who recognized my doubts showed me how our care and caring had helped the patient, the family, and the other medical students. To this day I remember that conversation and how he helped me grow in dealing with death and dying. Not long after that, Elizabeth Kübler-Ross came to our institution. I had a chance to attend her luncheon after the house staff lecture and to talk with her. She came at just the right time to reinforce what I learned from a caring physician who took the time to help me learn my role in death and dying.

There are cancer survivors and happy events that oncology nurses witness. Two of my patients come to mind. Both had acute lymphocytic leukemia; both were in their early 20s; both received treatment over four years on the same protocol and only a month apart in their treatment regimens. One is a young woman; the other is a young man. Both got married during their treatment years. Both are still in remission.

The young woman had twins, a boy and a girl, last year, one year after completing treatment (against medical advice—but what do we know!). The babies, who were premature, are healthy, lovable, and have distinct personalities of their own. There is no problem getting someone to babysit with them in clinic. Grandmother and mother get the babies back just before they are ready to leave. Mom has her hair back, Dad is working days, not nights, and they have a new home!

The young man is back to work after hounding the physicians to release him. He has returned to his old job in construction. Although he continues to have some neuropathy symptoms from his chemotherapy, they have lessened. He and his wife are expecting their first child.

A middle-aged lady with breast cancer who developed cardiotoxicity from her chemotherapy treatments is a wonderful fighter. She faces life with humor, determination, spunk, and faith, and instills these qualities in others. Another breast cancer patient told me that meeting this woman was one of the delights and benefits of coming to clinic. She has a way of cheering people up and lighting up the room. While fighting cardio-myopathy, she had to relinquish her busy farm life, social events, and housekeeping for six months. Not doing anything was a problem for her as it caused restlessness and boredom. But giving up activity with only minor cheating, such as "short time" quilt piecing, paid off. Although she gets tired now, she has resumed most activities and knows when to rest. Her fight against primary breast cancer, recurrence, and the development of cardiotoxicity before she could undergo a bone marrow transplant has been an inspiration to all of us. When I look into her face, I see the trust, faith, and confidence that she has in all of us who care for her and in her religious beliefs. She truly shines!

These patients and others like them are the reasons I stay in oncology. I have my blue days when someone whom I have gotten close to over the years relapses or dies, but I like to think that I have been a help to them and their loved ones during their crises. Some families and long-term survivors have continued to keep in touch with me over the years. Occasionally I will see a cancer patient or family member in another setting, and although I may not recognize them, they remember me.

Oncology nursing may not be for everyone, but those who practice in this field find that it is an addictive specialty. I know that I'm hooked on it! When people ask me how I can stand to work in this field, I can easily come up with answers. It is easy to get caught up in the challenges of what oncology offers, whether it is research, administration, clinical, social, educational, combinations, or some other related area. They are all directed toward one goal—providing excellent patient care!

These challenges are exciting and at times overwhelming. Choices between doing something in the work arena versus the personal life can often conflict. Being single does not necessarily negate home responsibilities, especially when you have family members living with you. Keeping a balance between work and home responsibilities and personal time becomes an art of juggling. My way of dealing with the juggling act is to set goals (which I may or may not keep), take a vacation day to do nothing, escape with a good book to the seashore when possible, and be a spectator sports fan at baseball, basketball, and football games.

I did not set out to become an oncology nurse. It was quite by accident. There have been many changes over the years in the treatment and care of oncology patients, all for the good! We still have, however, lots of room for improvement. It has been exciting to see the application of new research findings go from the lab to the clinical setting. I have given new drugs, cared for new technological products, and applied new knowledge and strategies to educational programs. Oncology nurses are like the frontier people going west to blaze a trail for future travelers. It is exciting and dynamic. I am glad that I have participated and, hopefully will continue to participate, in oncology nursing. Oncology nursing chose me! I'm happy to be hooked.

14

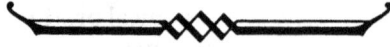

Mary Gerbracht

When I think about the reasons why I became a nurse, it's amazing that it has worked out so well! As a preschooler, I idolized my big sister who was 14 years older than me and a nurse. I have pictures of myself with my 1960s-era nurse's cap and cape, passing out candy pills. But in grade school my interests changed, and I decided I wanted to be an English teacher. At the Catholic school I attended, the English teacher was also the drama coach. I loved the stage, and decided that was the "job" for me.

I remember a conversation with my dad at the end of my junior year in high school. He mentioned that it would be tough to get a teaching job when I graduated from college, but there always seemed to be a need for nurses. My boyfriend at the time also wanted me to be a nurse. So I looked into entrance requirements for nursing degree programs. I dropped the English, drama, and literature courses for which I had preregistered, and added more science classes to my senior year schedule. I'm sure my dad thought we were just having a casual conversation, but it was a turning point in my life.

I was first attracted to oncology nursing the summer after my freshman year in college. I was working as a nurses' aide in a nursing home. Mrs. S. was a patient with cervical cancer who lived there. She was usually in a lot of pain. She was particular about who took care of her, and made it known when a staff member did not care for her the way she wanted. Frankly, I was afraid to take care of her, intimidated that I could not live up to her expectations. Another aide, Jan, who worked the same schedule I did, was always assigned to Mrs. S. My only contact with her was to occasionally answer her call light, or help Jan turn her.

That summer Jan planned a vacation for August. She had a difficult time telling Mrs. S. that she would be gone a whole week and that someone else would be assigned to her on the day shift. When Jan came out of the room after breaking the news of her vacation, she also had news for me: Mrs. S. had requested that I take care of her in Jan's absence! I remember feeling very flattered, yet scared that I couldn't live up to the responsibility. By the end of Jan's vacation, Mrs. S. and I were getting along well, and I felt confident in my ability to take care of her to her satisfaction. After Jan came back, we were able to trade off being assigned to Mrs. S. I learned an important lesson about oncology nursing: Jan had found it very stressful and at times emotionally draining to care for a terminal, pain-ravaged patient every day, and needed the break I could provide. I found caring for Mrs. S. very challenging, but very satisfying.

After that summer I returned to college and was assigned to an oncology unit for my first hospital-based med/surg rotation. I was impressed by the care, compassion, and knowledge of the oncology nurses. I was fascinated by the patients. They were so sick, and so in need of all nursing skills—what our faculty called "biopsychosocial man" at his most vulnerable. During that semester, my instructor offered a lot of encouragement. I'll never forget when she told me I was "graduate school material." It was the first time I considered making a career out of oncology nursing, as opposed to thinking of it as something to do just until I got married and had kids.

The rest of my college experience cemented my commitment to oncology nursing: the summer I spent working in orthopedics, which I didn't find very satisfying; the summer I spent "floating" to nine different med/surg units, where I found myself drawn to the cancer patients. I would go home and read more about their diagnoses in my med/surg book. Two patients stand out in my mind from that summer.

A woman was admitted to the renal unit with renal failure of unknown origin. She had been seeing a chiropractor for "arthritis" for several months. I had to collect a specimen for Bence-Jones protein. I had no idea what that was until I looked it up and found it was a marker for multiple myeloma. Later that week the patient was informed of her diagnosis and prognosis, which in 1979 was a death sentence. I remember being shocked that this relatively young woman who thought she was fairly healthy was actually dying. I remember being angry at her misdiagnosis by the chiropractor. I didn't know at that time how many, many patients I would eventually care for whose diagnoses had also been delayed, and the grief and guilt that that would cause them and their families.

I met Mrs. R., a patient of about 50, on a surgical unit. This was a unit where, to my dismay, nursing assistants and technicians were not allowed to listen to the change-of-shift report. We clocked in and were given a handwritten list of the room numbers of patients whose vital signs we were to obtain; we were not even given their names, and we certainly knew nothing of their diagnoses. When I went into Mrs. R.'s room, I could see that she and her husband were very anxious. Before I even finished her vital signs, the OR staff came to get her. As it turned out, I ended up being assigned to Mrs. R. for the rest of the shift. I was surprised when at about 10 A.M. the charge nurse told me Mrs. R. was returning to her room already. The patient's family members were all crying when they brought her back to the room. It had been an "open and close" surgery. They were told the pancreatic cancer was inoperable and that nothing could or would be done. For the second time that summer, I had a sense of shock and bewilderment that someone who seemed so well could be struck down in the prime of her life by cancer. It was a formidable enemy. I wanted to help with the fight.

I learned a few other lessons from Mrs. R.'s case that have served me well in my 14 years of oncology nursing. When the system doesn't work, I question it! Approaching the head nurse of the surgical unit and requesting that the nurses' aides/techs be given more information about patients before entering their room took all the courage I could muster. I basically got no for an answer. However, I was proud of myself for having been assertive enough to ask.

I have also come to deplore phrases such as "inoperable," "open and close surgery," and "nothing can be done." These were all used to describe Mrs. R., and left her and her family with little hope. I believe patients shouldn't be denied their hope, although what is hoped for may change after the diagnosis: hope for a comfortable existence, or hope to live for a landmark event such as a wedding or the birth of a grandchild. To present information in such a way that a patient feels a complete loss of hope is unnecessary and cruel.

In my senior year I had the opportunity to choose my own patients and units for our critical care, advanced med/surg, management, and community health experiences. I took care of people with cancer throughout the year. I requested and was allowed one observation day with the oncology clinical nurse specialist. I vowed that someday I would be one too.

I got my first glimpse of how others view oncology nursing as I started looking for a job. I was fortunate to graduate during one of nursing's cyclical "shortage" years, and was recruited by many hospitals. Time after time, I would hear from recruiters things like, "You're so young to want to go into oncology nursing. It's so depressing." I quickly decided I would not consider working at any institution where the recruiter thought my chosen specialty was depressing! Of course, since that time, I've been asked dozens of times if oncology nursing is depressing. So it was refreshing to talk to the recruiter for M.D. Anderson Cancer Center where I ended up working after graduation.

I had started looking into graduate programs in oncology nursing also. At the time, there were only eight! M.D. Anderson was across the street from the University of Texas Health Science Center, which offered very low tuition for its M.S.N. program in oncology nursing. The only problem was that M.D. Anderson and UTHSC were in Houston, a thousand miles away, and I didn't know a soul there. So when my boyfriend (now my husband) called to say that he had been unexpectedly transferred to Houston during my senior year, I took it as an act of fate that I was meant to move there too.

My first day at Anderson was awesome. There I was, a 24-hour drive from where I'd lived all my life, in a huge city where I knew only one person, in a huge hospital. There were patients with obvious alopecia in the halls and cafeteria and clinics—a site I was not used to seeing. It was a place where cancer was part of normal life.

I had a great need to talk about the sometimes horrifying things I saw at work as a way of coping with oncology nursing. I talked to my boyfriend for hours on the phone about patients, never revealing their names or confidential identifying information, but talking about their situations. Somehow, verbalizing what it was like to see tumors growing out of breasts or abdominal walls, to see a person hemorrhage to death or die of septic shock, or vomit 17 times in an hour after getting cisplatin, helped me to deal with it. I didn't want or need answers; I just needed someone to listen.

I found myself going home every night and looking up all of my patients' diagnoses in the American Cancer Society *Clinical Oncology* book. At that time, there was a dearth of oncology nursing references, so I used a medical text. Because I experienced the patients' case histories every day at work, and because we saw such a wide variety of diagnoses, this method helped me learn a lot about oncology in a relatively short period.

One personal frustration about my job there concerned the role of the clinical nurse specialist. We had two CNSs for the service. They were both very good, and in fact I became good friends with one of them outside of work. But it seemed that whenever the parts of nursing that were really interesting came up, such as extensive pre-op teaching, management of complex wounds, postmastectomy counseling, or complex discharge planning, it was the CNS who intervened, not me, the staff nurse. I felt that if I had the CNS's education and experience, I could do the job myself! So I started back to graduate school just nine months after getting my B.S.N., so that I could be either a staff development instructor or a CNS myself. I might not recommend going back to school so soon after graduation to anyone else, but it has worked out well for me.

Oncology nursing has made me question a lot of my own beliefs. After being an oncology nurse for about 18 months, I went through what I call my "atheist period." A patient I was caring for at Anderson looked up at me and said, "If there is a God, why is this (cancer) happening to me?" Something clicked in my head; the patient was right, there must not be the all-knowing, ever-present God I had heard about all my life, or my patients wouldn't be suffering so much. I had been asked the question so many times, but now was feeling uncomfortable. I read books on religion and spirituality to try to gain insight into my thoughts and feelings. I went to church a few times, but just felt empty. At the time I was going through this, I was sort of ashamed and didn't tell too many people. I really *wanted* to believe in a loving God, but just couldn't. When patients identified feelings of hope about their cancer situation because of their strong faith in God, I would nod and smile and try to appear supportive, but I was thinking otherwise. When my older sister heard about my change in religious attitude, she figured it was time for me to get out of oncology nursing. But that was something I never considered.

I stayed at the comprehensive cancer center for two and a half years. I worked on two different units, in addition to doing all my clinical for graduate school there. I knew a lot of staff and had met hundreds of patients. When I married, Bob was in graduate school in another city, so as soon as I finished my graduate studies, I left. I am still grateful for the opportunities and experiences I had at M.D. Anderson, and keep in touch with several of the staff.

I took a job as a staff nurse in oncology at a tiny community hospital. I felt like a fish out of water. I missed the hustle and bustle of a 500-bed cancer hospital, and the specialists and subspecialists for every problem or situation. Because I had worked at a research-oriented institution, I was very concerned that the patients at my new job were not getting adequate medical care. I now believe I was wrong to think this, but at the time, whenever a patient was managed in a way different than we had managed patients with a similar diagnosis at Anderson, I wanted to secretly tell the patient to pack his or her bags and go to Houston. I later learned the difference between "standard care" and clinical research, and that different physicians have different opinions about what constitutes the best treatment for a patient. Contrary to what the public (and young nurses!) thinks, medicine is not an exact science, and human judgement must play a large role.

Needless to say, feeling that way, I left that job after only two months. I took a position as a charge nurse on an 11 P.M. to 7 A.M. shift at the county hospital. It didn't have an oncology unit, but the surgery unit where I worked was about 25 percent occupied with cancer patients. Every night I would make my "cancer rounds," checking on all the cancer patients' care, talking to those who were awake (many were), and making sure their care plans were updated.

After about six months, I left that position to take a teaching job. In my interview at one of the largest universities in the country, I don't think the panel knew what to make of me. There I was, 25 years old, with three years of nursing experience and a new master's degree, being interviewed by 40-year-old Ph.Ds. I felt as if they didn't take me seriously. After the interview, the Dean smiled very kindly, and said that she enjoyed offering opportunities to young, inexperienced faculty with potential, to give them a chance to see what they can do. I got the job at the University of Texas at Austin.

I worked very hard to do a good job in my instructor position. I took my responsibilities with the students very seriously. In looking back though, I was probably too demanding of the students, with expectations that were very high. Hopefully, they learned some things from me. One interesting side effect of the teaching experience was that I got a taste of the CNS consultant role. My students were at a hospital that didn't have an oncology CNS. Because I had been a hospital staff nurse that dealt with students, I tried hard to treat the staff and students as I wished the faculty had when I was in their situation. As the staff got to know me and my oncology specialty, they asked for my advice on nursing management of oncology patients even if my students weren't assigned to them.

I remember one particular student's frustration, a pattern that I have seen repeated by new oncology nurses several times. This student had as her goal for the day to "get the patient to open up" and talk about his feelings about cancer. A couple of times that day the student expressed frustration that she wasn't getting anywhere with her patient. When the oncology chaplain came out of the patient's room after making rounds, the student immediately asked, "What'd you get out of him?" I remember thinking, it's not an inquisition! So I decided to assess the patient myself. During the first visit, I established a rapport with the patient. The second day of clinical, the patient did share a lot of his feelings about cancer and death with me. The student was surprised, and wanted to know how I had "done" what she had been unable to. I really don't remember what I said to the student, but I have seen that behavior many times. An inexperienced nurse who has been taught that cancer patients should be allowed and encouraged to verbalize their feelings, pushes too hard and actually makes patients uncomfortable in talking about any of their feelings! There is a fine nursing art to assessing the patients' readiness and need to talk about their feelings so that the nurse can offer support, versus meeting the *nurse's* need to feel that she has been helpful.

After three semesters of teaching, it was time to move again. My husband finished graduate school and got a job in Dallas. Again, I was fortunate to be in the right place at the right time, and was offered an excellent oncology CNS position at a teaching hospital, St. Paul Medical Center.

I attended my first Oncology Nursing Society Congress a few months after starting the position. I was overwhelmed by the sheer number of nurses in the Houston Convention Center. I remember the wonderful feeling of—I'm not alone in my love of oncology nursing. I couldn't believe I was surrounded by thousands of nurses who were interested in the same thing I was. In my five-year oncology nursing career, I'd heard some really strange comments. It was as if people wondered what was different about me, that I liked oncology nursing. My least favorite was: "I could never be an oncology nurse, I'm too tenderhearted" (or sympathetic, or other similar descriptors). It was as if the only reason I could cope with oncology nursing was because I was coldhearted. Others would comment that I must be a "strong" or "special" person to work in oncology. Again, I don't feel particularly strong or special—just challenged by a disease that affects 30 percent of the population and kills half of those; challenged by a disease and career that demands the most of my intellectual and emotional resources; and challenged by a disease whose outcome is uncertain, whose treatment has nasty side effects, but one in which a good oncology nurse can make all the difference for the patient.

The 1985 Congress kicked off my involvement with the Oncology Nursing Society. About that time, the president of the Dallas chapter of ONS called me. She was an experienced oncology CNS whom I greatly admired. She said that I had leadership qualities and encouraged me to get involved with the chapter board of directors. So I did. Two years later, I became chapter president. Looking back, Jeanne's call to me was very important in my career, just as my instructor's encouragement to attend graduate school had been earlier. There are many other opportunities I would not have explored without the encouragement of other oncology nurses along the way. I am grateful.

I learned how to incorporate my early childhood interests into my CNS role. I had done a few inservices and professional talks in my career, but did not consider myself to have a lot of ability in that field. Almost immediately after starting my CNS job, I was involved in planning a CE seminar with the staff development department of the hospital. I identified pain management as a timely topic. I was new to the institution and didn't know who the good speakers were. The other members of the planning committee couldn't identify anyone either. So I tentatively volunteered. I got a lot of support from the committee, and it was decided I would do the talk.

The night before the seminar, I was so nervous I could hardly sleep. I felt like a zombie at the seminar. Once I started talking though, I loosened up. When the seminar was over, my talk had been evaluated by the participants as the best of the day! I was thrilled and surprised. That gave me the confidence to pursue other speaking opportunities.

Now I've done dozens, and stage fright, for the most part, is a thing of the past. I often feel like an actor before a performance, trying to size up an audience, trying to deliver what it is they came for, trying to keep them engaged and entertained. So even though I'm not a teacher or drama coach as I thought I would be in grade school, I am teaching, and I do get to act!

One of my "success" stories at my CNS job involved a cancer screening program. In my first couple of years on the job, I had been involved in a lot of health fairs. We would give away sunscreen, stool blood test cards, information on cancer prevention techniques, and have breast and testicular self-exam models available for practice. But the cancer booths never attracted as much attention as those testing percentages of body fat, blood sugar, or cholesterol. So I thought about asking physicians to volunteer to perform no-cost clinical breast exams at the next big health fair, scheduled at a local mall. One of the physicians on the hospital's cancer committee told me it was a terrible idea, that a woman would never wait in line at a mall to go behind a curtained-off area to have a breast exam performed by a doctor she didn't know. My medical director and supervisor were more supportive. Like me, they weren't positive women would participate. But we had nothing to lose, so they authorized it.

The rest, as they say, is history. The first year, nearly 200 women were screened. After eight years, more than a thousand women have been screened, with the provision of free follow-up diagnostic mammograms added more recently. Several cancers have been detected. Although financial data aren't assessed, the participants appear to be from a wide array of socioeconomic groups, although many appear to be in the lower income groups. It is a service that the involved hospital staff feels good about every year, knowing that we've performed a valuable service women might otherwise not take advantage of. And every year when I see the crowd outside the exam area, I smile to myself, and remember how I was told the program would never work.

I had been an oncology nurse for nearly eight years before our first son, Steven, was born. The pregnancy was complicated by pregnancy-induced hypertension, bedrest, and subsequent labor induction ten days before my due date. Although it was scary, I remember thinking that I was pretty lucky. I had a self-limiting illness. My patients had a potentially life-threatening one. Steven's birth also erased my "atheist period." After seeing so much pain and suffering and death at work, the miracle of childbirth and new life reestablished my faith in God and my religious beliefs. It was good to be back.

At different stages of my own life, I've noticed that I've had different emotional reactions to patients. Fresh out of college, it was the patients who were female, young, and single, like me, that I would take home with me in my mind, wonder about when I was off, and regard as my "favorite" patients. Five days before my wedding, I left a dying patient's room in tears. He had metastatic melanoma in his gut, and was bleeding rectally. I had changed his underpad every 30 to 60 minutes for the previous 14 hours. His wife began to reminisce about their 49 years together, and expressed regret that they wouldn't have a 50th anniversary. So conscious of my own upcoming marriage, I found the situation incredibly sad.

Since becoming a mother, however, I find myself identifying with and becoming attached to not just certain patients, but the patients' mothers as well. Such was the case with Chris and his mother Elizabeth.

A bright, articulate high school senior with an ironic sense of humor, Chris was diagnosed with a mediastinal yolk sac tumor. As clinical nurse specialist, I was asked by the staff oncology nurses to help with patient education. My first visit with Chris and Elizabeth lasted nearly an hour, as I answered multiple questions. I think they had an immediate trust in me when they learned I was the only nurse on the staff who had ever taken care of a patient with the same rare diagnosis. I was glad at the time that they had not asked about the outcome of that patient's disease; he had died less than a year after diagnosis.

Over the next eight months, I saw Chris and his family multiple times as he was in and out of the hospital for chemotherapy, complicated by bone marrow depression. Because of an ongoing problem with refractory nausea, Chris was often sedated while in the hospital. So most of my interventions were accomplished through his mother. I taught about oral care, central line care, infection prevention. I suggested various antiemetic combinations which the oncologist would order, to little avail.

A warm, open, generous person, Elizabeth began to ask me about my own family during the many hours I spent with hers. Although in nursing school I was taught to redirect inquiries about my personal life back to the patient with statements like, "I'm here to talk with you about your health concerns," I was never comfortable with that. It seemed to me that if patients bared their souls to me, I could at least answer when they asked if I was married or where I was from. Especially in oncology nursing, where interactions with patients frequently occur over a long period of time, establishment of a more reciprocal relationship seemed natural. And so it was that I began a relationship with Elizabeth based on our common experiences as moms. So often when I would tell her about then three-year-old Steven, she would say, "He sounds just like Chris at that age."

During most of Chris's illness, I was pregnant with our second son, Kevin. I had to cut back to part-time work when I was six months along, and by seven months was on complete bedrest due to pregnancy-induced hypertension. It was scary again and I worried about a possible premature baby in addition to fearing that I might have a stroke. But again, 11 years of oncology nursing experience helped to put my own problems into perspective. They were probably self-limiting and not likely fatal. I had seen hundreds or thousands of patients face significantly worse odds with courage and grace. I tried to learn from their examples. And with the help of my mom, the baby and I ended up fine.

I came back from a four-month maternity leave to the sad fact that Chris was back in the hospital with massive brain metastases. Despite aggressive treatment, it soon became obvious Chris was going to die, although of course no one knew when. One afternoon I was making rounds late. Elizabeth sought me out and said she'd been fighting an urge all day to call in the family to tell Chris good-bye. I immediately got the chills. Although physically there was no detectable change in Chris's condition, experience had taught me that when a patient or family member feels that death is near, they are usually right. I took Elizabeth's hands and encouraged her to make the call.

The next day I came to work and was told Chris had just died. I went to his room and Elizabeth's first words were, "I was right." She thanked me for encouraging her to call the rest of the family. I touched Chris's arm and silently said good-bye. Elizabeth and I hugged and cried for a long time. When we finally pulled apart I told her that I did not usually cry so much over a patient's death. "It's mother love," she said. "It's mother pain."

I cried throughout Chris's beautiful funeral service too. I cried for a promising young life cut too short. I cried for his family, left without their beloved brother and son. I cried from my own feelings of guilt, that the health care team had been unable to control all his cancer-related symptoms. But mostly I cried tears of mother pain, feeling that bond that so many nurses share with their patients and their patients' families, and each other.

"Take care of your babies," Elizabeth had whispered to me after Chris's death, knowing she could no longer take care of one of hers.

I vowed I would.

Having two children and an oncology nursing career has been stressful. It's not that I find oncology nursing particularly stressful, but I think having any career, a house, a husband, two kids, and a long commute is a balancing act for many women. The first year after Steven's birth was hard, and I ended up physically ill (including meningitis) several times. I think these illnesses were stress induced. It got easier in subsequent years, until Kevin came along. Both my obstetrician and internist told me I needed to exercise more. I had always hated to exercise, although I had done it sporadically since I was 14. But I started exercising regularly 3 to 4 times a week when Kevin was four weeks old.

I've kept it up now for two and a half years. I think that without that I wouldn't have the energy or strength to cope with my life. I've also found that shopping is a great stress release for me too!

I sometimes wonder if I enjoy being an oncology nurse because of my basic personality, or if my character traits today have been shaped by having been an oncology nurse since I was 22. Maybe it's a little of each.

I think what I brought to the role was an acceptance of death as a part of life, and a philosophy that there is always something that can be done to improve a bad situation.

What I have learned from oncology nursing is what a real problem is. Bad traffic? The baby not sleeping through the night? This too shall pass. As one of my patients, now dead of his disease, said, "If all your problems could be fixed with money, you have no problems." It's a cliché, but when you have your health, you have everything.

The best part of oncology nursing, of course, is the people. To be able to share in patients' lives when they are experiencing a health crisis, and hopefully help them with it, is a privilege, a sacred trust, a gift. The lives of both patient and nurse are enriched.

Oncology staff members are wonderful. Three times in my career I've moved to cities where my husband was the only person I knew. But I have always been able to make good friends working with oncology social workers, dietitians, chaplains, physicians, and nurses. I've marveled at the volunteerism in ONS. Employed nurses with families giving up their weekends to attend a committee meeting? Yes! The wonderful feelings of camaraderie, and the sense of what can be accomplished by bringing together talented nurses from all over the country working toward a common vision, are addictive.

Recently, one of the radiation oncologists at work noticed the ONS button on my lab coat that says, "No, oncology nursing is NOT depressing." He smiled. "They ask that about my job too. But it's not. You meet some pretty wonderful folks."

I couldn't agree more.

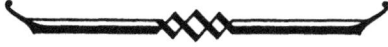

15

Elaine Glass

Beginnings

"Choose a job you love, and you will never have to work a day in your life."

—Confucius

I grew up in the country, outside of Springfield, Ohio, with many assorted animals—dogs, horses, pigs, ducks, geese, rabbits, and the like. I loved animals and spent a lot of time with them since there were not many kids my age in the neighborhood. When people would ask me what I wanted to be when I grew up, I answered, "I want to be a vet." However, when I was in high school, I started going to a church in the city. It was then I decided that people were more important than animals and that I should be a nurse. I contemplated being a doctor, but I was afraid that if I made a mistake that resulted in a patient's death, I would not be able to live with myself. Since there was a diploma nursing school three miles from my house, I planned to go there.

My dad was a carpenter who worked hard for a living. He insisted that I go to college to "catch a better husband." So I sold my horse, cashed in my $1,000 life insurance policy, applied for a scholarship, got a summer job as a waitress at the local truck stop, and enrolled myself in Ohio State University's school of nursing.

My first weekend at college, I looked up the sister church of my church denomination that was closest to campus. A very unique individual kept talking to me there. When he found out that I wanted to be a nurse, he assured me that I would change my mind. (He had changed his major several times and he was a junior.) Although he was the most eccentric person I had ever met, he was nice and we started dating. As the relationship became more serious, he was not enthusiastic about my pursuing a nursing degree. He said he was worried I would fall in love with a dynamic doctor or a wealthy patient. However, I was enjoying nursing school and

161

I could not think of anything else I wanted to do. So I reassured Steve that I loved him and we were married at the end of my sophomore year, the day after he graduated with a B.A. in sociology.

"Accept the challenges, so that you may feel the exhilaration of victory."

—*General George S. Patton*

While I continued to work on my nursing degree, Steve continued in college to get his M.B.A. We both had to work to make ends meet. I can still remember my first day on the job as a nursing assistant at the Ohio State University hospitals. They assigned me to a unit that specialized in people with gastrointestinal disorders. The head nurse was there that Saturday morning to make sure I got oriented. She assigned me *eight* patients! I immediately approached her and told her that I could not care for eight patients. In my two years of nursing school, I had never taken care of more than one patient at a time. There was no way I could do eight! Well, the head nurse reassured me that I could do it; I just needed to get started and try to do my best. She told me she would help me later in the morning if I needed it. So I rolled up my sleeves, took eight vital signs, made eight beds, and helped eight people do their A.M. care. When I came up for air, it was not even noon yet! I was so proud of myself I could hardly stand it. My self-confidence soared. I could do just about anything now.

". . . the luckiest people in the world"

—*Bob Merrill*

Once I had become an experienced nursing assistant on the gastrointestinal unit, the supervisors kept pulling me up to the general medicine/oncology unit. This unit was always short-staffed and morale was quite low. I thought to myself, "How awful—having cancer and no one wants to take care of you." I really felt needed there. Besides, this unit did not have a "BM Board." (The gastrointestinal unit had a "BM Board." Every weekend that I worked, it was my responsibility in the afternoon to visit each patient and ask them how many BMs they had had that day. The patients and I were both embarrassed with this routine task—especially when visitors were present in their Sunday best.) Therefore, when I graduated from nursing school, I applied for a position on the general medicine/oncology unit. They were pleased to have me work there.

"I've lived a good life."

—*John*

I hadn't been on the general medicine/oncology unit more than a few months when a medical student with Hodgkins disease was admitted to our floor. He was the same age as I was and he looked pretty sick. I was afraid he might die and I wasn't ready to deal with that. I told my head nurse, Norma Selders, that I didn't want to take care of John. I suggested she assign him to the older nurses. Norma told me that I couldn't back away from uncomfortable situations. She said I had to learn to deal with my feelings. I had to take care of John.

I didn't know what to say to John so I just kept my comments focused on his physical care. After I cared for John for a few days, he started to talk about his impending death. I marveled at the ease with which he shared his feelings. I was awed by his courage and the sense of peace he had with himself. He told me: "Sure, I would have liked to have been a great doctor—like Albert Schweitzer—but not too many 22-year-old men can say they've done what I've done. I lettered all four years in high school, I dated all the cheerleaders, and I got myself into medical school. I'm satisfied with my life. I've lived a good life."

I was the only one with John when he died at 4:00 in the morning. He died peacefully and without pain. John's death was the first I'd ever experienced. Thanks to John, I was not afraid. After I did morgue care I called the supervisor. I asked her to cover the unit while I took John to the morgue. She was appalled at my request and told me that the transportation aide would take John to the morgue. I told her that I didn't trust the aide. The rumor around the hospital was that the last body he was supposed to take to the morgue, he had parked in the men's room while he took a coffee break. A late night visitor was quite traumatized when he went to relieve himself and discovered a dead body in the toilet with him. I was not going to have that happen to John. I was going to make sure he made it straight to the morgue. Well, the supervisor thought I was nuts and told me I had to let the transportation aide take John to the morgue because she would not cover the floor for me. I refused to comply and told her John would stay in his room until I got off duty to take him safely to the morgue. The supervisor was furious with me. Luckily, one of my favorite hospital aides from our unit came to work early and volunteered to take John to the morgue for me. I trusted Mike. I knew he liked John too, and that he would make sure that John made it to the morgue without any mishaps.

After John died I thought a lot about what he had said. I reflected on my own life of 22 years. My goal from then on was to make decisions and choices that I could feel good about if my life were to come to a sudden halt. I aspired to be like John—always to be ready to say: "I've lived a good life."

"You can't get a bedsore."

—Elaine Glass

Nearly a year after John died, I was still working on the general medicine/oncology unit. I was on nights when I first walked into Barbara's room. My first impression of her is still very vivid. She looked like a defeathered chicken, one of those joke rubber ones. She was nothing but skin and bones, and she was bald except for a few strands of fuzz atop her head. Her appearance was ghastly. I told her I'd be her nurse for the night and after I took her vital signs, I turned her on her side to check her back. (The report I'd received from the evening nurse was that Barbara's backside was breaking down because she refused to turn on her side. Since she was dying anyway, most of the nurses did not fight with her about turning every two hours. This was in the early 1970s before high-tech beds and mattresses were available.) Her lower back was reddened and there was a small area of skin breakdown on her coccyx. I rubbed the area with lotion and began to place a pillow behind her back. Barbara panicked and told me to turn her back onto her back, that she couldn't breathe. I reassured her that she was breathing fine and that I intended to leave her on her side for at least two hours. I told her that her backside looked bad and that it would become very painful if it were allowed to break down further. Barbara didn't care, she wanted to be back on her back. She told me that if I left her on her side she would stop breathing. I sat on the bed next to Barbara, looked her in the face, stroked her back, and told her that I would stay right there beside her until she fell asleep. I would also come back in two hours and turn her back over onto her back. I can still remember the stupid comment I made next, "If you stop breathing, I'll wake you up." Surprisingly, Barbara was reassured by my approach and within about ten minutes, she was asleep. I woke her up at 2 A.M. and turned her onto her back. She was pleased. At 4 A.M. I woke her up to turn her to the other side. Barbara again protested, but complied—she had to, she weighed less than 100 pounds. At 6 A.M. she was happy to be on her back again.

The next night when I came on duty, Barbara's husband was still there. After I took her vital signs, I turned her on her side and checked her backside. I could tell she'd been on her back most of the day. As I placed the pillow behind her back, Barbara cried out to her husband. I can still see the look on his face. If looks could kill, I would have been dead. But I knew that one of my former nursing instructors, Lee Mourad, would kill me if I ever let one of my patients get a bedsore. So, I reexplained my rationale about skin breakdown and pain and made

Barbara as comfortable on her side as possible. I told her that her husband and I would be right outside her room talking. I reinforced to her husband my plan of care for Barbara to prevent a painful bedsore. I reassured him that she had done well the night before and it would just take her a while to get used to breathing on her side. He bought into my plan of care and the next night Barbara gave me no trouble at all. As it turned out, Barbara's husband began making her turn on her side throughout the day and she finally became reasonably comfortable with breathing on her side.

By the time I got back on day shift, Barbara was even sitting up in the chair. Her husband decided he could handle Barbara's care now that she was no longer completely bedridden and he wanted to take her home. When we discharged Barbara later that week, we were pleased that she did not have to die in the hospital and would be able to spend her last days at home.

Several months later I transferred to the hospital's chemotherapy clinic. I was drawing a patient's blood in the hallway when I heard a yelp. The next thing I knew, some woman was hugging my shoulders from behind me. I tried to steady myself so I didn't harm the patient's arm that I was drawing blood from. I turned and told this enthusiastic person I'd be with her in a second. I had no idea who she was. I quickly finished drawing the blood and turned to see what this excited woman wanted. Standing beside her was her husband with a smile on his face. It was Barbara! She'd gained 25 pounds, she had a gorgeous head of hair, and she could walk—and squeeze—really well. I couldn't believe my eyes!

As we talked, Barbara caught me up on what had happened to her. She credited me with saving her life. I asked her what I had done. She said I was the only nurse who always made her turn over in bed to prevent a bedsore. She said, "Everyone else thought I was going to die so they were nice to me. You weren't. You made me turn anyway. I thought to myself, 'Maybe I won't die.' So I started to try again." I chuckled to myself, because I had thought Barbara was going to die too. I just couldn't let her die with a bedsore since that would not be good nursing care.

"Can I chew on your ear a minute?"

—Debbie

Debbie was one of the reasons I transferred to the chemotherapy clinic. Our head nurse had quit and I had been assistant head nurse for less than a year. Administration was trying to get me to be head nurse. I'd been out of school less than two years and with what I'd seen of management's duties, I was not interested. One afternoon when I was in charge, the nurse caring for Debbie said that Debbie wanted to see me. Debbie was a young woman in her 20s with leukemia. She was angry about being sick and cooped up in the hospital. She rarely talked about how she felt. She just sulked. So I was surprised that when I entered Debbie's room, she asked me if she could chew on my ear. I said, "Sure," and sat down on the corner of her bed. Just as Debbie was starting to talk, the supervisor stuck her head around the corner of the curtain. She told me that I had to come to an administrative budget meeting. I told her I was busy. She told me that if I didn't come to this budget meeting, our unit would not be allocated any more nurses and we'd always be too busy. I felt I had to go, so I apologized to Debbie and told her I would speak with her when I got back. When I returned, Debbie was asleep, so I didn't wake her. Debbie was still asleep when my shift was over, so I decided to wait until tomorrow to talk to her. Debbie died that night unexpectedly. I was sick. I vowed then and there that I would never allow anyone or anything to come before patient care. Patients would always come first. Twenty years later, I have never regretted sticking to this rule.

"You'll never find the right card for Wally,"

I said to my husband.

Wally had been coming to the clinic for chemo for a couple of years. He was a spirited soul—a little like John. He was a truck mechanic and he loved to tell me stories about the latest rig he'd souped up. He had Hodgkins, too, and he was not doing well. However, he told me he'd rather take chemo once or twice a month than have diabetes like his mom. She had to check her urine four times a day (the days of Testape®—before Accucheck®) and he thought that was totally gross.

One day I was sitting in the living room and Steve brought in the mail. As I opened a letter addressed to me, tears came streaming down my face. Steve asked me what was wrong. Between sobs I told him that one of my favorite patients, Wally, had died. His sister had written the letter and described how impressive the funeral procession was with 30-some jacked-up trucks following the hearse. Poor Steve didn't have a clue how to comfort me. As he headed for the door, he told me he was going down to the drugstore to get me a sympathy card for Wally's family. I was irritated by his offer, since I thought only I could pick out the right card for Wally. Nonetheless, I pulled myself together by the time Steve returned. I even liked the card that he had selected. We talked then, and I was able to tell Steve that what I needed most at times like these was to be held and given special treatment—like dinner out or at least an ice cream outing.

Since then, to help Steve better understand my work, at the end of the day I have always shared with him the interesting stories and dramas that I have with my patients. I use only first names to respect their confidentiality. Through these stories, Steve has really come to appreciate and value the work that I do. He even helps the patients by helping me—such as stopping by the library to get a video or going by Cheryl's to get some gourmet cookies for a special patient.

Changing the System

Rules For Radicals

—*The title of the book the chemotherapy project's clinical nurse specialist gave me.*

It was in the chemo clinic that I first took an unpopular stand with administration. There were three nurses working in the clinic giving chemotherapy. We mixed and gave all the chemo. We did not wear gloves, goggles, or gowns. We had no hood or special ventilation and we mixed the drugs in the hallway where patients and other staff passed behind us. We squirted excess drug into the wastecan. We stored prepared syringes of saline in an empty Maalox box for the busy times during the day. It was really archaic by today's standards.

I believed that we nurses were spending an inordinate amount of our time doing the pharmacist's task of reconstituting drugs. So I contacted the state board of pharmacy. They told me we were practicing pharmacy and that we should stop doing so. I told my director of nursing what I had found out. She told me that administration was not pleased about these findings—especially since hiring a pharmacist would be so expensive. However, we eventually got a pharmacist and he negotiated a "mixing" room and, later on, a biological safety cabinet. At that time, I was glad I had taken the initiative to make these changes because we had more time to do nursing care. Now I am glad that my exposure to the hazards of the chemotherapy was decreased because I was able to get the system to change.

The Oncology Nursing Society

"To promote excellence in oncology nursing . . ."

—*ONS Mission Statement*

Since I am "Type A," I always have to be doing something. So I used to keep professional journals under my chair in the hallway of the clinic to read during "down" times. My head nurse initially scolded me for sitting and reading. She said it made me look lazy. She suggested that

I stand in readiness for when a doctor came out of a room and needed help. I laughed to myself at the generation gap between my head nurse and me, and I sat and read anyway. Since I was a hard worker otherwise, she finally left me alone. It was during one of those quick minutes of reading that I saw a news clip in *AJN* about a group of nurses that had just formed a new professional organization called the Oncology Nursing Society. I sent away for an application and joined.

> **"Friendship adds a brighter radiance to prosperity, and lightens the burden of adversity by dividing and sharing it."**
>
> —*Cicero*

I attended my first Congress in Colorado in 1977. I was so excited and motivated to be with this group of nurses who did what I did. Although I was exhausted at the end of the second or third day, the evening program on death and dying looked too good to pass up. (I still wear myself out at Congress, going to breakfasts at 6 A.M. and dinner meetings until 10 P.M.) During this evening presentation on death and dying, we were asked to sit on the floor and find someone in the group whom we did not know. I paired up with a nurse named Shirley. As we talked and shared our feelings about death, we discovered we were both from Ohio. We bonded instantly. We exchanged addresses and phone numbers and continued our friendship after the congress. At the next Congress we made arrangements to room with each other. We have both attended every Congress since then and have been roommates every year with few exceptions including the times when our husbands came along. Needless to say, I count Shirley Gullo as one of my best friends and nursing colleagues. She is one of those people you feel very comfortable with and look forward to having fun with.

> **"It is the greatest of all mistakes to do nothing because you can only do a little. Do what you can."**
>
> —*Sydney Smith*

In 1979 I agreed to run for the national ONS Nominating Committee. It was my first national election. I never thought I had a chance to win. I was shocked and thrilled when I was elected with the most votes. My husband had a special red T-shirt made for me to commemorate the occasion.

After I served a two-year term on the Nominating Committee, I was asked to chair the Executive Director Search Committee. When we had completed interviewing all the candidates, we had a lively discussion about which of the excellent candidates we would recommend to the

ONS Board. Some of the non-nurse business people were very talented and experienced. However, we noted that although Pearl Moore, R.N., M.S., did not have the business experience and training that the other candidates did, we believed she could learn that. What Pearl had, which was not as evident in these other people, was a very strong commitment to oncology nursing. After reflecting on this discussion, we unanimously recommended Pearl as our first choice candidate. I have been more than pleased with that decision ever since.

> **"People rarely succeed at anything unless they have fun doing it."**
>
> —*Author unknown*

Next I served on the Oncology Nursing Forum's editorial review board for four years. After that I was asked to be a member-at-large on the strategic planning subcommittee. Well, I knew nothing about strategic planning, but it sounded interesting so I said, "Why not?" I soon fell in love with the strategic planning process. Since I liked it so well and was continually developing skills in it, and it was a subcommittee of the board, the board allowed me to reup three times. During my fifth year, the incoming president, Carol Curtiss, asked me to co-chair the subcommittee with her since I was now the ONS volunteer "expert" on strategic planning. I was thrilled. I was also grateful to Carol for recognizing me as an ONS leader by allowing me to share 'his important leadership role with her. The next year I chaired the structure task force (an outcome of strategic planning). I really grieved when I was told that after six years, the board could no longer renew my membership on the subcommittee because others needed the opportunity to serve in this capacity. I understood—and agreed with the rationale—but I knew I would still miss strategic planning at ONS. Not to worry though, I am now on the Columbus Chapter strategic planning task force, and I am in charge of the James Cancer Hospital's nursing strategic planning process. From novice to "expert"—thanks to ONS's volunteer opportunities.

The Evolution of a Clinical Nurse Specialist

> **"Unless you try to do something beyond what you have already mastered, you will never grow."**
>
> —*Ronald E. Osborn*

One day while working in the clinic, I noticed an RFP (request for proposal) from the college of nursing. The topic looked interesting, so I drafted an outline and submitted it for review to the nursing director of the clinic, Fran McNew. I can still remember the diplomatic way with which she told me that my outline stank. She told me that I had a good idea, but my writing reflected my lack of knowledge of the research process. She suggested I enroll in a graduate school research course. I did and had so much fun in the course that I decided to get my master's degree in nursing.

While in graduate school, Dr. Mary MacVicar became my mentor. One of the things she made me do was volunteer for the American Cancer Society (ACS). I did not mind serving on the nursing committee; that was fun. I began to learn the art of networking there. However, she insisted that I become a member of the public speakers bureau. I had never done public speaking and I was scared to death. My first speaking engagement, at a local nursing home, was on the seven warning signals of cancer. I knew the topic well, prepared a detailed outline, read pamphlets and took them with me for backup, and showed up early to get familiar with the room set-up. Was I relieved! There were only about 40 people in the audience. Some of them slept through my whole presentation, some could not hear, and those who did hear what I had to say smiled a lot. The part I dreaded even more than giving the lecture was the question and answer period at the end. Luckily, there were only a few questions and they were all ones that I could easily answer.

After this positive experience, I did more nursing home presentations and I eventually became more and more comfortable with public speaking. When I took my first job as a clinical nurse specialist (CNS), the physician I worked with, Dr. Jim Neidhart, told me that if I submitted an abstract to ONS that got accepted, he would pay all my expenses to go to the Congress. After that, I submitted and presented a paper every year for five or six years.

I have given scores of presentations since those early nursing home days. Now I am very comfortable in front of all kinds of audiences. My largest audience to date has been at the 1992 ONS Congress in San Diego where I presented to almost 2,000 ONS colleagues on the topic of humor. It is rather humbling to see yourself projected on two of those huge screens so everyone in the audience can see you. If you would have told me 15 years ago that I would have been able to speak in front of such a large group and that I would have enjoyed it, my response would have been, "No Way!"

Dress for Success

—*John T. Malloy*

As I was nearing the end of my graduate studies, I began looking for a clinical nurse specialist position. One choice was with the state department of health and the other was on the inpatient interdisciplinary oncology unit (IOU) at OSU Hospital. I chose the latter because patient care was my first love and the other position was a desk job.

One of my friends during this time was working on her M.B.A. in business. We talked about my upcoming new position, particularly about what I should wear. Having read Malloy's book, *Dress for Success*, we decided that a white lab coat would serve as the "business jacket." The clothes underneath should be a conservative dress or skirt/blouse. A briefcase would also be necessary to give that "professional, business" look. I was excited and a bit scared since every nurse in our hospital, including the CNSs, directors of nursing, and the administrator for nursing, still wore white uniforms. Fortunately, I made a positive impression, and in less than a year, other clinical and administrative leaders began to wear "street" clothes as well.

"Courage and perseverance have a magical talisman, before which difficulties disappear and obstacles vanish into air."

—*John Quincy Adams*

My first 18 months as a CNS on the interdisciplinary oncology unit (IOU) went quite well and I was able to function effectively in the role. However, the next six months were very stressful, as the full effect of the nursing shortage of the early 1980s hit. We had three head nurses quit during this time and there were only three staff nurses and myself left who were capable of giving chemotherapy. Everyone else was new or from the agency. Since the IOU was in crisis on a daily basis, I could not function as a CNS—I felt more like a firefighter, putting out one crisis after another. So I decided to be proactive. I developed a proposal that I would be the CNS/head nurse of the IOU if I could have three assistant head nurses to help with scheduling, precepting, and monitoring chemotherapy on 3–11. Administration accepted my proposal and I rolled up my sleeves to begin building up the unit. Within 18 months, I had recruited and educated a staff of 34 nurses and 21 of them could give chemotherapy. I also developed a proposal for a weekend work program, which was implemented housewide and was very effective in retaining nurses and improving morale. Because I had never been in management before and had not taken any courses in graduate school in administration, I was flying by the seat of my pants. So when the unit was stable, I began intensive self study and became one of the few nurses in our hospital to be certified in nursing administration.

I really enjoyed the six years I spent in this combination management/clinical role. One of the highlights of this time was a comment made to me by one of the best staff nurses on the unit. She had worked at a number of other places and had been a nurse for several years. She told me that this was the first job she had ever had where she really felt that she knew what nursing was and what good nursing care was all about. Her words were the best evaluation I ever had.

Another special outcome of this time is the number of current leaders at the James Cancer Hospital who used to work on my unit. One of my former assistant nurse managers, Phyllis Kaldor, was promoted in 1994 to director of oncology nursing—and is now my boss! Another former staff member, Bertie Ford, president of the Columbus chapter of ONS and coordinator-elect of the ONS clinical trials SIG in 1994.

> **"When you become reluctant to change, remind yourself of the beauty of autumn."**
>
> —*Author unknown*

My six years as leader of the IOU ended after a new nursing administrator was hired. I was the only CNS who was in a management role. So I had to choose one or the other. I could either be a head nurse or a CNS, but I could no longer be both. It was an extremely difficult decision for me. I had done a good job in the combination role, and I thought it was unfair to make me change my role now, after all I had done to build up the unit. I could not convince administration to let me stay in the combination role, so I finally chose to be a CNS.

> **"Things turn out best for the people who make the best of the way things turn out."**
>
> —*John Woodson*

I felt traumatized having to make this role change. Six things kept me together and functioning:

- Steve. He was behind me all the way. Almost every night we strategized and problem-solved on how I could keep my combination position.
- My faith in God. Prayer and meditation were a great inspiration to me. They helped me keep my attitude positive.
- My ONS and ACS colleagues. Because of my volunteer activities, I was able to maintain my self-esteem and self-confidence. Even though I felt unappreciated by management in my job, I was receiving recognition and positive feedback from others outside of work. I was on the board of the

Franklin County unit of the ACS. Their executive director, Mike Segal, whose wife had died of breast cancer, had taken me on as a mentee. He groomed me, encouraged me, and inspired me with his enthusiasm. I eventually became the second female president of the Franklin County unit. One of my graduate school professors, Dr. Grace Sills, was also a tremendous support. And lunchtime walks with one of my best nurse friends, Diane Eleftherakis, were very therapeutic.

- The staff on my unit. When I told my staff I had to change my position, my staff gave me a recognition dinner at a fine restaurant. I framed the card they gave me. This card, a plaque, and sundry "gag" gifts still sit atop my desk eight years later.
- A sense of humor. My favorite expression during this time was that I had developed immune antibodies against administrative decisions. I wholeheartedly agree with the person who said that every survival kit should include a sense of humor.
- People with cancer. I felt the patients still appreciated my efforts. Nelson was one of those special patients who made the struggle all worthwhile.

"You gals are like daughters to me."

—Nelson

Nelson was a short, pudgy fellow who battled lymphoma for 12 years. He spent many weeks during those years on the IOU unit as he tried new research drugs and kept one step ahead of his disease. Whenever Nelson was in for treatment, he would get up early, go into the research office, and make fresh coffee for the day shift before we came in at 7 A.M. He always asked to have nursing students assigned to him so he could "teach them the ropes" from the patient's perspective. One night he was up until 2 A.M. cutting out shamrocks for our St. Patrick's Day door decorations. After that he got his wife's elementary school class to make seasonal decorations for us, and he brought them in with him when he came to be admitted. He appeared on local TV after being on the "con" side of not taking the soon-to-be released marijuana pill. He would have nothing to do with anything that resembled street drugs, even if it meant being sick.

One day a young intern with the sniffles entered Nelson's semiprivate room without a mask. Nelson yelled at him and ran him out of the room, pointing out the big red sign on the door that indicated you were to wear a mask. Then, within the next few minutes, Nelson's roommate passed out in the toilet. Nelson dragged him back to bed and then ran outside into the hall and hollered for help. The intern that he had just reprimanded was in earshot and came running to the rescue. The intern ran into the room and seconds later ran back out to get a mask and then ran back in again. Nelson was so upset. He could not believe the intern did not have enough sense to forget the mask in the midst of an emergency. We teased Nelson a lot about scaring the intern to such a degree that he feared for his safety if he entered their room again without a mask.

Nelson was a special guy. We all loved him. And especially since his own family lived three hours away and could not visit often, Nelson was truly a member of the unit family.

"A door closes and a window opens."

—Author unknown

For a year after my combination CNS/head nurse position on the IOU was dissolved, I was depressed and uncertain about what I should do next. I went to a career counselor. I did a lot of introspection and reflection about what had happened. It was a "veg" year for me and I needed it badly.

My new supervisor had an idea for a new role for the CNSs. She wanted to place us on one of the hematology services to work collaboratively with the attending physician and housestaff. Her proposal was approved and the other CNS, Molly Moran, and I ventured into the loosely-defined role with more than a bit of trepidation. We developed the role as we went along and it gradually evolved into a case management-type position. We have both continued in the role for nearly seven years.

Although Molly and I have been doing very well in our roles, health care reform with its restructuring, re-engineering and rightsizing is worrisome. Both of us have enrolled in the OSU college of nursing's nurse practitioner program to prepare for new possibilities. In the meantime, I have been documenting and sending to administration how my interventions have resulted in cost savings to the hospital. I've been collecting data for less than four months and so far my cost savings estimate is $66,000. I hope administration decides I am worth it. I only have ten years until retirement.

"Good-bye Jim. I'll miss you . . ."

—Carol

I really enjoy my collaborative practice CNS role because of the intense, in-depth patient/family care opportunities that it offers me. Almost daily

I am able to make an impact on people's lives, which gives me a great sense of satisfaction. The following story exemplifies the difference I am able to make.

Jim had had chronic leukemia for a couple of years and now it was in blast crisis. Knowing his prognosis was poor, he asked to be a DNR. This time he had been admitted for fever and was diagnosed with pneumonia. He was not doing well and could not make his own decisions because he was too short of breath and hypoxic. The housestaff asked his wife, Carol, if they could transfer him to the ICU and put him on a respirator to get him over this pneumonia. Since it was going to be a temporary thing to treat the pneumonia, Carol agreed. As his bed was being wheeled out of the room, Jim stopped breathing. They wheeled the bed back into place and began to bag Jim as a Code Blue was called. Carol was asked by the housestaff to leave the room. She did not want to leave Jim, so I stayed with her as she sat in a chair by the window, about three feet from Jim's bed. We watched as the onslaught of doctors and nurses came to the code to try to save Jim. I sat on the arm of the chair and Carol clung to my arm and hand like glue and said little. I explained to her what the doctors and nurses were doing as well as translated what they said as things happened. When the nursing supervisor arrived, she tried to get me to get Carol out of the room. I told her that Carol did not want to leave Jim and that I thought she was doing all right. Next, the attending physician came into the room just before they were getting ready to intubate Jim. He assessed the situation. He then turned to Carol and said that he couldn't do this to Jim. Jim would probably never get off the respirator and we would not be doing him any favors by putting him through this. Carol told the attending physician to do whatever he thought was best. The attending physician instructed the team not to place the endotracheal tube. He called the code and they stopped bagging Jim. Several of the unit staff stayed in the room.

I told Carol it was time to say good-bye to Jim and I walked her up to the head of his bed as I politely asked a doctor to step aside. At this point, Jim's heart was beating erratically at only about 30 beats per minute. Carol told Jim that she loved him. She said she would miss him a lot, but would be all right with support from family and friends. Carol then commented to Jim that he would now be able to go fishing with Eric. There was a period of silence, so I asked who Eric was. Carol stated that he was their godson who had been killed in an auto accident the month before. She said that Eric and Jim were fishing buddies. As we spoke, Jim lay totally motionless, without any response. I then glanced over at the cardiac monitor which was still hooked up to Jim's chest. I was amazed to see that his heart rate was now in the 80s in normal sinus rhythm. I could not believe it! And neither could the others in the room from the looks on their faces. I told Carol that Jim must have heard her because his heart was back to normal (and he was breathing on his own at this point). Carol got excited and told Jim he could stay if he wanted to—she would help him keep fighting his disease. Within seconds, Jim's heart failed, he stopped breathing and died. Carol gave him a kiss and cried. It was a special moment I shall always remember.

Awards

"Let another praise you and not your own mouth."

—Proverbs 27:2

Some other memorable moments for me have been the awards I have received. A few of the most special to me include:

- The Lane Adams Award from the American Cancer Society in 1988. I received $2,500 and Steve and I were treated to an all expenses paid trip to New York City, including a stay at the Waldorf Astoria. We had a fabulous time and the award meant a lot since my friend Diane Eleftherakis nominated me, and several peers wrote letters of support.
- The Outstanding Staff Award from Ohio State University in 1992. This award was of special significance because my boss, Nancy Davis, RN, JD, nominated me for it. I received $1,000, a poster that was hung in our hospital lobby for a month, and a recognition luncheon with President Gee. My husband and my friends Barb Fersch and Dr. Eric Kraut attended the ceremony in my absence, since I was at the ONS Congress in San Diego.
- The Outreach Ohio/Amgen Mentorship Award on nurses day in 1994 at the Cincinnati ONS Congress. Recognition from my peers and colleagues for mentorship was one of the most meaningful experiences I have ever had. I received a gorgeous glass plaque, a huge lead crystal vase, a dozen red and white roses, and a $250 check. Plus, the incoming ONS president, Linda "Burnie" Johnson, gave me a dog sweatshirt and some cat socks. I was so delighted with the awards ceremony at the recognition reception. Over a hundred Ohio and national ONS leaders and colleagues were in attendance. It was terrific!

Thoughts About Oncology Nursing

"Ask not alone for victory; ask for courage. For if you can endure, you bring honor to yourself; even more, you bring honor to us all."

—Bud Greenspan

As you may well know, oncology nurses are often asked by friends, family, and professional colleagues, "How can you stand working with people with cancer? Isn't it depressing?" My quick response is usually something along these lines: "No, it's not depressing. It's sad when people don't get better and die, but it's not depressing. In fact, I find working with people who have cancer inspirational. They demonstrate tremendous courage, optimism, and hope. Many are positive thinkers and appreciate each day of life that they have. They have learned how precious life is and they're grateful. It is indeed an honor to know them."

Although the above is my quick response, I would like to share some of the insights I have gained about what has helped me continue to practice oncology nursing in various clinical roles for more than 22 years. (Please note that my thoughts appear in sequential order and not in any priority.)

"The family is the nucleus of civilization."

—Will and Ariel Durant

I was raised in a loving home by two wonderful, Christian parents. Dad was hoping his first born would be a son, so he built goal posts in the backyard in preparation for my arrival. Since I turned out to be a girl, he turned the goal posts into a swing set and he turned me into a tomboy. He spent hours coaching me and my brother, who finally arrived three years later, in sports, gardening, carpentry, and bible teachings. My mom was a good homemaker, and she took good care of us. In summary, I feel I am extremely fortunate to be blessed with such a loving childhood.

"The greatest happiness in the world is the conviction that we are loved, loved for ourselves, or rather loved in spite of ourselves."

—Victor Hugo

Steve and I have been married 24 years. I would not be as happy, as effective or as professionally accomplished as I am without Steve. He listens, he supports, he helps me problem-solve and strategize. He appreciates what I do for patients and families. He is an avid reader (something that I, unfortunately, am not). He copies articles for me and cuts out newspaper clippings of items of interest to me. On many occasions this has resulted in my having the advantage of being on the forefront of new ideas or knowledge. The information has really helped me grow and develop professionally.

When a favorite patient dies or I get an award, he takes me out to dinner. If I am super busy working on an ONS project or studying for school, he does the dishes. He has done the laundry for years. He always cooks for himself as we each eat at different times and like different foods.

Steve is my most helpful critic. He challenges my decisions and actions at work and in my volunteering. His perspective has redirected me on several occasions, resulting in more satisfying and acceptable outcomes. He also edits my writing—and this is always a major struggle for us. Knowing that we will be arguing over words and phrases, we both get psyched up to duke it out. Although it is an arduous process, the final product is much better than my original. In sum, Steve is a special guy, with an ego strong enough to be supportive to a professional spouse.

I am not an advocate of separation of work and home. Instead, I believe that sharing your stories about your care of patients and families helps your family understand and appreciate the special work that you do. Over the years, Steve has come to really value what I do. I believe this is partly due to patient and family stories that I have told him. On several occasions, I know he has been touched by these experiences.

Because Steve provides me with so much support, I try to support him as well. One of the things I do for him when I'm away is to leave him a pile of "miss you" cards. Each one is labeled to be opened the morning and evening of each day that I am out of town. Also, he gives me my wake-up calls when I am on the road. A couple of years ago when I was in Sante Fe, I told him to wake me up at 5 A.M. I meant Sante Fe time and he thought I meant Ohio time, so I was rudely wakened at 3 A.M. in Sante Fe. Needless to say, I now am very clear about which time zone's time I'm referring to.

Steve has always hated being alone, so he has a tough time when my trips last more than a few days. He has done a lot better the last six years since I surprised him on his 40th birthday with a beagle-mix puppy from the Humane Society. At first he thought I was crazy for getting him a dog, but within 24 hours, he and Ollie had bonded. Now Ollie is a great joy to us both. In fact, one of the things we find most rewarding as a threesome is taking Ollie to the OSU rehabilitation hospital to visit patients there once a month. Ollie even has his own business card: OLLIE, CANINE VISITOR, PET PALS.

"To get the body in tone, get the mind in tune."

—Zachary T. Bercowitz, M.D. (1895–1984)

I work at taking good care of myself. I never skip meals, and I try to eat low-fat foods (although I am easily tempted by anything chocolate). I exercise daily by walking Ollie three to five miles and by going to a weight-lifting class once a week. I do some of my best thinking while walking the tree-lined streets of our neighborhood with Ollie. I spend 15 to 20 minutes every morning reading devotions and I pray every morning while walking Ollie and every night while holding hands with Steve in bed. I love to take naps and to lie on the couch and cuddle with Steve and Ollie. For fun, I shop for the perfect greeting card, flip through home-shopping catalogs, visit with family and friends, and travel whenever I can. Keeping my life balanced has paid off for me. I have had perfect attendance at work for 14 years. Establishing daily habits that provide for your physical, mental/emotional, social, and spiritual fitness is critical to stress management and personal well-being.

"Where, oh Death, is your sting?"

—I Corinthians 15:55

I have a strong faith in God. Belief in a spiritual, higher being and an afterlife provides me with a perspective that does not fear death. Instead, death is another state of being that leads to a better life. I feel at ease about death, so I am comfortable talking with patients and families about it. Writings by Raymond Moody on near-death experiences and by Callanan and Kelly on pre-death experiences offer reassuring insights into the death experience. Sometimes I share these ideas with patients and families. They seem to find this information comforting and helpful in the dying process. Not everyone believes in God or an afterlife, but because I am comfortable with my own mortality, I am able to help people, whatever their beliefs. One of the most comforting thoughts about death was written by Thomas Campbell, "To live in the hearts we leave behind is not to die."

Regardless of your religion or spiritual beliefs, I believe that oncology nurses must come to terms with their own death or they will not last in oncology nursing. There is a lot of suffering and grief in oncology nursing practice and nurses must be able to integrate these negative experiences into philosophical beliefs that have a positive, meaningful frame of reference.

One of our night nurses died of breast cancer. At her funeral, we filed out of her church singing these words from a song by Eliza E.

Hewitt: "When we all get to heaven, what a day of rejoicing that will be." One day I look forward to reuniting with family, friends, and hundreds of patients and family members who have touched my life.

> **"To teach men how to live without certainty and yet without being paralyzed by hesitation, is perhaps the chief thing philosophy can still do."**
>
> *—Bertrand Russel*

In conclusion, I love being an oncology nurse. It is rewarding, fulfilling, exciting, and full of touching moments. The essence of my philosophy for practicing oncology nursing can be summarized by the following:

"To affect the quality of the day, that is the highest of arts."—Thoreau
"Be flexible and you won't get bent out of shape."—Argus Communications
"Humor: Never leave home without it."—Argus Communications
"Grant me a willing spirit to uphold me."—Psalms 51:12
"Attitude is everything."—Successories

Notes

Accucheck is a registered trademark of Boehringer Mannheim Corporation.

Testape is a registered trademark of Eil Lilly Corporation.

16

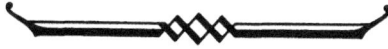

Janith Griffith

Both my love for nursing and for writing began in my childhood. As a small child during World War II, we lived with my grandparents in a small Iowa town. My grandfather was a dentist and had his office in our home. From the start, I was "Doc's helper" and learned to provide for the comforts of strangers.

Probably because of the gas rationing, "Doc" would take me along on errands each day by pulling me in a wagon instead of using the car. During these walks, Grandpa would tell me stories and share his love of nature. He often recited poems to me he had learned by heart. Since both my great-grandfather and great-uncle were published poets, poetry always was present in my life. My grandfather's bookshelf always contained poetry among the classic volumes. I was never discouraged from using these books and read at an early age.

My parents continued to encourage my love for books, poetry, and nature. We were all active in Scouting and camped outdoors often. My childhood attempts at writing stories and poetry were always supported. As a result, I grew up with a deep love of books and the worlds they are able to open up to me. To this day the combination of love for nature and poetry is strong. Rarely can I take a walk in nature without being inspired to write several stories or poems.

I feel lucky to have grown up in a close-knit family of artists, writers, and musicians. Family get-togethers always included readings and a sing-along around the piano. As a result, the creative therapies of art, music, and writing coupled with renewing nature walks have come naturally to me over the years. As I faced the challenges of a nursing career, I turned to these therapies not only for my patients, but for myself as well.

While growing up, my parents took care of each of our grandparents in our home as the need arose. It was natural to care for and to comfort these loved ones. Carrying supper trays, helping with walkers and urinals, and changing beds were just part of the daily routine starting in junior high. During high school, my Girl Scout volunteer work was

spent doing candy striper and nurses' aide type duties at the Methodist
Hospital in Sioux City, Iowa. This same hospital was then my choice for
nurses' training in 1961.

In those days women had few choices for a professional career and
I found I could pursue both choices—nursing and teaching—by attending nursing school and becoming an RN. The nursing schools of the
1950s and early 1960s had the philosophy that there was only one correct
way to do things. Furthermore, students should never question authority
figures, designated as almost anyone else in the hospital system! Being
a child of the times, I outwardly went along with this. However, inwardly
I questioned some of the responses I was expected to make. The most
difficult times came when patients would ask about their prognosis. We
were expected to be bright, cheerful, and encouraging even if the
prognosis was grave. The answer to "Am I going to die?" was never to
be "Yes." The following poem was written after looking back at those
training years from today's vantage point.

Nurses' Training: Then and Now

As a young teen
Overflowing
With questions and excitement
Nurses' Training beckoned,
And I followed
Into the mysteries
Of body and soul.

In those days
We didn't talk about
Despair or disappointment
Or especially
About death.

We were trained
To be cheerful, bright, and helpful,
Respectful, reverent, and kind.
Never questioning authority,
Never allowing
Emotions to be seen.

Trained
To duck from surgeon's fury
As instruments came flying.
To turn away

As tears stain the Dr.'s face,
His skill not strong enough
To save this young one's life.

Trained
To simply smile
And say
You're getting better
Day by day.

This new calling
Beckons me along a path
Where I must look inward
To find new strengths,
Sharing my emotions
Along with my new skills.

Training now
Changes
To educate me.

Over the years, learning to "untrain" myself from giving only those "correct" responses has been a difficult learning experience. The old ways were deeply ingrained. My best teachers for learning to honestly and bravely face death have been my oncology patients. With the opening of our oncology unit in 1983, I began that learning process.

I went to oncology from management and critical care. A divorce and a move back across the state had placed me in a night shift on a big medical unit. The opportunity to be part of a new unit and to learn exciting new things was irresistible. In my innocence, I never dreamt how much I truly had to learn. During the learning process, I again turned to music and poetry for strength and to nature for renewal. A strong inspiration has been Deanna Edwards, a music therapist from Salt Lake City, Utah. Her words and music were my strength and guidance during my first years as an oncology nurse. One of her songs in particular, "Teach Me To Die," inspired the following poem early in my career.

Teach Me How to Live

The doctor's words were foreign,
And you looked to me to translate.
But I couldn't make you hear me,
The knowledge had come too late.

You dream of the snow next winter,
And the sunsets never to see.
You smile at me so sweetly,
But you're not really listening to me.

Your ears are hearing the laughter
Of a grandchild yet unborn,
And try to capture the birdsong
Of a warm September morn.

Time suddenly changes,
A minute is worth a year.
All I can do is smile,
And brush away your tear.

I came into this blindly,
With so much knowledge to give.
While I teach you of dying,
You've taught me how to live.

As I grew both personally and professionally, one of the most important things that I learned was to continue to use the creative therapies. Art, music, and writing are helpful not only for myself, but also for my colleagues, patients, and the significant people in their lives. I was able to apply these therapies in many ways. During the first few years that our unit was open, I provided art supplies, posters, and music cassettes for the unit. We encouraged patients and families to use these, plus individual journals for writing. Encouraging the use of a journal in our family room has been a wonderful method of expression for many family members. It is left open on the table with an invitation to write anything you want, signed or unsigned. There have been expressions of love, anger, poetry, letters to loved ones, and words of hope and inspiration for others. I would encourage other nurses to try this in their family room areas.

Over the past ten years that our unit has been in existence, I have written many poems about my own feelings and about the special patients whose lives have touched mine because of my choice to work in oncology nursing. This has been a very satisfying method for me, recording memories of specific patients and dealing with the stresses of this very demanding specialty.

All nurses have those special patients they can really relate to. They are the ones who have become special teachers or friends. One of mine is named Red. He was just my age when he presented with myelodysplasia, progressing to leukemia before his death. I work the night shift. I consider this a distinct blessing. It provides a quiet time for communication without doctors, tests, or visitors for interruption. We would talk during these late night quiet hours. One of the things we shared was a love for music and art. I once made Red a calligraphied copy of the words to another of Deanna Edwards's songs, "Walk In The World For Me." He framed it and gave it back to me one day. I was in denial about losing this friend, one of the first oncology patients I was to lose. At the time I didn't realize it was his good-bye to me. A few days later I burst in, full of that old nursing school enthusiasm, telling him how good he looked with his suddenly bright rosy cheeks. The next autumn I wrote this poem.

Autumn Blush

The maple stands,
A bright yellow ball of sun
   Sent from heaven
   To brighten the brown of fall.

Weeks go by,
The bright sun
breaks into sunbeams
   Fluttering through the woods,
   Carpeting the ground with gold.

The palest trees
Enjoy a bright red flush,
   The false blush of fever
   Before death.

I believe these experiences can either turn caregivers away from oncology or make us stronger to carry on. Luckily, I have felt stronger for knowing Red. Some nights his voice still echoes down the corridors reminding me of that special bond that can be established with patients. His memory helps to focus me as I "walk in the world" for him, and to remind me of my mission here.

Other poems and patients have brought out my sense of humor and helped me to maintain that important balance between laughter and tears. One of those patients was a middle-aged guy with lymphoma named Gary. He had been in and out of the unit many times. Suddenly one day he said, "You know, after all this time you guys still never say my last name right!" We quickly apologized and reassured him we didn't want to make that mistake again. Luckily the correct pronunciation rhymed with easy. We laughed about that but never said it incorrectly again. I wrote this to help me remember him always.

Easy

His last name
Rhymed with easy.
"A good choice," he said,
Considering
All the exwives
Collecting alimony.

We all found him
Easy, too.
Easy-going, easy to laugh,
Easy to care for,
Easy to love.

A vivid contrast
Watching him decline
And fade away
In midlife,
All too soon.

Loving him
And caring,
Was the easy part.

Traveling the road
Together
Through treatment,
On toward cure.
Then parting,
Coming back alone.

These things
Are never
Easy.

An older woman was particularly stoic as she lay dying. I spent many hours with her those last few days and marveled at her peace and strength. I offered to call family or friends, but she preferred that I not call anyone. Over the next hours she laughed with me and told me many stories of her life. This trust and sharing is another sacred privilege offered to oncology nurses. Among her stories was this one which was only a small part of a long struggle that had contributed to her individual strength and growth.

Growth

They all have a story to tell
Those last few days of life.
Hers was of a mean and angry man
Named Husband.

Every morning
He would urinate
On the flowers that she loved.

She laughed,
And told how they had grown,
Tall and beautiful.
Rooted strongly,
Abundant with new growth and blooms.

From my school days, two mentors stand out. The first is a high school teacher, Edith Pollock. Her love of poetry and her encouragement were invaluable. She died recently in her 90s, and former students read poetry at her funeral celebration. For many of us she instilled a lifelong love of literature and poetry.

Another professor, who has been a mentor and friend, is Dr. Nick Mason-Brown from Coe College in Cedar Rapids, Iowa. I managed to squeeze several of his Latin American Literature classes into my B.S.N. completion curriculum recently. I found him an excellent teacher, also able to instill that love for his subject. He is an excellent poet and perhaps understood me better for that. I felt I could go to him with any problem and could always find encouragement for the struggle to return to school in my "grandmotherly years."

From my nursing career, two nursing mentors stand out in my mind. Mary Blomme was night house supervisor at St. Joseph's Hospital in Ottumwa, Iowa, when I worked there. When she retired after a long career, she oriented me to her position. Always encouraging and instilling confidence, she never once allowed this young nurse to think she couldn't do the job. This was a period of both professional and personal growth for me. She was always just a phone call away, no question too unimportant to be answered. During a time of personal crisis, she was like a second mom to me and for that I will be always grateful.

Following a divorce and relocation, I met my second nursing mentor,

Susan Primrose, nursing supervisor at St. Luke's Hospital in Cedar Rapids, Iowa. Susan embodies all of the qualities I look for in a nursing leader. During a crisis, she is efficient but calm. Her clinical skills remain excellent and she has worked closely beside me through several critical events on the night shift. From her I have learned to improve my critical thinking and problem-solving skills. She always maintains a pleasant, positive attitude and open lines of communication with staff nurses. One of the things I appreciate most from her is the expectation for excellence in me as a staff nurse. This expectation keeps me current on all of the patients on the floor and keeps me growing both personally and professionally.

When I decided to return to college for my B.S.N. completion, Susan continued to encourage me throughout the long struggle. As I received my degree after many years of full-time night shift work and part-time college classes, she was one of the important colleagues and friends cheering me on. Outside of work we share a love of art, music, literature, and nature. This has strengthened our friendship. Susan encourages my use of creative therapies and recognizes their benefits in both personal and professional life.

Thinking of colleagues has led me to think of those who have faced cancer and its treatments. Caring for nursing friends is difficult both for them and for us as caregivers. Suddenly we are faced with our own vulnerability. For them the roles are reversed and they look to us as their patient advocates. If we are to be useful in our role as advocate and caregiver, we must first learn to put our vulnerability in perspective. Once again our patients are often our best teachers. For me, the use of creative therapies has centered me time and again. Writing about the funny or tender moments and allowing myself free time with nature's healing powers has restored me and allowed me to do valuable grief work.

One colleague, a nurse manager, came to our unit for pain control and palliative care in the last stages of her disease. She and I had only a brief, business-like acquaintance before this admission. Perhaps this was to her advantage. With me she could let her guard down and let me comfort her inner vulnerable self. The end was very difficult with both the high doses of morphine required and the advanced stages of illness robbing her of her brilliance. As I continue to work through the fairly recent loss, one image of those days makes me smile. One night she insisted I find her a pen and wrote in the air as I sat by her bed charting. That urge to document is buried deeply within us!

For Sharon

Nursing was your life
Your focus.
Now cancer has taken

Even that love from you.
The colleagues come,
Well-meaning,
But it's too close to home,
When one of our own
Is in that bed.

In this dark night
I am the only one left,
To kiss the head
Where hair no longer grows.
To understand
There are voices and terrors
In narcotic dreams.
And to help you find the pen,
To write frantically
In the air,
Finishing one last chart.

Rest well, my friend,
The shift is finally over.

Another colleague, a breast cancer survivor, is also a dear friend. I wrote this for her.

For My Friend

The bilateral scars
Somehow balance you
And make you stronger,
Your female self
Now centered deep within.

My softness,
Without visible scars,
Is allowed closer
To your heart.

Many emotions must be dealt with as an oncology nurse. The most difficult for me is anger. Patients, families, friends, and caregivers are all angry—at the disease, at God, at each other, and at our inabilities even with modern technology to make much headway in this battle. Two of the writings I have included here followed my frustrations in dealing with 30- to 40-year-old men whose wives were dying. One lashed out at me in particular, one at the world in general. The first writing describes my own feeling.

Battered

Over and over and over
Anger
Pounds into me.
Yet I stand tall.
Protected by
Position, education,
Understanding, patience.

Slowly,
As minutes turn into hours,
the Anger
eats into
My protective cover,
Yet feeds and strengthens
Itself.

Withdrawn,
I curl inward,
Surrounding the ball of hostility
Forming deep
Within my center.
Trained not to let it show.

Suddenly
I am diminished.
Exhausted
Lost
Devoured by this
Overwhelming power,
Unleashed by the
Red
Lashing tongue.

The next writing is for Sal. The anger kept her from being able to talk honestly with her family. She kept looking to me for answers. I was there for her as best as I could be but never seemed able to reach her husband.

Running

He runs
Before and after
Visiting hours.
The anger
Pounding deeper
And deeper
Into the path
With every jarring stride.

How many miles
Of pounding steps
Must be endured
Before he can
Look at you,
Growing weaker
And further away
Each day?
Before he can
Answer your questions
And fears
And reassure you
He'll find you again
One day,
And you will
Still be
His love?

I see him still
Long after you've gone.
Running along the river
Pounding and hammering the
Anger
Into the ground.
Turning still
Away from me.

The nurses on my unit have had to endure, though on a smaller scale, many of the same emotions that our patients and families face with a critical illness. These include turmoil, change, and grieving over the loss of nursing family members. In 1983 our hospital decided to open an oncology unit. This involved restructuring one wing of our medical floor and redistributing management and personnel. Our nursing family was split without choice. Unfortunately for us our unit opened at the same time as a large same-day surgery area which overshadowed our open house celebrations. That following Christmas I wrote my first poem about patients and the emotions connected with the beginning of our oncology nursing careers. It was published in our hospital newsletter and distributed at our unit retreat.

Ten years later in 1993, to accommodate health care changes, our unit moved again. Once again a former unit and management team were dissolved. We all suffered the loss of former colleagues and the change of gaining new colleagues into our nursing family. This time there has been no open house. However, we continue to grow in our chosen specialty. We are all very different individuals but have the common bond of caring well for very special people. We share laughter, hugs, and tears, and a deep understanding of what it takes to continue this work. We truly do believe we make a very important difference in many people's lives.

Over the years my special friends, children, and grandchildren have all put up with my sleeping after working nights when they are all wide awake, and with my studying when they have wanted me to play. My parents and sister have all been encouraging and proud of my B.S.N., even if they had to wait to celebrate it 30 years after the R.N.! They all have thought nursing was a wonderful profession but have not been sure of my latest choice of oncology nursing. Those seeds of childhood were planted deep and have taken root strongly. With their support my growth has taken me firmly into a very meaningful specialty and back into my love of writing.

For my family and friends and for my oncology colleagues, I have rewritten that first poem. Hopefully my writing will help them all understand the importance of oncology nursing in my life.

Beginnings

TV news trucks
Block the drive.
Important appearing
Strangers
Scurry to and fro,
Excitement and busyness
Fill the air.

We hurry upstairs
Eager for our open house.
But our hallway
Is quiet,
Subdued.

Relaxation music
Fills this air,
Broken only by
Quiet tears,
Washing over
A grief stained face.
Prayers and hugs
Communicate here.

Save the bright lights
And musical fanfares
For the "money-makers"
Down the hall.

Here
Bright smiles
Light up our way,
Hugs provide the warmth,
Caring and laughter
The music,

And I am home.

17

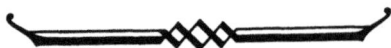

Mary Magee Gullatte

As an African-American child growing up in rural Mississippi, one of ten children and the oldest daughter, I learned quickly the art of caring for and nurturing my younger brothers and sisters. I am the progeny of a rich heritage of support, service, and commitment from my family and my community.

When I graduated from nursing school, one of the first females in my family to have had the opportunity to go to college, one of my uncles proudly said to me, "Do you remember the letter you wrote to me when you were in the third grade?" I thought to myself, What letter? Third grade? "No, I don't remember." He replied, "You wrote me and said you wanted to be a nurse when you grew up. I knew you would make it." Another big smile beamed from his face and he gave me a big hug.

Later that night I began to remember what sparked my choice. In the rural black communities of the 1950s and 1960s, public health nursing and family practice were the norm. We received our immunizations at school. I vividly remember the image of a most beautiful, tall, slender black woman dressed in white, who came to our elementary school to give us "shots." Her clothes were so white and perfect; she wore a white cap and white shoes. She was soft-spoken and the splendor of her white uniform looked dim when compared to her warm smile and gentle, caring eyes. While the others were afraid and crying as they received their immunizations, she would speak softly and try to distract those of us who stood lined up one behind the other waiting with our arms down and sleeves rolled up to the tops of our shoulders. She would say, "Be brave, it will only sting for a few seconds and it will keep you well; I wouldn't do anything to hurt you bad." I had almost forgotten that that was the beginning of my dream to become a nurse, so many years ago.

Upon graduation from high school, I knew my parents could not afford to send me to college, with so many younger brothers and sisters. In my parents' eyes they had already fulfilled their goal of having me graduate from high school because it was more than they had achieved in their formal education.

I enlisted in the United States Air Force after high school graduation in 1970. The Air Force would afford me the means to obtain a college education. While in the Air Force I traveled and excelled in skill and knowledge, receiving several recognition awards for outstanding leadership. While stationed at Eglin AFB in Florida, I enrolled in the local junior college where I obtained an associate of arts degree in pre-nursing. During my enlistment in the USAF I worked as a volunteer at the base hospital. I assisted the staff on the pediatric and female surgery unit. Some of the surgeries were related to a cancer diagnosis. I was taught to do wound care, simple dressing changes, and post-op care. Because I told the staff I was pursuing a nursing degree, the nurses and orderlies taught me a number of technical clinical skills which strengthened my novice nurse background.

Following an honorable discharge from the Air Force, I returned to Mississippi and enrolled in the B.S.N. program at the University of Southern Mississippi. While a student at Southern I again had the opportunity to work with cancer patients. As part of our medical/surgical clinical rotation we went to Charity Hospital in New Orleans for our experience with leukemia patients. I recall that the primary treatment was immunotherapy with BCG. We observed patients in the laminar flow units. I found myself being drawn more and more to the cancer practice specialty. For me, working with cancer patients meant providing holistic care for both patients and family, which included providing psychosocial as well as spiritual support.

Following graduation and marriage, I relocated to the Atlanta area where I sought employment on the hematology unit at Emory University Hospital. My commitment and devotion to oncology nursing care blossomed and exceeded my initial interest. Because of my enthusiasm and thirst for new knowledge and skills, I quickly transitioned from novice to expert in providing care for the leukemia patients and their families. I had some great role models, such as my head nurse Nelza Levine, and a staff nurse who was my mentor, Edith Honeycutt. They were both wise, knowledgeable, and skilled. Even more important, they were easy to approach and always took time to provide instructions and training in medical/surgical skills and holistic patient management. Another staff nurse, Jane Clark, was always encouraging and complimentary. She provided support and guidance in day-to-day nursing practice. As a novice nurse it is important to be surrounded by nurses who are confident, knowledgeable, and positive, and have a strong sense of self-worth. I believe I was very fortunate to have worked with what I consider to be a group of committed, informed, and caring professional nurses early in my career.

As I became more confident in my skills and knowledge I began to contemplate graduate school. Initially I had planned to attend part time. Jane Clark, who had just completed her master's, was a "one-woman recruiter" encouraging me to go full time. But I was pregnant with our first child. At that time, my head nurse was asked to take an interim position as assistant director of nursing, which would leave our unit without her calming presence. Surprising to me, I was asked to assume the position as acting head nurse on our hematology unit while she was in her new position. This was my first brush with management in nursing other than being charge nurse. I had a great deal of support from Nelza and Edith. I remained in the acting head nurse position for six months until the blessed event of the birth of our first child, a son, Rodney, Jr., on April 17, 1980.

I stayed home with the baby for five months before returning to work. I chose not to return to the management position because of the extended hours. I again began to plan for graduate school when Rodney was six months old. I went on educational leave from Emory and started school full time. I continued to work PRN with a nursing agency to help supplement lost income. Because I had been in the air force, I was also able to receive financial support through the GI Bill educational program.

In graduate school I majored in adult health with a clinical specialty in oncology. Again, I was blessed to be connected with a great professor, Dr. Rose McGee at Emory's Nell Hodgson Woodruff School of Nursing. Rose was actively involved as a volunteer with the American Cancer Society. Part of our clinical education was to become involved with, and knowledgeable about, ACS. This was the beginning of my interest and volunteer involvement with cancer prevention, screening, and early detection through ACS. Rose also schooled students about the importance of being involved in professional nursing organizations, such as the Oncology Nursing Society. Thus, another turning point occurred in my oncology nursing career.

Balancing graduate school, work, home, and motherhood was not an easy task. But thanks to divine intervention I was able to maintain a measure of success in all endeavors.

Following graduate school, I returned to full-time employment at Emory on the hematology unit. After a year I felt a need to seek new challenges in oncology. I applied for the job as head nurse of the medical oncology unit at Emory Hospital. This promotion was to be a pivotal point in my present career path. Another blessed life event was the birth of our daughter Ronda in 1984. After a few months of leave, I returned to full-time work, now a mother of two, but with much help from my husband, and best friend, Rodney, Sr.

There are numerous patient situations that are so memorable for me. Caring for my patients was extremely gratifying. The bonds of trust, friendship, and compassion were an ever-present force in my interactions with patients and their significant others. There was a great sense of fulfillment as a professional nurse in being able to provide personalized and expert care and teaching to my patients and the people who loved them. There were numerous initial successes which were only to give way over time to exacerbation of disease and death. The loss of a patient I had worked so hard to help get well was difficult. It did not take long for me to get in touch with my own mortality and come to accept death as the final stage of life. There was still pain, grief, and a profound sense of loss for the patient's significant others as well as for the care giver. However, there was a sense of gratification in helping the patient and family prepare for the journey from life to death. When the patient expired, it was time to refocus 100 percent of my energy on comforting and supporting the family as they grieved for the loss of their loved one. Even amidst loss and grief there was a sense of satisfaction that I was there for the patient and family, and that in some not-so-small way I had made a difference in the quality of their life and grief.

As I have grown professionally I have also grown spiritually. I recently read a passage that has stayed with me and by which I base my life and practice:

> I shall pass through this world but once. If, therefore, there be any kindness I can show, or any good thing I can do, let me do it now . . . for I shall not pass this way again. . . .
>
> *Étienne de Grellet*

My passion for oncology nursing encompasses practice, education, and participation in community and professional activities. My active participation in ONS began with my appointment to the nursing administration committee in 1988. I have also been involved as a faculty member with the series of cancer prevention and early detection workshops for African-American nurses and nurses working with African-American clients. Dr. Sandra Millon Underwood, R.N., Ph.D., is a mentor in research and community involvement in cancer prevention education activities.

My life and career as an oncology nurse has been personally and professionally gratifying. There have been some tough times, but I have become a stronger, wiser, and better person and nurse. I enjoy sharing with students and colleagues what I have learned, and supporting them in their endeavors.

I have been fortunate to have published in numerous journals and several books. I have found supportive and encouraging colleagues as I have strived for yet a different and higher level of professional practice.

Through my many activities in cancer patient care in the community and in acute care I have been blessed to be recognized with several professional awards, a few of which include: the 1991 ACS Lane Adams Award for excellence in cancer nursing practice; the 1993 Georgia Division Ruby Life Saver Award; the Chi Eta Phi 1993 Community Service Award; 1993 Mother of the Year from Turner Chapel African Methodist Episcopal Church; 1992 Manager of the Quarter at Emory University Hospital; 1992 Family of the Year at Turner Chapel A.M.E. Church; and certificates of Appreciation from the Boy and Girl Scouts of America, the Oncology Nursing Society, and the American Cancer Society. Most of these awards and recognitions were a direct result of my work as an oncology nurse, in practice and in the community.

I love nursing. I am pleased with my decision to choose nursing as a career and oncology nursing in particular. I have a loving family, including my mother Hazel and father Bilbo Magee who still live in Mississippi, and many brothers and sisters. I am especially blessed to have a loving and caring husband and healthy and talented children, who are the center of my life, with God being the light of my life. Whenever possible I like to share my knowledge and skills with other colleagues.

A message to all who follow:

Dare to dream, to be creative and committed to making a difference and touching a life. Dare to care and give of yourself. You will receive more than you can possibly give. Oncology nursing is rewarding, challenging, and filled with the hopes, dreams, and desires of your many tomorrows.

18

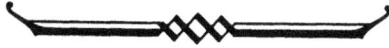

Shirley Gullo

As long as I can remember I have wanted to be a nurse. At the early age of ten, I accompanied my mother and her church group to feed ice cream to patients in the county nursing home. I wanted to do more for the people I met there, especially those with the "scary" disease called cancer. I felt close to these patients and was in awe of their courage and spirit; I am still in awe. This was my initiation into volunteerism.

In 1969 I was a single mother of three boys, ages 5, 9, and 12. I had worked for 12 years in a new field of analytical chemistry called gas chromatography. After my divorce, I felt more than ever that I wanted to pursue a career in nursing but because I was the sole support of my family that seemed to be a dim possibility. I prayed about it and felt that if it were to be then the resources would be there. They were. I applied for and received a scholarship to cover educational expenses but I had to continue my full-time job. It took five years to complete a two-year nursing program. As with any educational endeavor, there were sacrifices of time and family. I often had doubts and wondered if I was doing the right thing for my sons by continuing my education to become an RN. This was *my* dream, *my* goal, but was I being fair to my young sons? I continue to hear these same concerns from other mothers seeking further education in nursing. Each of us has to make our own decisions but I know that I could not have made it through without the support from friends. My sons remember their mom going to classes as an adult and striving for educational goals. This has been a lesson that no one else could have taught them. I continue to believe that if God wants me to do something, He also provides the resources . . . and He has. I continue to maintain this philosophy.

In 1975 I married a man with four children. We merged our families together. My husband Joe continues to be a blessing and has been supportive of my efforts to continue my nursing education to acquire my B.S.N. and then my M.S.N. in 1990. I often joked that I didn't know if I would retire first or graduate first. What kept me striving in my educational endeavors? Support from colleagues each step of the way.

Their faith and confidence in my ability to succeed provided me with the inspiration to continue. Their support came in many forms: notes of encouragement, sharing of information resources, listening and helping me sift through projects and issues, and last but not least, financial assistance. As an undergraduate I received a scholarship from the Oncology Nursing Foundation. When I pursued my master's degree in nursing, a scholarship from the American Cancer Society made it financially possible. These were the "knots on my rope" that I held onto and I will always be grateful. My gratitude was expressed in service. I served on the Oncology Nursing Foundation board years later and I have continued to be a volunteer for the American Cancer Society.

Most of my nursing career has been at the Cleveland Clinic Foundation. I first entered the oncology specialty in 1972 as a chemotherapy nurse. At this time we weren't called oncology nurses, we were "chemotherapy nurses." The Oncology Nursing Society was not formed until three years later. When I read a small notice in a nursing journal that a group of cancer nurses were forming a new group, I was excited. At last I would find other nurses to network with! At that time, there was a great deal of discussion over the title "cancer nurse" versus "oncology nurse." Some felt that oncology was incorrect because "people don't die from oncology, they die from cancer."

My key job responsibilities as a chemotherapy nurse in the early 1970s were mixing and administering chemotherapy and performing bone marrow biopsy procedures. I mixed the chemotherapy drugs in a small room on the unit. The room had no ventilation and the mixing involved up to 100 drugs per day. Our main concern was the safety of the drug mixture. We didn't wear gloves, or take any precautions to protect ourselves because we were unaware of any hazards from the drugs.

After a while I developed a rash on my face and neck. It had an unusual pattern; in the summer when I wore an open-neck top, the rash extended to include my neck. In the winter when I wore clothing that covered the neck area, I didn't have any indication of a rash there. The rash was a puzzle to the dermatologists who could only say that I was "allergic" to something in the environment. The usual patch tests didn't reveal any allergies. While in an elevator during an Oncology Nursing Society Congress I noticed other nurses on the elevator with the same rash. They also mixed chemotherapy drugs in the same manner that I did. I began to suspect that there may be a connection between the mixing of chemotherapy drugs and this rash. Suzanne Miller, a colleague I had met at ONS in 1975, and I began to discuss our concerns and asked questions of other nurses and pharmacists. The Oncology Nursing Society actively supported our endeavors and a resolution was passed in 1983 to explore the issue. ONS also provided funds for this early inquiry. Today we are aware of the potential hazards of these drugs and health care providers take necessary precautions to protect themselves and the environment.

Bone marrow biopsy procedures were a challenge primarily due to the equipment that we used. The aspirate portion of the procedure required the use of an Illinois needle; after the aspirate was taken, a Jamshedi® needle was used to obtain the biopsy. This two-step method required entering the bone twice which prolonged the discomfort for the patient. Today the added expense of the two-step method would also be scrutinized although in all honesty that was not a major issue at that time. Another drawback was that the Jamshedi needle used for the biopsy had a handle that was spot-welded on. The needles became dull from the sterilizing procedure following each use. My husband Joe assisted me when I shared with him the frustration I was having with dull needles during the procedure. Joe kept them sharpened for me and I thought that all was well until I ran into another predicament while performing a bone marrow biopsy on a young leukemia patient.

Young patients generally have harder bone and require more strength to core the sample. I had given chemotherapy to Randy and knew him well. During the procedure, the handle came off the instrument as I was coring the sample. I looked up at the laboratory technician with shocked disbelief. The needle portion was firmly lodged in Randy's post iliac crest and I had no handle to get the leverage needed to remove it. The technician searched my eyes for direction. I explained what had happened to Randy and assured him that I would stay with him until I could get additional help to remove the needle. Just days before, I had watched Joe use scissor-grip pliers at home. I immediately thought that may be our solution to removing the needle. I asked the technician to call both the physician and the machine shop to obtain scissor-grip pliers. Randy, a religious young man, asked me to pray with him while we waited. I did. After what seemed like hours but was only minutes, I had the pliers and began to work the needle free. Surprisingly, we were able to use the core specimen obtained. Randy had remained very calm during the whole incident. I think I was more upset that he was.

I decided there must be a better way to do this procedure. After several months of inquiry I met a man who was developing a new tool for doing the procedure. His name was Pete Lee and his needle was called the Lee needle. It had several advantages. It could be used to obtain both the aspirate and biopsy in one step. The aspirate was taken and then the biopsy from the same instrument. This device was not spot-welded together; it was assembled each time. The needle part could be discarded when it was dull, thus eliminating the need for sharpening. As chemotherapy nurses, we did the clinical trials on the instrument and helped work out the "kinks."

Now, years later, the concept of the Lee needle is still used and they are all disposable instruments. Randy and I were bonded in many ways and this young man never ceased to amaze me with his equanimity and grace under pressure. He was not verbally articulate but he liked to draw. He used his drawings to tell me what he was feeling. He would explain each drawing when I asked him to. Our discussions of his artwork disclosed many of Randy's unspoken emotions. He was pleased when I would ask him to describe through his art a feeling he may be experiencing. The drawings were very basic but they opened a door from him to me, and I continue to expand on this in my work today. It was Randy who opened this door by demonstrating the value of using art to communicate difficult feelings.

Out of necessity, the major issues we faced were those of treatment and symptom control. Quality of life concerns were always there but it was not until years later that I was able to focus my practice on this aspect of oncology nursing. The joys I have received from this work have exceeded my expectations. The sorrows are inevitably blended in this tapestry of oncology nursing but the sense of fulfillment has surpassed my hopes. The patient experiences have made it a "revered gift" to be an oncology nurse.

All patients are special in some way but there are always those that are indelibly engraved on our hearts. They are the ones that we never forget no matter how many years may pass by. One of the joys of oncology nursing is sharing these patient stories with peers. As oncology nurses we all speak the same "heart" language.

Patients have challenged my life and made it more significant. They fortify my belief that, as nurses, we often learn valuable lessons in life from our patients and that we never stop learning. The priceless value of these special patients is not from any extraordinary acts or any truly unusual achievements on their part or mine. They are special because of the bond we had and how they influenced my oncology nursing practice. We all have been blessed with these special patients that stay in our hearts and memories. They are like rare gems, never losing their radiance.

Fred, a true diamond, with his dry country humor, taught me the therapeutic benefits of humor. When I met Fred, the familiar quote, "One can take the boy from the country but not the country from the boy," took on a new meaning. From the first few minutes that we spent together, I knew Fred was unique. His face was weathered with smile lines around the corners of his mouth and eyes. His tall frame, like a majestic mountain, was topped with a shiny bald peak with bits of snowy white hair on the sides. His eyes had a glimmering sparkle within them and I felt that he looked deep into my soul whenever he talked with me. His infectious laugh and quick wit never took a recess or missed an opportunity to be expressed.

During his admission interview I asked him where he was from. He said he was a "buckeye," which is a common slang word for an Ohioan (the buckeye is the state tree and bears an inedible nut). Within minutes he fired his first zinger question: "Do you know what a Buckeye is?" This was my initiation into biting the bait for his jokes. I replied, "Well, the buckeye is our state tree." Before I had a chance to say anything more, he zapped the punch line: "Well my dear, a buckeye is a worthless nut, you can't *use* it for anything can you?" As Fred slapped his knee with roars of laughter, I stood there wondering what kind of a nut this patient was going to be.

Both Ohioans by birth, Fred and I shared a common heritage and loved the Ohio countryside and rural life in the Midwest. Fred had spent all of his 75 years on an Ohio dairy farm. My fondest childhood memories were of summers on a small dairy farm with my aunt, uncle, and cousin. For those who may not be familiar with Ohio, let me explain that it has a diverse topography, flat in some areas and hilly in others. Our part of Ohio is graced with rolling hills and curling fields of corn, hay, and wheat. These hills remind me of notes of a fine harmony melodiously blending into each other. Over the next days, as I taught Fred about his chemotherapy treatments, we shared stories about the long, hot summer days in the fields, strawberry socials, swimming in the local "swimming hole," picking blackberries, and the joy and toil of haying season.

When Fred was first diagnosed with colon cancer in 1973, he left his farm and came to the "big city" of Cleveland to receive his five-day treatment of 5-Fluorouracil infusions. In 1972 this was a new method of administering 5FU which previously had been given orally in juice. I was a fledgling oncology nurse in 1972 and eager to learn all that I could about cancer as a disease and these "chemo drugs." Fred and I were learning together. Each day I was challenged as Fred presented me with questions that I had to seek answers for. I wondered if other nurses were so motivated to learn. As I taught Fred about his disease, treatment, and drug side effects, he taught me about effective coping and the therapeutic use of humor.

Fred approached life as a gift. He stated that he was used to dealing with circumstances beyond his control and that cancer was "very much like the weather in that respect." I too had often struggled with things beyond my control. I am totally deaf in my right ear, a hearing impairment I have had as long as I can remember. As a child I attended a special school for the deaf and I seldom told others of my hearing deficit since I didn't want to be seen as different from those with normal hearing. Fred also had difficulty hearing. I could sympathize with him and shared the secret of my own hearing deficit with him. I have total nerve deafness in my right ear and only 80 percent hearing in my left ear. I often rely on lipreading to supplement what is heard. Fred quickly summed it all up. He rubbed his chin, looked straight into my eyes, and slowly drawled, " I guess you could rightly say that you never hear right and you only have one ear left." We both roared with laughter after a painful pause on my part as I let his words sink in. From then on I began to realize that humor was an excellent way to handle the awkward circumstances of informing others of my handicap (which avoids assumptions by others that I am ignoring them). This was a lesson in reframing a situation.

Fred's caring philosophy was also contagious to other patients on the unit. He was a support group before support groups for cancer patients were more formally established. Each morning Fred would wake at the crack of dawn, dress in his bib overalls, sit in the solarium for "his time with the Lord," and then visit his "neighbors" (other patients). He offered them words of encouragement: "You're looking better today," or: "One more day to go." He provided hope: "Sometimes I feel that way too, but it passes." He often told them he would be keeping them in his prayers and added, "and I have lots of time to pray." He honored all feelings with his humor, including hair loss concerns. When he saw a fellow patient despondent over the loss of her hair, he rubbed his now completely bald head and told her that "only the sexiest people had bald heads" and that "smooth heads are amazingly sensuous." He reassured her that her hair would come back but he was enjoying being this "sex symbol" so much that he was going to figure out how he could keep his "sexy bald head." He added with a grin that he was certain that it was his bald head that was attracting all the younger women to him.

It was obvious that Fred missed his farm life while he was in the "big city hospital." One day he commented about how much he enjoyed feeling the cool summer breeze and the warmth of the summer sun, the feel of the rich dark earth in his rough hands, and most of all, he really missed the smell of freshly mown hay. As I left work that day I had my car windows rolled down and could smell that beautiful aroma of freshly mown hay. On impulse, I stopped and scooped up a mound of it and put it in my lunch bag. This was to be my special gift to Fred the next day.

Fred was delighted with this unusual present. He gleefully told me this was the "best hay he ever did smell!" Whenever he felt homesick he would breathe in the aroma as if it were a rare blend of coffee. This would summon fond memories of his farm and let him mentally escape there. This was my first introduction to the positive use of imagery. During one of these sessions of breathing in and using imagery, Fred was interrupted by a group of oncology physicians. One of them asked him what he was doing. Fred dryly smiled and said that he was "just enjoying the grass." The medical group looked at each other in bewilderment. One of the physicians asked Fred where he got this "grass."

Fred very calmly stated it was from his oncology nurse and he provided my name. Within a short time I was questioned about bringing in "grass" to Fred. At first I wasn't sure what they were talking about. I was a single mother with three sons and prided myself on teaching them high values and "grass" wasn't part of my lifestyle. Where did they ever get the notion that *I* was providing grass to one of our patients?!

This part of the story has a happy ending. Upon investigation, the physicians realized that this was a bag of fresh hay, not "grass." When I told Fred of this mix-up, he roared with laughter and slyly said, "Now how you suppose they got that so mixed up?" Fred lived for an additional three years and during that time he never forgot his "special gift." When he came back for his check-ups or was in "this part of the woods," he would bring me a small bouquet of flowers, a jar of home-canned peaches or tomatoes, and he always enclosed a note that stated, "In payment for the grass of '73, the best crop of hay ever!"

Geraldine was another "patient gem." It is not usually a matter of our choice to work on Christmas eve, but one particular Christmas eve at Cleveland Clinic will stand out as a star that shines in my memory. I was in graduate school, working as a weekender staff nurse on the oncology unit. At first I was less than enthused that I would not be with my family on this special evening but I was grateful that I had an employer and a work schedule that would accommodate my classes.

I recall that certain echo that permeates the halls of a unit on holiday evenings after the visitors have gone. There are empty beds since many patients are discharged to be with their families. The vacant beds and quiet halls seem to echo the despair of those unable to leave the hospital. One particular patient, Geraldine, had no home. Her aged family and sparse friends were unable to care for her multiple needs. Geraldine was 87 years old with metastatic cancer and deep decubiti that had required surgical intervention and frequent wound care and dressing changes. Geraldine was confused much of the time as her mind wandered and she would not answer questions with much clarity, if she answered them at all. After washing her and changing her dressings, I heard the faint sounds of voices singing Christmas carols in the distance. As the voices came closer, the familiar words of the Christmas carols were tugging at my thoughts of family and the season. I began singing to Geraldine (or myself, for she did not respond to conversation). My scratchy, off-key voice singing the words "Away in a manger, no crib for a bed" was soon fortified by a clear and beautiful voice in perfect pitch. To my surprise, I realized that it was Geraldine's voice! The words were sung with exactness and as the carolers sang the next song, she continued singing with passion and perfection, every note in perfect tune, and every word in exact distinctness! I reached out and took her withered dark hands in mine and looked into her hollow face. Her eyes were bright and glistening as she stared into my tear-filled eyes. We sang together until the carolers reached the room and came in to join our voices. As they gathered around her bed they allowed her to take the soprano lead and what a performance—every perfect note and every melodious word sung in exact precision and without hesitation! The carolers stayed for a while and as they left and their voices faded into the normal din of the hospital, Geraldine continued to sing as I listened, until she motioned for me to join her in song. I don't remember how long we sang or how long we held our hands together, but after the last hymn I asked her how she remembered all the words and notes to so many hymns. With beaming eyes and a smile I'll never forget, she looked at me and said, "My dear Shirley (I didn't know she even knew my name), I was the choir director for my church for over 40 years when I lived in Alabama." The carolers were there but a brief time but they were instrumental in helping Geraldine communicate. I wish I could have thanked each one of them. Although Geraldine died later that night, she sings in my heart every Christmas. I didn't want to be there that Christmas eve but it was a wonderful experience that I will never forget. The lesson I learned from Geraldine is that each person deserves dignity regardless of their ability to respond.

During the past few years I decided to keep a journal of some of the significant patients in my life as an oncology nurse. I don't write daily or even weekly but as frequently as I feel inspired to document my feelings. I seldom write more than one page but it is a way of "finalizing" some of my feelings. Once they are written down I feel a sense of closure.

Seeing Beyond the Surface

Daniel, age 24, was diagnosed with Hodgkins lymphoma; he also had cerebral palsy. He was considered a demanding and sarcastic young man. He was also HIV positive. When I was assigned to him I wasn't sure what to expect. He was in need of a bath and shampoo. His long, thick brown hair was dirty and covered his eyes. He didn't want to leave his room and kept the shades drawn and the door closed.

I have a son also named Daniel, the same age as my patient. My first internal question was, "How would you treat your son Daniel if he were in this situation?" I began by finding out what his interests were. Reluctant at first, he slowly began to open up when we talked about his favorite TV show. I sought his permission with almost all the direct care I provided. I wanted to empower him with control over any areas that I could. I asked him if I could help him wash. Reluctantly he allowed me to assist him in this endeavor and each day we did more. Then one day, with his consent, I cut and shampooed his hair. I jokingly told him

I would shave him if he trusted me. He scowled at me and said that I might as well or I would only find some other way to make his life miserable. I laughed and told him that I was staying up nights to think of ways to aggravate him. He smirked at that. He seldom ever expressed any gratitude or smiled. I reasoned that he probably never had much to celebrate in his brief life. His mother and father divorced when he was six and his mother "disowned him" when he was 18 because he chose a "different lifestyle." During the haircut he yelled that I wasn't doing anything right (but made no suggestions for change). Finally I finished the "renovation." As he examined his new hairstyle in the mirror he paused and he actually smiled. I saw in his eyes a young man who was a frightened child, a young man who never walked, nor ever would walk, a young man who wanted to be accepted and loved but didn't know how to go about it. I momentarily closed my eyes and envisioned him tall and straight with his dark clean hair neatly groomed, with a smile on his face as he said "Thank you." When I returned to reality, I heard him demanding that I get him some ice cream *now*.

Each time he was admitted I asked to be his nurse—not much argument on that from my colleagues. He asked for me when I wasn't there and quickly told them how things were to be done the way Shirley showed him. I then convinced him that the others had really great ideas and he should give them a try. As he felt more accepted with his new neat physical appearance, his self-esteem soared and he demonstrated a new personality. He began wheeling down to the nurses station to talk with the nurses. He flashed his ever-brightening smile and found that others responded favorably to him. Eventually Daniel gained self-acceptance and opened up to others. He found friends who also had cerebral palsy and when he died several years later he was surrounded by people who cared. Daniel was a tarnished nugget of gold that needed a bit of polishing to see his true radiance and value. Sometimes we have to look beyond the obvious to see the person within.

Simple Joys Lighten the Darkness

The laughter of a small child is a delight on the oncology unit. I usually trace it to the source to offer a small toy and see the glow on his or her face. I carry small toys with me at all times for both little and big children. One day the laughter was from the three-year-old grandson of one of the patients. He took the toy, giggled, and quickly flew back into his grandfather's room. Hours later he emerged with his grandmother tightly holding his small hand in hers. She walked so slowly and seemed to carry a heavy weight on her shoulders. I commented on her beautiful grandson and she beamed with pride. Her posture lifted as we began to exchange "grandmother stories" about how bright, energetic, and smart our grandsons are. She seemed to grow a foot taller and walked down the hall with a new lightness to her steps. I guess we grandmothers are all alike; we have a special sisterhood of joy. Sometimes caring takes the form of listening and helping others see the uncomplicated happiness of a grandchild, and lets some light into the darkness.

Listening With the Heart

Sarah, age 76, was diagnosed with metastatic cancer with an unknown primary. She was Jewish and her family was looking for a placement in a nearby Jewish home. I loved Sarah from the first time I met her. She was a teacher and volunteered in her retirement years. In assessing how she was with acceptance of her current situation, I asked her how she felt she was doing. Her reply was, "My mind is alive and active but my body is dying and I'm trapped inside it." During our sessions, she shared that she firmly believed that cancer was from stress. Slowly she confided that she had had 25 years of continual stress and pain. She shared her story with me in segments: Her 29-year-old son had committed suicide in New York City 25 years earlier and she was carrying this secret burden in her heart. He was homosexual and was fired from a job he enjoyed when he was "discovered." He went from job to job until he could no longer face any further rejection and he ultimately killed himself. Through her tears of anguish she blamed herself for his death and society for not dealing with him "humanely." While she was volunteering she met a 25-year-old man who looked like her son. For some reason she had felt compelled to tell him, "I know what's on your mind and don't do it, just hang on!" The young man quickly left and when he returned the next day he asked her, "How did you know that I was contemplating suicide last night?" Sarah cried as I held her and she shared this secret that had been locked in her heart all those years. She thanked me and said she felt as though she had been released from confinement. She asked me please to see her again. The next day when I returned I was informed that she had died peacefully during the night.

Ginny was my first patient in my role as an oncology clinical nurse specialist. She was a jewel that never lost its brilliance. Ginny was a teacher with sarcoma. Her left arm and shoulder were amputated and she was having difficulty coping. Her husband had died five years earlier and she kept saying that she "just wanted to join him," that life had no meaning for her anymore. At first I was honestly scared of this challenge and wondered if all my great book knowledge and education was going to help me now. Initially we met on a daily basis and as time and Ginny's self-sufficiency progressed we met less frequently. The first goals we worked on together. Once these were accomplished, new ones were identified and Ginny continued to set her own pace. Over the months that followed, Ginny made her own goals and constantly placed new challenges in front of her. The mailbox difficulty was her first "baby step," as she called it. How could she carry in her mail, and what if she saw a neighbor? Being a private person, she wanted to keep all this to herself and didn't want any sympathy. Use of a basket and other aids helped her adjust to independent living, and meeting her neighbor face to face over a cup of coffee helped "break the ice." Eventually she took her grandson Justin on a trip to Washington, D.C. without any assistance. It was a trip that he will remember for a lifetime. Two years after we first met, Ginny came for an appointment. She explained that she had recurrent disease and that there was no further treatment. She tearfully thanked me and said that life had had great meaning to her the past two years and that I had been instrumental in helping her achieve that quality of life. We kept in touch with phone calls and notes and when she died her grandson Justin called to tell me that his grandmother wanted him to call and thank me for her. He also wanted to thank me for the trip they had shared years earlier. Ginny had always had a warm glow to her and I truly wanted to thank *her*, for we had both learned new skills together.

All of my experiences in oncology nursing were not as joyful as those I have already shared. Just as steel is made from iron and high heat, perfume from pressed flowers, my morning juice from squeezed fruit, and the soil in my garden from pulverized rock, so has my oncology nursing experience had its trials and tribulations. There were many frustrations and heartaches. Shortly after I began my career in oncology nursing I almost left nursing altogether. I was being sued for negligence by a patient who had suffered injury resulting from an extravasation of doxorubicin. In 1974 we didn't have the benefit of current knowledge about extravasation of vesicant drugs. We were administering this drug without an understanding of the potential for tissue damage. The drug was infused by piggyback method. Following an extravasation, the patient had complained of pain. Hoping to relieve the pain, the medical oncologist and I had applied heat and gently massaged the affected arm. The resulting tissue damage was extensive and a shock to all of us. At that time, we had no indications that this type of damage could occur; therefore it was dealt with as a routine extravasation. I remember talking with a physician in Italy seeking answers that might help us to understand what was happening to this patient. The drug had been developed there and it wasn't commercially available yet. He had no insight or suggestions to offer us except that there was reason to believe from dog studies that tissue damage could occur with extravasation.

The patient and his wife were understandably upset and angry. I was the target of their anger. Prior to going to court, I experienced physical symptoms of diarrhea, insomnia, and lack of appetite, but the mental anguish was worse. I felt that I was no longer a competent nurse and that I would surely burn in hell for eternity for what I had done to this patient. The verdict of the case supported our actions which were based on the knowledge at the time of the incident, not at the current time. All this made little difference in my mind; I had caused this pain to another human being and I felt great distress. I wanted to leave nursing and go back into chemistry where I didn't have to assume such responsibility.

After much prayer and support from new acquaintances I had met through the newly formed Oncology Nursing Society, I realized that my feelings were not unique and that there were other similar situations that nurses were able to grow from. Suzy Miller, Juanita Garrison, and Elaine Glass were a few of those new supportive colleagues, and we have maintained our friendship and mutual respect for almost 20 years now. I feel good that I have been in the position of supporting other nurses in similar situations since this happened to me many years ago. By telling them of my experience they knew that I truly understood much of what they were painfully experiencing. In efforts to help others in the prevention of extravasations, I have published on this topic and have lectured to other nurses throughout the country. I didn't leave the profession I love but my experience enabled me to help others to learn, understand, and in some cases, forgive themselves and go on.

Listening to the Unspoken Words

Sometimes we listen but may not be hearing unspoken concerns. Joe's wife helped me to understand that sometimes the question asked is not the real concern. Joe, age 25, had received chemotherapy for his parotid tumor. The tumor size was visibly reduced after treatment. His wife came into my office and after general conversation she asked me, "Where does the cancer go?" Concerned with metastasis, I proceeded to gently explain the usual pathway of metastasis. The phone rang and I was called to another area. The next day she returned. This time she closed the door and began to cry. Upon further discussion it was clear that her real question was, "Can I get cancer from Joe's tumor if I kiss him?" She saw the large tumor mass "melt away" and she was afraid that she would "catch it." I had completely missed the meaning of her question. This was a lesson in listening for me, one I have not forgotten. I often use this as an example when I am teaching other nurses about communication with cancer patients and families. All questions should be clarified and after an answer is given there needs to be an evaluation to assure that all issues related to the question have been addressed.

Although I have mostly addressed my relationships with my patients, I am also deeply inspired by and indebted to my colleagues. To use an analogy: We are similar to coals in a fire; we gain heat and energy from our closeness and if we drift too far away we lose our power and ability to produce warmth.

In closing, I hoped that I would have a son or daughter to follow my footsteps in the nursing profession. At this point in time, it doesn't appear that it will end up that way. I have two new granddaughters. Maybe . . .? However, bonds of shared values and common directions can be more powerful than those dictated by genetics. There is tremendous joy in nurturing and mentoring new nurses and watching them grow. They are the foundation of our profession; they are our future. They will need our support to help them through the troubled waters of change in our health care system. Whatever transformations may occur in this system, the elements of the human spirit will still require compassion, empathy, humor, and caring, all the arts of our oncology nursing profession.

Notes

Jamshedi is a registered trademark of Pharmaseal Division of Baxter Healthcare Corp.

19

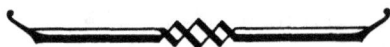

Pamela J. Haylock

Many nurses and doctors are steering their children away from health care professions out of skepticism over the future of health care. Many say they'd go into another field if "they had it to do over again." I am at odds with people who think like this. Nursing in particular offers women and men an opportunity to take on any number of roles—some yet to be defined—in health care in the future. I have been lucky to experience just a small sample of the opportunities available to nurses. Nursing has allowed me to live in big cities and small towns in health care roles beyond what is (at least until recently) generally thought of as nursing. Mostly, nursing has allowed me to help others and to contribute to my community—which is why, I believe, most of us become nurses. I'd definitely "do it over again."

I know many nurses who've become "burned out" and have fantasized about working in a flower shop! I'm sure these fantasies have become even more prevalent over the past few chaotic years in health care settings. Still, I think that many who consider leaving nursing have not thoroughly explored all of the options their nursing education and background offers. If one position no longer fits, another setting or avenue might be just right, or at least a step in a better direction. Career goals should be adaptable to what opportunities are available at the time and place.

I'd always wanted to work in a major cancer center—somewhere like M.D. Anderson or Memorial Sloan-Kettering. I've now been a nurse for 23 years, and I still have not made it to a major cancer center. One problem could be that I've never lived in a city where a major cancer center exists. I lived in Baltimore and worked at Johns Hopkins Hospital before Hopkins developed its cancer program. When I moved to San Francisco, several hospitals pledged that a cancer center was in their future. Seventeen years later, there still is not a comprehensive cancer center in the San Francisco Bay Area.

If I'd waited for a cancer center, I'd still be waiting. Instead, I found an oncology clinical nurse specialist position in a small community hospital. While I think I was good for the hospital, I was by far the greater beneficiary. Because it was a small hospital, the team included every employee: the housekeepers, the people in the linen room, the man at the copy center, the pharmacists, unit clerks, nurses, doctors, and technicians. We knew each other, knew our strengths and weaknesses, knew who to call to get tasks completed most efficiently. I had the chance to learn and grow. I got to see what other disciplines could offer, and what we could accomplish when we worked together. The community hospital setting allowed us to follow our patients and families, to experience the peaks and valleys of the many and varied journeys. Not everyone gets to have that experience. I've been so lucky!

Neither of my parents had gone to college. My father had not graduated from high school. My parents wanted me to go to college. In the mid-to-late 1960s, there were still few career options open to girls. I thought that I would probably be a teacher, mostly because I thought I could get away with the least amount of post-high school chemistry. My dad was opposed to that idea. He wanted me to be a nurse. Dad thought nursing education offered the most security, especially in case my future husband couldn't support me.

I went to Ellsworth Junior College in Iowa Falls for my freshman year. Ellsworth was one of several Iowa community colleges with a planned transfer to the University of Iowa for the B.S.N. program. In a work–study program, I worked as a secretary in the science department. That job helped me get extra help with chemistry and also helped with expenses.

I transferred to the University of Iowa after the first year. My experience and empathy with people affected by cancer probably started during my junior year medical/surgical experience. One man in particular stays with me. He was fairly young—I suppose he was maybe 40. He was going to die. He was probably the first patient who I knew was going to die. Death was not frightening to me. My grandfather had been a mortician. The highlight of visits to grandpa's house had been a tour through his embalming room topped off with seeing the newest line of caskets. Lots of people I'd known, as well as relatives, had died, and I usually went to the wakes and funerals. But this man was different; he wasn't a relative. I wasn't sure how to relate to him or his wife. He was in excruciating pain. His doctor had ordered "daily weights." For this man, the daily weight meant being pulled and pushed to the bedscale. It seemed senseless to me and I waited to question the doctor before weighing this man. It turned out that the daily weight order had been written much earlier and had not been discontinued by the intern. It was so simple! The doctor agreed with me and thanked me for advocating on behalf of his patient. The patient and his wife were relieved—and more comfortable. It was the high point in my medical/surgical student experience.

The 1970 shooting of Kent State's antiwar demonstrators by national guardsmen caused political upheaval on college campuses across the country. The University of Iowa, then a stronghold of several antiwar groups, was featured on the evening news each night with film footage of arson fires, picketing, and other forms of antiwar demonstration. The local Ramada Inn was converted to what looked like a barracks for the Iowa Highway Patrol and the National Guard. To avoid more violent altercations, university officials tried to get as many students as possible off the campus. Various options allowed students to leave, including taking grades as they stood or taking incomplete grades and planned completion during the next semester. The daily confrontation with picketing students was threatening. I decided to start my summer early and I left campus. I blame my sketchy understanding of liver function on the fact that this was course content left uncovered because of my early departure from campus.

Despite a rocky start to the summer, I had one of the most memorable experiences of my life. The University of Iowa offered a public health nurse traineeship. I worked under the supervision of the county nurse in my home county. Mrs. Wilma Scherrer had been the county nurse (there was only one) during my childhood. She routinely visited the schools to coordinate and carry out vaccination programs and schoolwide growth and vision checks. I accompanied Mrs. Scherrer on her trips throughout the county. This was a public health position which, I learned then, is very different from a visiting nurse position. The county nurse was responsible for follow-up of clients who had gone through any of the university's clinics. We visited families where a family member had been discharged from the state's tuberculosis sanitarium. Families with children who were not immunized were visited and gently encouraged to go through with recommended vaccinations. Babies born after complicated pregnancies or births were followed by the county nurse. The county's head start program was a frequent stop for the county nurse. There were a few home care assignments, mostly bedfast elderly people who had limited caregiver options. Eventually Mrs. Scherrer entrusted these patients to me. All of these visits opened up parts of my county I'd never known existed. It opened my eyes to the ways in which some people are forced to live. There were many homes in the county that had no indoor plumbing (they still exist to this day). Many children did not know what they looked like because there were no mirrors in homes. In Iowa, where winter temperatures routinely drop below zero degrees Fahrenheit, many homes have no floor other than the packed dirt surface.

My public speaking debut occurred that summer. Mrs. Scherrer asked me to give a presentation to parents of grade-school children. I was supposed to encourage parents to comply with immunization recommendations. The event took place in a church basement in Andrew, a small farming community. It had been a typical hot, humid summer day. Nevertheless, fathers, mothers, and some children were in the audience. From the sunburned faces with the border of white skin on foreheads—signs of the famed "farmer tan"—it was clear that most of the fathers had spent the day in the fields. It didn't take long before most of the men in the audience, and a fair number of the women, were dozing—a few audibly snoring. I thought I'd never get up in front of an audience again.

Other than flat tires at inopportune times, that is my only negative memory of that summer. I really loved the work, and appreciated the hardy and self-sufficient people I met. Not only did I want to be a county nurse, I wanted to be *the* county nurse in Jackson County, Iowa. That was my goal in 1970.

In 1971 new graduate nurses were in great demand: we could go just about anywhere and get a staff nurse job. I wanted to leave Iowa to experience life in a real city. The classified advertisements in the *American Journal of Nursing* provided enticing descriptions of the wonderful life young nurses could have in any of hundreds of world-class medical centers. The ads showed pretty, young nurses in white uniforms and caps talking to handsome, also young, attentive doctors. Or they pictured an attractive young woman, supposedly on her day off, sitting next to the ocean or under a tree sharing a picnic lunch with equally attractive, happy friends. A friend had moved to Baltimore and invited me to be her roommate. Based on the image of the famous Johns Hopkins Hospital and their advertisement in *AJN*, Baltimore and a job at Hopkins seemed like a good choice.

Johns Hopkins Hospital in 1971 was a huge disappointment. The Marburg building where I was assigned to work was part of the original Hopkins hospital. It housed two medical and two surgical nursing units. It seemed to me that the only thing that had been added since the building was new was electricity. (What a shock to realize how modern the University of Iowa really was!) There was one other nurse in the Marburg building who was close to my age: she'd been a new graduate one year earlier. The other nurses were at least my mother's age—some much older. The older nurses still wore white stockings, starched uniforms, and the ruffled caps that identified them as Hopkins graduates. While I was not required to wear white stockings or my cap, not wearing them was cause for ridicule and, more difficult for me, ostracism. Nurses' schedules (at the time, one weekend per month off with rotating shifts) gave me little chance to see the country or develop friendships. I spent my coffee breaks locked in the stall of the ladies' room crying. I was utterly miserable, yet too proud to admit it to my father (who never understood why I would leave Iowa) by going home.

Despite my unhappiness, the Hopkins experience was good for me. I developed good skills, and learned from nurses who were literally from an earlier generation. They were great mentors. Then, as now, Hopkins attracted patients from around the world. I loved talking to people from foreign countries. It was almost as good as going there myself, and I never dreamed I'd get to see these places. Famous doctors were on staff, and many of the patients in the private Marburg units were their private patients. I met Dr. Hugh Jewett who had achieved prominence in genitourinary cancers. He was a kind man who was impressed that I had come from the University of Iowa, where his friend, Dr. Rubin Flocks, was acclaimed in the same specialty area. He caused me to reconsider my opinion of Iowa.

After two years I returned to Iowa. I did, in fact, apply for a job as the county nurse. Mrs. Scherrer was planning to retire in a few years and I hoped to be her replacement. But the candidate selection process was lengthy and I needed a paycheck. I found a position in the Linn County Health Department as a public health nurse. Linn County encompasses one of Iowa's major cities, Cedar Rapids, and several rural communities. My job involved enforcement of public health statutes regarding communicable disease and monitoring compliance of the county's subacute nursing facilities with state regulations. I went to public schools to look through kids' hair for lice, conducted clinic interviews of clients with diagnosed sexually transmitted diseases, initiated communication with people named in these interviews as potential infected contacts, carried out school- and work-setting tuberculin testing and follow-up, and followed and monitored compliance of tuberculosis patients after discharge from the state TB sanitarium. I inspected the county's skilled, intermediate, and basic nursing homes. Inspections involved visits—some scheduled and some surprise—with other county officials, including the fire marshal, food service inspector, and building inspector. During my four-year tenure, I forced closure of a basic nursing home. I was quite uncomfortable with the responsibility and questioned my expectations of these facilities. What if I was unreasonable? What if I was too "easy"? It was tough: I put the proprietor out of business and displaced elderly people who had few housing and care options. Still, these concerns were outweighed by the experience of going into facilities that smelled of urine and feces, seeing pressure ulcers that needed attention, finding residents' doors locked, substandard diet preparation and service, and in general, unacceptable conditions.

Epidemiology was the other half of my job. I went to the Centers for Disease Control in Atlanta for a short course in epidemiology and discovered a fascinating field. The investigative aspects of tracking down the source of infectious disease can be like reading an intriguing mystery. (Indeed, some of the same methodology is applicable to cancer control.) Very often, the "VD" clinic clients were "repeaters"; they have been infected numerous times. Many were teenage girls who clearly needed help. There was no counseling involved in my role, and no referral mechanism even if a need for counseling were recognized. Other than getting infected people treated, there was little I could offer. I began to feel like a broken record when I'd conduct interview after interview with clients who more often than not, told the same story. It was more difficult still to contact unsuspecting people to inform them of their potential infection. Quite clearly, I was not a welcome sight! I couldn't picture myself going through life in this sort of job. I was not exactly sure what I wanted my future to be, but I did know that I didn't want it to be head checks, VD clinics, or the tuberculosis registry.

My county health department boss encouraged me to go the University of Minnesota's public health program, but I lacked the resources to pay out-of-state tuition. I thought about going to a nurse practitioner program: I still had hopes of finding my place in an underserved, rural area—if not Jackson County, at least a similar setting. Iowa did not offer a nurse practitioner program. I started taking graduate level courses that matched my interest and which I could apply toward a graduate-level minor. I took courses in anthropology, women in American history, sociology, and photography. Much to my surprise, I got my best grades ever and was admitted to the graduate nursing program at the University of Iowa in 1975.

Ann Whidden, R.N., M.S., chaired Iowa's graduate program in medical/surgical nursing, officially called "nursing care of the adult." She was a vibrant, inquisitive, thoughtful older woman with white hair and twinkling, smiling eyes. She always wrote with a nub of a pencil and took endless notes during interviews, conversations, and classes. She was an inspiration for all nine of us in the program. She believed in me and challenged me to value my ability.

There were some discouraging experiences in graduate school. One particular faculty member was anything but supportive. Her negative example gave me many ideas about how I would deal with students or colleagues looking to me for support. But with the support of Mrs. Whidden, Dr. Laura Hart, my faculty advisor, and my classmates, I discovered the understudied concept of fatigue. With Dr. Hart's collaboration, I designed a study, and found myself doing data collection in a radiation therapy department in Cedar Rapids in 1976. At this time, few nurses were working in radiation oncology, and this department was no exception to the rule. The technical and secretarial staff were very supportive and cared for patients going through treatment. The physician was a respected radiation oncologist. The department served patients within a 150-mile radius in eastern Iowa. The staff was skeptical of the hypothesis of my study and they also wondered what I would do in their department. My fatigue study was one of the first to describe the fatigue phenomenon in people going through localized radiation in the treatment of cancer. Through the continual prodding and mentoring provided by Dr. Hart, our paper drawn from this study was published in *Cancer Nursing* in 1978. I was proud of this achievement and hoped to continue to study the concept of fatigue in people with cancer. Another meaningful outcome of that experience was that after I left the radiation oncology department, a nursing position was created!

During graduate school I took courses beyond traditional nursing education. I was exposed to other disciplines, diverse populations, new ideas, and gained a new appreciation for the arts. I particularly enjoyed sociology, anthropology, and history courses, all of which continue to serve me well. As a teaching assistant, I supervised senior students in various clinical settings. I was a research assistant for faculty interested in oncology nursing. These practical experiences helped me develop beginning teaching and research skills. Equally important was my new appreciation for my women friends and colleagues. Each of my graduate school colleagues was brilliant in her own right, even though we had vastly different career goals and interests. These women remain an important part of my life. They taught me that I too could make a contribution. That was an enlightening discovery.

During the summers of my graduate education, I indulged myself. Again, the *AJN* classified ads fueled fantasies and I applied for a job as a camp nurse at a children's camp in Maine. These two summers, the kids in camp, the counselors, Maine's picturesque coastline, the camp's doctors, and my counterpart nurses combined to create treasured memories.

After graduate school I wanted to leave Iowa. Based on my fondness for Maine's coast, I decided to live at an ocean—I didn't particularly care which ocean. That is, until I got snowed in one last time in Iowa. It was while I was lying on the ground putting chains on my tires—in April—that I decided I never wanted to live in that kind of climate again. I found a job as a nursing instructor in an associate degree program at Southwestern Oregon Community College (SWOCC) in Coos Bay, Oregon.

I worked harder and more hours at this job than any I've held. During my year at SWOCC, I taught five courses in five quarters. My students were first- and second-year students. For the most part, I started from scratch—course objectives, course outlines, exams, assignments, and lectures all needed to be developed. I was responsible for students' clinical supervision, for reviewing assigned papers, and evaluating students. The community college experience was both rewarding and frustrating. My students represented the community spectrum. Several students were young women who had just graduated from high school; two men and several women were entering nursing as a second career; some women students were my mother's age. The students varied in ability as well. An especially painful dilemma involved an older student who did not function at the expected competency level after her first three quarters in the program. Even after remedial work, it was also my opinion that she lacked the ability to function at a registered nurse level. Students were angry when I failed this woman: some boycotted class and others resorted to confronting me openly. I was accused of being cruel and unfeeling. To add to the drama, the student disappeared from the community for several days. I was totally unprepared to handle this situation, and I muddled through. The question each of us faced was whether this student was capable of handling the expectations and role of a registered nurse. Eventually, class members agreed that their peer indeed was unlikely to reach these expectations.

Even though it is likely that the second year would have been easier than the first, I decided it was time to pursue my interest in oncology. I started looking for oncology positions in the San Francisco Bay Area. I interviewed for positions at the University of California at San Francisco, and Letterman Army Hospital. Neither position was offered to me, and I accepted a staff nurse position at the Veteran's Administration Medical Center in San Francisco (VA). I was told there were plans to develop the oncology clinical nurse specialist role and I hoped I would be a candidate.

At the VA, a large percentage of the medical and surgical patient population had cancer diagnoses. Because of the VA's relationship with the University of California at San Francisco (UCSF), many patients were on experimental protocols. The VA system also fostered continuity of care. We followed patients throughout the cancer experience. Many veterans in our care were elderly and had no family, few friends, and limited supportive resources. The nursing staff became a source of support and encouragement. Most of us developed really special relationships with our patients. It was the long-term relationships and the opportunity to make a difference in the lives of these men—or even to make a moment better by doing some comforting intervention—that drew me to oncology nursing. I was hooked for good.

At the same time, I found the Oncology Nursing Society. A VA nurse–colleague told me about an oncology nursing interest group that had recently been formed in San Francisco. The interest group was composed primarily of oncology nurses from the university, and in oncology clinical nurse specialist and management positions in various hospitals throughout the Bay Area. The interest group eventually became the tenth interest group to receive a chapter charter from the Oncology Nursing Society.

In 1979 my mother was diagnosed with a brain tumor. She was scheduled for craniotomy at the University of Iowa. While there with my mother, I met Roberta (Bobbie) Scofield. Bobbie was a clinical nurse specialist and had been working with my mother. She introduced me to my mother's surgeon, went over X-rays and test results with me, and included me in conferences during which plans were being made. Bobbie supported Dad and me during the lengthy surgery, and continued to give us updates as the long day went on. The tumor was diagnosed as a meningioma. Even after I returned to San Francisco, Bobbie continued to keep me informed of Mom's progress. Five years later, Bobbie invited me to participate in the Oncology Nursing Certification Corporation's "cut score" committee for the first oncology nursing certification examination.

Nurses from the ONS local chapter were the best resources for those of us who were job hunting. After a year there was still no oncology clinical nurse specialist (OCNS) role defined at the VA and I began looking outside. I interviewed for OCNS roles at several community hospitals (and was turned down) before finally being offered a position at St. Francis Memorial Hospital in San Francisco. I was ecstatic! St. Francis is an old, traditional, and relatively small community hospital in San Francisco. Of the community hospitals in San Francisco, St. Francis had the longest track record for the OCNS role. The physicians and nurse managers seemed to be supportive of the role and were anxious to fill the position being vacated. The OCNS position seemed to offer everything I'd wanted in my career, and I felt like the proverbial kid in a candy store. There were so many possibilities, so much potential. At the same time, I was surprisingly reluctant to leave the VA hospital. I hesitated to leave this group of nurses whom I'd grown to love and respect. During my exit interview at the VA, I was offered an OCNS role on the condition that I "find a replacement for my staff nurse role." I was furious, frustrated, hurt—any number of not-so-happy emotions! This condition, more than any other factor, convinced me to leave the San Francisco VA Medical Center.

On my first day as an OCNS, I walked to the cable car stop and took the cable car the remaining four blocks to the stop closest to St. Francis. To me, it was the ultimate San Francisco experience to actually ride the cable car to work! Breaking into my new role was not nearly so exhilarating. There were no other CNS positions at St. Francis. There was no nurse manager who knew what to do with the role, or me, or who would make the effort to explore the possibilities. The director of nursing who hired me became ill within weeks of my arrival and never returned to her position. Over the next year I reported to three different nursing administrators. I had few meetings with my supervisor. The nurses were distant, even hostile. I didn't know what to think but was hurt, frustrated, and felt rejected. Some weeks later, I discovered that my predecessor had told the staff that I had not been a CNS before and that I knew nothing about chemotherapy.

For several weeks I tried to hide in my office and managed to find lots of policies and procedures to review—anything but deal with the staff. One day, Fred Fanchaly, a nursing assistant, walked into my office and asked me if I really wanted to be there! He challenged me to get out of my office and do what I was hired to do. I love him for that. Fred, who had a degree in chemistry but had worked on the unit for several years, has since become a registered nurse, is a respected oncology nurse manager, and is an active member of ONS and our local chapter. He is also one of the best nurses I know.

I'm not sure if my strategy would work for others, but what I did worked for me. I planned a first project that would allow my strong suit to show. I coordinated a unit inservice program on radiation therapy. At St. Francis, patients undergoing brachytherapy were often included in our unit census. Members of the nursing staff were at one of two extremes in their knowledge of brachytherapy: some were cavalier about radiation exposure while others were unduly frightened and uninformed. The first inservice was a hit and evolved into a continuing education program that eventually became an annual oncology nursing offering.

A second project involved a staffing study initiated to determine appropriate staffing levels and skill mix for the oncology care unit in conjunction with a planned conversion to primary nursing. The study highlighted the additional nursing work load that occurred on the oncology care unit as a result of chemotherapy administration and monitoring, brachytherapy, patients' trips off the unit, and the need for intensive psychosocial nursing skills. The staff was involved in the study from the start, and I think enjoyed being part of a research project.

Even though I had attended two ONS Annual Congresses by 1981, I was thrilled to be invited to chair a round-table session on staffing for oncology care units. This was my first formal activity associated with the Oncology Nursing Society. During this ONS Congress, the San Francisco Oncology Nursing Interest Group received its chapter charter.

During my first two years as the OCNS, it was clear that patients being considered for ostomy surgery or those who had chronic or surgical wounds needed more timely access to an enterostomal therapy nurse. The system that had been used involved telephoning the university to request consultation with the enterostomal therapist on staff there. It was sometimes days before our patient could be worked into the ET's schedule. I proposed that I attend a professional enterostomal therapy education program and combine enterostomal therapy services with my existing OCNS role.

I went to Memorial Sloan-Kettering Cancer Center's professional enterostomal therapy education program in 1981. The course work was intensive, and the clinical experience was an interesting challenge. We were a small class of five students. A disappointment with the program was its total focus on cancer-related problems—for obvious reasons. I missed having student clinical experiences with inflammatory bowel diseases, nonmalignant genitourinary problems, skin care and incontinence, since many of these diagnoses formed the majority of cases I would eventually see in my community hospital setting. On the other hand, Memorial Sloan-Kettering offered me an experience in a major cancer center.

I've enjoyed enterostomal therapy nursing (recently changed to "wound, ostomy, and continence nursing"). Watching a wound heal, once it is properly prepared or managed, is a wonder of nature. Helping patients and caregivers learn and gain confidence in complicated self-care skills is, to me, a basic joy of nursing. The management of complex wounds and skin problems is a special and rewarding challenge. My knowledge base and skills were put to use during planning for the hospital's home care services, and I remained a consultant for that service throughout my remaining eight years at St. Francis.

For the next five years I functioned as an oncology clinical nurse specialist and enterostomal therapist at St. Francis. In a small hospital, limited patient volumes reduce the likelihood of creating two distinct positions. The radiation therapy department requested consultations quite often. Doctors with high geriatric patient volumes began requesting my help for patients with vascular and diabetic ulcers. People with cancer diagnoses often need a nurse with a working knowledge beyond the basics of skin and wound care, incontinence, and ostomies. At St. Francis, several staff nurses asked to create an "enterostomal therapy team" and planned a series of classes through which they could advance their skills in this area. Their enthusiasm, commitment to learning and providing skilled care, and their appreciation for what I could offer made me feel as if I had reached a turning point in my relationship with the staff.

In 1986 an oncology program director position was created at St. Francis. I was encouraged to apply for the position. I was hesitant: I'd never functioned as a manager—though again, in this small hospital setting, I was often involved in management issues. By 1986 I'd gained leadership skills through several avenues; most important was my involvement in the Oncology Nursing Society. Early in the San Francisco Bay Area local chapter's existence, I worked as membership chairperson, then secretary and newsletter editor. In 1984 I was elected to a two-year term as president. In 1985 Sue Baird, the editor of *Oncology Nursing Forum*, selected me as one of several new reviewers. Her writing and mentoring skills were tremendously helpful. My own writing abilities were enhanced and it was fun to help authors through the publication process. I'd become involved with the Association of Community Cancer Centers. One of my strengths was my knowledge of what was going on in cancer care circles in the local community, the region, and the country. I was aware of programmatic approaches that had succeeded, and some that had failed. I knew people who were key to the success of various programs. I think I have a realistic vision of what needs to happen for people with cancer and those people who love or care for them. I also know that these people are not always effective advocates for their own needs.

My decision to apply for the oncology program director position was ultimately fueled by fears of who might get the job if I did not! I got the job. I was responsible for the radiation oncology department, the hospital's cancer registry, inpatient and ambulatory oncology services, and services related to persons infected with HIV. The hospital's nursing educator and the infection control nurse also reported to me. With the team that had been assembled over the years, I believed we could offer a unique—for San Francisco—programmatic and holistic approach to cancer care.

It is a great disappointment that it didn't happen. In 1986 three San Francisco community hospitals began to explore plans for a joint venture cancer center. I was a member of the planning committee. It was an exciting time for those of us committed to cancer care. A year into the planning process, things started to unravel. The hospitals' board members were distrustful of their counterparts. Physicians were suspicious of colleagues' motives. There were disagreements about what services to offer and where the actual building would be located. For these reasons, the cancer center plan died in 1988.

A strike by staff nurses belonging to the California Nurses' Association (CNA) also occurred in 1988. Most community hospitals in San Francisco in 1988 were "closed shop"—staff nurses were required to belong to CNA. When the nurses walked off jobs for four weeks, staff and management relationships changed irreparably, I think. Cooperation and respect were replaced by skepticism and hostility. At the strike's conclusion, wounds inflicted by strike-related activities did not heal quickly. The scars are still present. For me, the strike was professionally devastating. It was impossible for me to forget that cancer patients entering the hospital were harassed by nurses on the picket lines or that nurses caring for patients "on the inside" were threatened. I was embarrassed by nightly television coverage of nurses shouting angry slogans from picket lines. After the strike ended, the level of nursing care continued to be compromised for some time. I know many nurse leaders believe in collective bargaining and strike action by nurses. I believe strike actions by nurses benefit no one. Certainly, the public image of nurses suffers during a strike. It continues to be a source of great frustration as I see staff and management disagreements lead to threats of strike. Someday I hope nursing leaders will devise more effective means of negotiation, where all sides—including patients in our care—win.

The year following the strike was equally chaotic. Like all hospitals, we continued to go through reorganizations. A consulting firm evaluated the hospital's programs and determined that cancer services was not a profitable service line. The hospital dropped my oncology position and offered me a position with more responsibilities for general ambulatory and AIDS-related services. I preferred that my major focus continue to be cancer care. My decision did not come easily, but I rejected the offer and resigned.

I didn't have a job and had no idea what I wanted to do. At the same time, a friend and colleague, Cynthia (Cindi) Cantril, was completing work on a master's degree in public health. Cindi has been involved in oncology nursing throughout her career, even as a candy striper. She is a founding member of the Oncology Nursing Society and I'd known her since she relocated from St. Louis to the Bay Area in 1983. We discovered that we share small midwestern town childhoods, stepchildren dilemmas, and a love for animals, especially dogs and horses. We both have a passion for patient and public advocacy, nursing, and quality cancer care. She and I decided to work together as consultants. We thought we were ideally suited to be business partners: we have different and complementary strengths and weaknesses. We envisioned helping community hospitals in planning cancer care services.

Our first and biggest job was the assessment of an existing cancer program in a San Francisco community hospital. We thought we did a great job. We gave the hospital administrators an objective review of existing services and realistic recommendations for building a cancer program consistent with community needs and the hospital's resources. To our knowledge, the report was shelved. That was a disappointment and a lesson. Consultants run the risk of being ignored. But as consultants, we could move on: we didn't need to continue to work with an institution whose goals were not consistent with ours.

Our partnership has tested our friendship and the strength of our commitment. Cindi has moved twice—not just across town, but to two different states. Despite the "geographic undesirability" of our respective home offices, Cindi and I maintain a business relationship, we share resources and ideas, occasionally get to work on projects together, and hold on dearly to a meaningful friendship.

The flexibility and freedom that comes with being self-employed allowed me the chance to do something I'd always wanted to do—write for the lay public. My public health experience convinced me that nurses need to do more to empower the consumer through public education. At a local ONS chapter meeting in early 1992, I met Kerry McGinn. Kerry is a nurse who has written two books for lay audiences: *The Informed Woman's Guide to Breast Health,* and *The Ostomy Book.* I'd first heard of Kerry when I bought my first copy of *The Ostomy Book.* Kerry also authored *The Ostomy Book for Nurses* to help generalist nurses work with various ostomies. Just after Kerry finished the first edition of *The Informed Woman's Guide to Breast Health,* she was diagnosed with breast cancer. Kerry is a survivor and is totally committed to consumer empowerment through information. Again, I've found someone to bolster my enthusiasm for public education. Kerry had been approached by a publisher to write a book on women's cancers for the lay public. Kerry wanted to write about breast cancer and wanted to give women information she wished she'd had during her own cancer experience. Given a short turnaround time for a completed manuscript, Kerry invited me to coauthor this book. I jumped at the chance.

For the next nine months I was immersed in "women's cancers." I reviewed the literature and completed my portions of the manuscript. Kerry is a patient and skilled mentor, and has become a special friend and colleague. Kerry knows about negotiating with a publisher, contractual specifications, and she has a master's degree in English! What more could a beginning writer want? Nearly 10,000 copies of *Women's Cancers: How to Prevent Them, How to Treat Them, How to Beat Them* have been sold. Kerry and I have been guests on radio and television shows and interviews, and are invited speakers in both public and professional educational forums. Our book has gotten really good reviews from the National Coalition for Cancer Survivorship, The Berkeley Women's Resource Center, *The Feminist Book Store News, Booklist,* and, among other newspapers, the *Maquoketa Sentinel-Press,* my hometown newspaper. At the 1993 annual assembly of the National Coalition for Cancer Survivorship, Kerry and I participated in an authors' reception. We sat with other authors and talked with cancer survivors, and signed copies of *Women's Cancers.* Many women stopped by our table to talk, and to thank us for the information and strength we'd given them. That's been the best reward.

What is next? I have no idea. In 1994 it looks like I'll be moving to Texas. For the first time, this move has nothing to do with my career. My husband, a native Texan, wants to move back to Texas. We've settled on Kerrville, a town with a population of about 18,000, in central Texas. Kerrville has lots of space for my horses and my other animals. I am interested in writing more cancer-related books and articles for the lay audience. I hope I'll be able to continue consulting. I'll need to establish a new network and put energy into marketing what I can offer. It certainly will be an adventure.

20

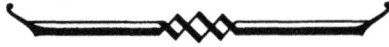

Laura Hilderley

As far back as I can remember, I always wanted to be a nurse. In the small Michigan town in which I grew up, my Aunt Helen was a nurse but she was the only role model I remember. I was very impressed by army nurses in the 1940s in their very smart uniforms and shoulder bags. Later my older sister became a nurse but long before that I wanted to be a nurse.

There was one brief episode, when I was about ten, when I really wanted to be a movie star. My best friend Janet and I thought we had talent. She could dance a little bit and had red hair and green eyes. I could sing, had blond hair, and blue eyes. So we wrote to MGM studios, described ourselves and our talents, and told them that we had a few hundred dollars in the bank. We suggested that if they could send us the rest of the money, we would be very happy to come to Hollywood and star in some pictures. We never heard from anyone, and after getting over the disappointment, we decided that the postman in our small town had intercepted this letter to Hollywood and returned it to one of our fathers.

In my early teens I volunteered as a candy striper at our local hospital. Then when I was old enough to have a work permit I was able to work as a nurses' aide. This was really exciting and I absolutely loved it. My aunt was then the head nurse in the hospital, a small 35- to 40-bed community hospital. My job as an aide mainly involved feeding the patients, changing beds, stacking linens, and doing anything that the nurses would ask me to do. In addition, I got to see an awful lot. I still remember watching my aunt very skillfully applying a hemostat to a spurting blood vessel on the scalp of a logger whose axe head had slipped from the handle, flown back and landed on his head, splitting it open. I also remember watching my first delivery right from the doorway—what a wonderful thrill! However, at the sound of an episiotomy, I became rather faint and light-headed; but I know that I didn't pass out. This type of an episode has repeated itself several times. I think the sound of an incision or the cutting or snipping of human flesh still causes my heart rate to accelerate and I get a big sense of light-headedness. I guess it's a good thing that I didn't become an OR or ER nurse.

All in all, my high school hospital duties and a friendship with a classmate, Bobby Olsen, who worked as an orderly, all helped to reinforce my desire and intent to go into nursing. My eagerness to be in the hospital put me at the nursing director's beck and call, especially during the summers. I'd work for two hours in the morning bathing and bed changing, then returned from 4 to 8 in the afternoon for the evening meal and to settle patients for the night. I felt very needed and loved this opportunity to be in the hospital. My Aunt Helen taught me how to give the best back rub ever. My friend Bobby worked a similar schedule and he was as happy as I for the opportunity since his intent was to become a doctor.

I can't say that my whole teenage life focused on the hospital and on nursing, but I will tell you that on the daily walks back and forth to school which took me past the hospital, I always imagined what was going on inside. I wished that I could cut through the corridors to see if there was anything interesting happening.

My older sister Marge left for nursing school in Marquette, Michigan, but after her first year she transferred to the University of Michigan in Ann Arbor. Fortunately for me that's where my parents wanted me to go and I never considered any other place. I consider this fortunate because in 1955 hospital diploma programs were the standard approach to nurses' training and through no initiative of my own I was able to start my nursing career in a baccalaureate program. I've always been grateful for that start.

My four years at the University of Michigan School of Nursing were invaluable. For a small-town girl from the upper peninsula, it was at first rather overwhelming. We were crowded four to a room in the dorm and our first year was spent taking courses such as chemistry, pharmacology, anatomy and physiology, math, and liberal arts electives. We had a few hours of nursing lab with "Mrs. Chase" to practice on, to remind us that we were nursing students. We wore blue polyester uniforms with removable aprons and those wonderful white caps to perch on the back of the head!

Marge had graduated the year I became a freshman and was working at the U of M hospital, so I had a support person to rely on when life at this big university became confusing. Graduating as a salutatorian (Bobby was valedictorian) in my high school class of 52 members had me feeling pretty confident, but I was totally unprepared for lecture halls filled with several hundred students and the sophistication of my big-city classmates. Marge also gave me her beautiful navy blue, red-lined nurse's cape which served as a confidence builder and security blanket at the same time. We wore our uniforms so seldom that first year that I often wished I could wear the cape with my street clothes.

In the spring of that year, organic chemistry threatened to be my undoing. I was struggling to maintain a passing grade when one of my nurse classmates offered to find me a tutor through her brother's fraternity. She knew there were many engineering and science students in this particular fraternity, and surely one would be able to help me. I did pass chemistry and within a few months became pinned, then engaged to my tutor, Dave Hilderley!

Summer session that first year was spent taking anatomy, physiology, and pharmacology. I believe to this day that that summer of total immersion in human anatomy was one of the greatest learning experiences of my life. We were fortunate to have human cadavers, which we shared with medical students, and our own "box of bones" to keep in our dorm to study. We nursing students may have reeked of formaldehyde on those hot summer nights, but the learning experience was invaluable.

During our second year we actually got to take care of real patients in the hospital. I looked forward to clinical days as a great reward for all the class work and studying. Just walking into that wonderful old institution made my heart pound. To this day, a hospital or medical setting intrigues and excites me even from the outside. In our travels over the years, Dave and I have taken many detours, just so we could drive past some well-known hospital or medical center (for me), or major manufacturing operation (for him).

My four years at the U of M School of Nursing were each better than the one before. Every new course seemed exciting and the faculty members were outstanding. One woman who impressed me was the assistant dean, Norma Kirkonnell. Dave and I planned to get married after my sophomore summer. I didn't expect this to be a problem with school since there were already two married students in our class. After notifying the dean's office that I would be moving out of the dorm and changing my name, a message came to my room that I was to meet with Ms. Kirkonnell immediately. I can still see her sitting behind her desk looking very serious and saying, "Laura, now that you have decided to get married we want you to know that from now on and forever, nursing will never be the number one priority in your life again. Your husband, your children, and family life will become your primary interest and rightly so." I left the dean's office stunned and confused, not sure whether I had been scolded or simply given some good advice. I recall protesting that nursing was still my great passion and that I would still be a good student and not slack off on studies or clinical just because I was married.

My dad reacted to our wedding plans much like the dean, saying something to the effect that all that wonderful university education was just going to go to waste. I didn't recognize it at the time but both the dean and my dad were probably throwing down the glove and challenging me to strive for a marriage and a career, something that wasn't too common in the 1950s. We were very young. I had turned 20 two days before our wedding and Dave had just turned 23.

Our junior and senior years in nursing were focused on three-month rotations in the specialty areas of medical/surgical, obstetrics/gynecology, pediatrics, psychiatry, and a choice between public health nursing in Detroit or three months as a team leader at the university hospital. One thing I regret is that I did not choose to do public health. There were many times later in my hospital nursing career when I felt inadequate in my knowledge of community health.

Psychiatric nursing seemed like the area I would want to specialize in, but after being assigned my "case" for the three months, I became turned off by the absolute powerlessness I felt trying to work with the fifteen-year-old incest victim. In my naivete, rape and incest were not a part of my vocabulary let alone my knowledge base. She was street-wise and profane; I wanted to cover my ears when she became loud and angry. As much as I *wanted* to work with her and offer support, she rejected my attempts to reach through that anger.

Medical/surgical nursing was never dull as I had thought it might be. The challenge of understanding the physiology of diabetes and other disorders, and then teaching the patients about their illness was really stimulating. My surgical case assignment was an inmate from the Michigan state prison admitted for a pneumonectomy for lung cancer. I believe this was my first experience in caring for someone with cancer, and it certainly left an impression. We started with pre-operative teaching and then observed in the OR. As the procedure was being completed, the temperamental chief of thoracic surgery was injecting nitrogen mustard into the thoracic cavity while the resident was closing. With so many hands working in a confined space, the chief was accidently jabbed with a suture needle and angrily pulled back, swinging the glass syringe onto the OR floor. Of course it shattered and we were all splattered with nitrogen mustard, my first "exposure" to chemotherapy! At the time it seemed more dramatic than serious but I have thought about it often in light of what we know today.

My prisoner/patient remained in the hospital for several weeks post-op. He was a convicted murderer who had not heard from his family in years. At his request, I wrote a letter for him to a daughter in California. He wanted her to know that he was dying and hoped to hear from her. There was no response, but after he returned to the prison, I was once again called to the dean's office. It seems the patient's daughter had written to the nursing school dean wanting to thank the anonymous student nurse who had befriended her father and taken the time to write to her. It was not difficult for the dean to check assignments and find out who that student was. Much to my relief I was not in trouble for writing the letter and, in fact, was commended for stepping over the normal boundaries of the student/patient relationship.

I shed a lot of tears over this incident—tears of relief that I wasn't in trouble, tears of joy and satisfaction that I had been able to help this man and his daughter, and tears of sadness because this gentleman had died shortly after returning to the state prison.

Cancer was a no-win situation in my student experience. There was little treatment besides surgery, and hospitalized patients were either trying to recuperate from radical procedures or were receiving terminal care. I focused my interest and energies on much more gratifying patients and even dermatology seemed interesting.

Obstetrics and gynecology placed second on my list of "nursing I would like to do." We had a patient to follow from the third trimester through delivery and postpartum care. By this time we had moved to an apartment very near the hospital. When my patient went into labor in the middle of the night, I was able to dress and dash right over to spend the next 12 hours with her.

When all of our rotations were completed and graduation drew near, I knew I was to be a pediatric nurse. I loved pediatrics. The children needed so much love and attention in this major institution, often isolated from family. Of course there were physical care and dressings and procedures to perform. I vividly remember working in the burn unit and wondering how these brave little people could manage a smile after all the painful dressing changes and baths we administered. But there was time to hold, to soothe, to sing, and read to these youngsters. Working with the parents to explain procedures and teaching them how to care for their own children was also very meaningful. I set my sights on becoming a pediatric nurse.

We were encouraged to work in medical/surgical nursing for a time after graduation rather than going directly into a specialty. However, I applied for a peds position at the university hospital and was thrilled to get accepted. My husband was now in graduate school with one more semester to complete so we knew we would be in Ann Arbor for a while longer.

Graduation in that first white uniform was a thrill. I realize now that it took me many years to get over my infatuation with the "trappings" of nursing and health care. Hospital buildings, hospital odors, uniforms, caps and capes, and even the patient charts with their wealth of information all seemed so important to me. Working as a graduate nurse, passing state boards, caring for babies, children, and parents, and thinking about my husband's career all made the next eight months fly by. I was offered a head nurse position on one of the peds units just as Dave accepted an offer from the General Electric Company for their marketing training program. We both knew I would give anything for that head nurse job, but the dean was right. Husband and family would always be first in my life.

For the next few years I was content to take part-time jobs wherever we lived. In those days, a nurse could specify the days and hours that she/he wanted to work and the director of nursing would agree. We moved frequently with the GE training program and I had opportunities to work in New York City, Syracuse, and Bridgeport, always in pediatrics.

After the birth of our son, I was completely content to stay at home and be a mom. It seemed that if I stayed away from hospitals, I didn't miss nursing. However, a neighbor asked me to "special" her husband for a few nights after surgery and since it wouldn't necessitate getting a sitter, I agreed. Just those three nights at Yale New Haven Hospital "turned me on" enough that my husband and I worked out a schedule so that I could work two evenings a week. My husband deserves great credit for his understanding and recognition of how much nursing meant to me.

I went to work in pediatrics ignorant of what this would mean in light of my new status of mother. The first few nights were fine, although I felt a little rusty after 18 months. On the third night, reality set in. I admitted a two-and-a-half-year-old to the unit with bruises all over his body, a fever, mouth sores, and lethargy. He had some lab work done and X-rays, while his mother hovered anxiously. In a few hours, the doctor arrived and delivered the bad news to this women. Her baby had leukemia. The mother cried and I cried, and I could do nothing but try to focus on my other patients. When pouring meds, I had trouble calculating doses and realized that I was in trouble. I called the supervisor and asked to be replaced for that shift. She understood and gradually so did I. After trying one more evening I realized that as a mother I could not be objective with pediatric patients and their parents. This was a bitter pill to swallow, and for a number of years I tried to place the blame for my failure in this situation on the always-fatal diagnosis of leukemia. It seemed my nursing career was to be rather limited, and never would I have imagined that 13 years later I would be an oncology nurse.

For a few months after the pediatric episode, I did work in medical/surgical nursing one or two nights a week, but always with an uneasy feeling of having failed at what I thought I should be doing. Fortunately, my husband was transferred again and I didn't consider working for several years.

Another move brought us to Rhode Island and after settling in, a friend asked me to consider volunteering with her at a local hospital. This was intriguing, so we met with the director of volunteers. She was very interested in my friend, but once she learned that I was a nurse she insisted that I meet with the director of nursing to see if she could use some volunteer help. The director and I talked at some length about my education, my experience, and my interest, and about some possible volunteer roles. I remember how this director of nursing leaned across her desk, looked at me directly, and said, "You will never make a good hospital volunteer. You are too much of a nurse and you would not be able to restrain yourself from jumping into the nursing role. Why don't you come to work for me?" This was flattering and very tempting, but my family was my priority.

Our second child, our daughter, was born that year, and I was quite content at home being wife and mother. I volunteered for the American Cancer Society, the United Fund, and our church. Meanwhile, I maintained my nursing license and membership in my professional organization. I eagerly awaited the arrival of every issue of the *AJN* and read it from cover to cover as soon as it arrived. My uniforms and caps stored away in plastic began to look yellowed, and at one time I considered throwing them away. But in the back of my mind I kept thinking that maybe someday when the children were grown I'd go back to work.

It happened much sooner than I expected. When Susan was 16 months old and David was five and a half, I wound up in the hospital for a cholecystectomy. My entire four days in the hospital were spent silently analyzing and being critical of nurses and nursing care. I was sure that we had done a much better job of post-op care at the University of Michigan, and I just knew that I could teach these aides, students, LPNs, and RNs a thing or two. Fortunately, I kept my criticisms to myself because a few months later I did go back to work part-time on the night shift on a gyn/surgical unit and immediately became "hooked" on nursing once again.

Two evenings a week became three and then four so that by the time our youngest was in school, I was almost working full time. Money was not the object. My desire to be a part of health care and to "do" nursing had been consciously suppressed as I had enjoyed being at home with my small children. As the years went by, I found that there was room for both family and profession, allowing me to respond to that need to practice nursing. Fortunately, my husband understood this (and still does today) and knew that nursing was a major part of my make-up.

During those years of part-time work as a charge nurse on an obstetric and gynecologic surgery unit, I had the opportunity to work with LPN students and hoped some day to become an instructor. I found that I could teach effectively and noticed that these adult students tended to migrate toward me for personal support as well as education. An offer to teach full time came along just as Susan started school all day and I eagerly accepted. Until then, my working hours had always been in the evenings so that I could be with the children most of the day. Dave had done a wonderful job with supper, baths, and bedtime stories for all those years.

For the next five years, I worked as a clinical instructor in practical nursing, realizing my dream of teaching while maintaining very close patient contact along with the students. During that time, I began work on a master's degree in nursing education/administration on a part-time basis. The local community college took over the state's vocational programs, including the practical nursing program, and as a college faculty member I had to become a member of the teachers' union. Although teaching was so very satisfying, the struggle between the administration and the teachers' union seemed to be creeping in and controlling what we as faculty were allowed to do. Attending mandatory union meetings, listening to angry and sometimes profane discourse from faculty, and the threat of possible cutbacks and layoffs made this job less and less desirable.

Opportunity once again came my way. As part of the students' outpatient experience, we would tour the brand new radiation oncology center at that hospital. This tour occurred several times a year as each new group rotated through and I became acquainted with some of the radiation oncology personnel. My students noticed that this center was advertising for a CNS and encouraged me to apply. The truth is that when the center had first opened, I had to look up the word "oncology." I now had to go searching the literature to find out what a clinical nurse specialist was! In 1975 there was little information available.

On our next tour through the department, I casually inquired about the CNS job and found myself being ushered into the medical chief's office for an interview. An hour later, I left filled with excitement over such an opportunity, curiosity about radiation, bewilderment over such a sudden and intense interest in me as a potential employee, and a realization that something new and unknown was out there for me to pursue. I was given a medical text to learn more about oncology and to help me make up my mind about the job. A few days later, I went back to the radiation oncology department to ask for nursing and patient care information, and left with more medical books and journals!

The year was 1975 and oncology was an established medical specialty. A joint medical and radiation oncology team was operational in this hospital and radiation needed a nurse. The chief of radiation oncology, Arvin S. Glicksman, M.D., had come from New York and knew what a CNS was and wanted that role filled in radiation oncology. My prior working experience had been entirely for and with nurses.

Nursing deans and directors had interviewed and made job offers to me. Nurses had always evaluated my practice. Now I was being recruited by a doctor who had the power and authority to make me an offer, negotiate salary, tell me unequivocally that I can take time as needed for completing my master's degree, and who would serve as my teacher, mentor, and boss. He also had the authority to hold this position for me for four more months until my teaching contract expired.

After much discussion with my husband and after searching for what information I could find in the literature, I decided that this was an opportunity not to be missed. There were a number of unknowns, primarily what was my job really going to be, what kind of patients would I be caring for, and what would I be doing. However, these unknowns were outweighed by the idea of going into a totally new area, by the feeling of absolute support and enthusiasm that I felt from staff in the department, and by what sounded like a real opportunity to expand my knowledge and my practice. Although I was reluctant to give up the teaching, I did accept the job and eagerly worked the next four months to complete my role as an instructor before starting as a clinical nurse specialist in radiation oncology.

The first three to four months were overwhelming. There was so much to learn, from the very language of the discipline to the real science of radiation oncology. As an employee of the radiation oncology department, I had no contact with the nursing department or any of the other nursing staff. However, on the first day that we had joint rounds with the medical oncology department, I was thrilled to meet the oncology CNS, Marcia Bliss. Marcia and I have remained colleagues in the truest sense of the word ever since. We were both new at our jobs and "babes in the woods" as far as oncology was concerned. Both of us had very supportive medical directors, who were eager for us to have learning opportunities. We both had enough experience in nursing to begin to carve out roles for ourselves in these new positions.

It took months to learn what radiation oncology was all about but once I got into it I was hooked! I found the science, biology, physics, and medicine of it fascinating and the work with radiation oncology patients was probably some of the most fulfilling that I had ever done. I also felt that I wanted to tell the rest of the world about radiation oncology nursing. I started on a reasonably small scale by inviting various groups of staff nurses from the units to come to the department and take a tour. Then we would sit down and I would give them a mini class on what radiation oncology was all about. The hospital staff development office recognized the value of these classes and thereafter a talk on radiation oncology was incorporated into all of the ongoing orientation programs for new nursing employees.

Working in a medical department with a physician as my director was my first real experience in working very closely with physicians. We were a team, along with the physicist, therapist, and social worker. It was an exciting revelation to me to see how these other disciplines practiced, and to learn from them, while teaching them what nursing was all about. For the first time I did not have a nurse as my employer/supervisor, and in spite of some initial reservations, I found that this was O.K. I made it a point to meet with the director of nursing services so that she would know of my existence in the radiation oncology department. We agreed that I would be professionally responsible to her or to her designee but that I would be managerially responsible to the medical chief of the department. This was never a problem. I had the freedom to interact with the other clinical specialists in the hospital as well as the staff nurses, and I served on relevant hospital committees and provided staff development classes on an ongoing basis.

Realistically, I do not believe that my professional life would have expanded as it did had I been employed by the nursing department. Unfortunately, nursing departments do not often have the funds to send a CNS or other staff on as many trips and to as many meetings as medical departments. When I first went to work in radiation oncology it was before word processors! But there was secretarial support available to type my manuscripts and speeches, which was also something that would not have been available through the nursing department.

A few months after starting this new position, my employer, Arvin Glicksman, M.D., told me about a group of nurses that was forming the Oncology Nursing Society, and had been meeting informally along with members of ASCO. He gave me literature on their first annual Congress coming up in Toronto and encouraged me to attend. This began my "love affair" with ONS.

I still remember walking into the huge hotel in Toronto and seeing a woman sitting at a small table in the entryway checking registrations and collecting dues. This was the ONS treasurer, Connie Henke Yarbro. Do you believe that registration was handled by a single person at that first ONS convention? The sessions were interesting, varied, and as I recall not altogether too sophisticated at that time. I also remember sitting at the business meeting and watching the struggle to get bylaws approved. Our membership even then spoke up and expressed itself and in this case caused the bylaws committee to go back to the drawing board and try once more to come up with an acceptable set of bylaws.

The next year in Denver, I submitted an abstract and presented my first national paper. I had been lecturing locally for the American Cancer Society nursing education committee and at other hospitals in the state but this was my first opportunity to talk to a broader audience. Following that Congress, I was invited to some other regional presentations and then my first publishing opportunity came along. Connie Yarbro was serving as guest editor for *Seminars in Oncology* (not *Seminars in Oncology Nursing*, which was launched much later) and asked me to write an article on the role of the nurse in radiation oncology. I am grateful to her for this chance to test new waters and to my employer for encouraging me to try. That article led to further networking and to many requests from physicians to help them incorporate nurses into their radiation oncology departments. It was exciting and very gratifying to have physicians asking for organizational advice, and to be able to show them that nurses were a necessary and vital addition to the radiation oncology team. Numerous nurses also contacted me for advice and information on working in radiation as a result of that article and from talks that I had started doing around the country.

I became quite active in ONS and was appointed to chair the local chapter committee as we struggled to make chapters a reality. As the membership grew, so too did the opportunities to meet and to learn from others. Through ONS I have met most of my nursing friends and colleagues, have been elected to two terms as national secretary, ran (and lost!) twice for president, and chaired the annual Congress two years in a row. There have been opportunities to present instructional sessions and workshops and to serve on committees. Best of all, I've had my wonderful subscription to the best journal of all, the *Oncology Nursing Forum*.

The ONS annual Congress is a major event on my calendar and I have not missed one since they began. I continue to plan and to look forward to this annual opportunity for networking and for professional renewal. As our membership grew and our Congress attendance increased, it became more difficult to catch up with everyone we had hoped to see. Groups of us with common interests began to make plans for a definite meeting place and time while at Congress so that we would be sure to meet. For a small subspecialty like radiation oncology, this preplanning was vital and provided not only an assured get-together for those of us who knew each other, but an opportunity for newcomers to radiation to find their colleagues. Thus were born the special interest groups (SIGs) and I believe that the radiation SIG was one of the first to be recognized. Hats off to Roberta Strohl who served as the first chairperson and helped get the group organized and focused on some significant projects.

Paralleling my involvement with the Oncology Nursing Society, I began another "career" as an American Cancer Society volunteer. Actually, I have been a door-to-door crusade volunteer since my children were in strollers, and I had also served on a local unit board for some time. However, when my professional "job" became full-time oncology nursing, it was a natural transition to increase my ACS volunteerism role. Before long, I was on the nursing education committee and we began to lay the groundwork for an ONS chapter. The Rhode Island division of ACS (as was true of many others) facilitated the ONS chapter development and has remained our ONS partner in many respects.

After serving as a member, then chair of the Rhode Island board of directors of ACS, I had the opportunity to be elected as a delegate to the national organization and another whole new world in oncology opened up. While nurses represented only a minute percentage of the national delegates and committee members, we were a strong and unified voice and had been strengthening our bond through ONS. Under the able leadership of Trish Green, Gen Foley, and others, a major change occurred when the national American Cancer Society voted to include nurses as medical (as opposed to lay) members.

This opened even more doors to leadership positions within ACS both locally and nationally. For me personally this has meant election as the first nonphysician president of the Rhode Island division of the American Cancer Society, and as a director-at-large on the national board and executive committee.

I happen to believe that volunteerism (a healthy mix of scouts, church, school, ONS, ACS, or any combination of worthy organizations) is essential to strengthening professionalism in nursing. It provides a whole other dimension to one's life, and can provide respite from the intensity of work. I also believe that volunteerism is an obligation, a means of giving back some of what we have been given.

After ten happy and fulfilling years as a CNS in radiation oncology at a teaching institution, opportunity once again came my way to explore a new direction. The story of my move into a private practice setting has been chronicled in the *ONF* (Volume 18, No. 3, 1991). Therefore, I won't review the details here. However, I do want to tell anyone who might be considering a change to carefully weigh the pros and cons, then go for it! I've always felt that great opportunities have just come my way; I have not actively pursued them. My husband points out, however, that the decision or choice has been mine to make, and that professional as well as personal goals come about through the decisions that one makes.

The choice I made in 1985 was the right one. It involved some serious negotiation concerning salary and benefits, as well as gaining the assurance that professional time would be available to continue my schedule of travel, committee meetings, speaking engagements, and writing. Philip Maddock, M.D., has been a fair and generous employer, and a really great person to work with. He has taught me a great deal about the science of radiation oncology, and has stimulated my thinking in the process. We have both learned to work with each other's "quirks," and to appreciate our separate as well as overlapping practice roles.

We've reached another milestone with the incorporation of an additional radiation oncologist into the practice. I will admit that I was uncertain as to how the two physician/one nurse team would work, but I'm happy to report that it does. Victoria Cividino, MD, has brought skill, experience, and a fresh perspective to this successful collaborative practice relationship.

Over the years there have been many, many nursing colleagues and other friends who have had an impact on my professional growth and "staying" power in radiation oncology nursing. Some have already been mentioned and I would like to tell you about a few others, what I admire most in them, and what I have learned from them.

Susan Baird—She taught us all how to cope and how to avoid burnout in our stress-filled lives. Her sense of humor is wonderful; ask her about her story of "green beans or broccoli." Sue's lasting legacy is the *Oncology Nursing Forum*, a journal that in many ways has helped to shape our nursing lives.

Nancy Berkowitz—From the early days as the Oncology Nursing Society's only staff member, through some turbulent developmental stages, and into the present maturity of ONS, Nancy has been a steadying presence, a source of sound advice, and a keen observer of human nature. I hope she writes her book.

Jennifer Dunn Bucholtz—The smartest "student" I ever had the opportunity to precept, and now an expert radiation oncology CNS, and dear and brave friend.

Connie Engelking—Persistence, perseverance, perfectionism, all wrapped up in intelligence and coated with a great sense of humor!

Arvin Glicksman—The radiation oncologist who first enticed me into this field, truly stimulated and supported my professional development, and taught me that there will always be more to learn.

Shirley Gullo—The personification of kindness and true friendship. A caring nurse who gives to her patients above and beyond the call of duty.

Karen Hassey Dow—A marvelous blend of intelligence, beauty, and collegiality. I am grateful to Karen for insisting that we do the book.

Ryan Iwamoto—A gentleman and a scholar, expert radiation oncology nurse, fluent writer, and friend.

Philip Maddock—He challenged me to take a chance on the private practice role, expanded my clinical practice horizons, and generously supported the fulfillment of my professional needs as well. A truly caring physician who puts patients first.

Connie Henke Yarbro—Connie exemplifies the utmost in leadership skills and professionalism. She was there from the beginning and remains an example of achievement for all to follow.

For all of us in oncology nursing there have been some significant turning points, when choices had to be made, events or moments when we knew that what we were doing was right, and that we would keep doing it in spite of the difficulties and downtimes that are inevitable in nursing. Recently I had such an experience, one that involved a patient and her family, my family, and my colleagues. I think that this is an example of the oncology nursing network at its very finest.

Susan, my daughter, called me one evening from her home in California. One of her friends and fellow attorneys, Kathleen, had expressed great worry and helplessness over the sudden admission of her mother to a major hospital in St. Louis with stroke-like symptoms and an inability to walk. Kathleen's mother had been successfully treated for breast cancer ten years earlier, had a recurrence approximately four years ago, was treated again, and had been doing well ever since. Kathleen had just been told that the diagnosis of cord compression from metastatic disease had been established and radiation treatment would be started. Her parents were devastated and overwhelmed by the sudden change in their lives. The patient was to start radiation therapy and be discharged to her home very quickly. She would need transportation for treatment and would need help at home because her husband had to return to his job. Their only other child was away at college in Michigan.

Susan told Kathleen that if her mother were only in Rhode Island, "my mom and Dr. Maddock would be able to take care of everything." She told her friend that I would probably be able to help anyway even by phone. Apparently, the patient and her husband had good contact with their doctor, but could not identify an oncology nurse. Susan couldn't remember the name of the hospital but was able to recognize it after I listed a few. I promised her that I would be on the phone first thing in the morning and would find help for Kathleen's parents.

Because I was home without my precious ONS membership directory, I couldn't start looking up St. Louis colleagues that night. But I called Karen Hassey Dow in Boston since I knew that she had lived in St. Louis and could probably give me some names. She immediately identified Paula Goldberg as an oncology CNS at Barnes Hospital. Early the next morning at work, I found Paula's number in the ONS directory and placed a call. I had never met her, but it was like talking to a longtime friend. She did not know this particular patient but identified how this patient had probably slipped through the "oncology cracks"; she promised to link up with Sandy Siehl, and together they would find the patient and offer help. I knew this was going to work out, and I couldn't wait to call Susan with a progress report.

At noon (9 A.M. California time) I called my daughter at her office and before I could even tell her help would be coming sometime that day, she excitedly told me that Kathleen had just heard from her father about these two terrific oncology nurses who appeared in her mother's room early that morning, had provided all the missing information about the diagnosis and treatment, had begun the discharge planning, and left her mother laughing for the first time in weeks! Later that day, Sandy called me with a progress report. As Paula had correctly guessed when I first called her, this patient had been admitted directly to a neurology unit because of the diagnosis of cord compression, thus bypassing the oncology team.

This story does have a happy ending. Kathleen had flown immediately to St. Louis and had met with, I believe, Sandy. Sandy oriented her to her mother's plan of care, directed her to the patient information resource library in the hospital, and generally facilitated this family's transition from hospital to home. The patient's physical condition improved with treatment and physical therapy, her husband was able to return to work, and at this writing (approximately one year later) the situation is stable.

I've thought about this whole episode many times. And I've told the story to numerous colleagues. Thinking about it brings a lump to my throat and sometimes tears to my eyes. These are tears of mixed joy and sadness, sadness that patients and their families should ever have to feel alone and bewildered, but joy to think that there are oncology nurses like Sandy and Paula out there caring for people in need. I'm so grateful that I have the privilege of knowing them. I'm also content in the knowledge that there are people like my daughter out there who know us and know what we do, who seek that help from us, and who have confidence that nurses will provide the care and caring that people need.

Norma Kirkonnell was right back in 1956 when she told me as a young nursing student about to be married that my husband and family would be number one in my life and nursing would have to take second place. There have been periods when family demanded much more of me than nursing and, at times, nursing and professional commitments have upstaged family life. I'm thankful that I've been able to enjoy the best of both worlds with the love, support, and companionship of my husband and partner of 37 years.

21

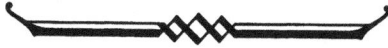

Renilda E. Hilkemeyer

I am frequently referred to as an internationally known pioneer in the specialty of cancer nursing. I have been actively involved for 34 years in cancer nursing. I began my career as a consultant in nursing education with the Missouri Division of Health, assigned to the Ellis Fischel State Cancer Hospital in Columbia, Missouri, in 1950.

After five years I was recruited by R. Lee Clark, M.D., as the director of nursing for The University of Texas M. D. Anderson Cancer Center in Houston, Texas. I served as director of nursing for 22 years and then was promoted to staff assistant to the president where I remained for seven years until retirement in 1984.

I have lived through and participated in many of the dramatic changes in the field of cancer, which resulted in changes in cancer nursing practice. I was so fortunate to be at these two renowned cancer hospitals where the patient was the focus and care was excellent.

These have been extremely rewarding years. I have had an opportunity to work with caring, sensitive, knowledgeable nursing staff, expert physician oncologists and researchers, and many other staff such as nutritionists, pharmacists, medical social service workers, and chaplains.

I have met and interacted with so many wonderful, courageous, hopeful patients who put their trust in the staff to do the best that could be done for their cancer problems. Many believed their faith in God and all the staff and resources at these cancer hospitals would cure them. Actually, in the 1940s and 1950s only about 25 percent of all patients survived, compared to 70 to 80 percent now for adults with lymphoma, breast, uterine, prostate, and bladder cancer, and acute lymphocytic leukemia, as well as for children with acute lymphocytic leukemia. Following are a few more comments on the status of cancer prior to 1950 to provide background for comparison with present cancer nursing.

In 1851, the first cancer hospital, the Royal Marsden, was established for the care of cancer patients in England. In 1884, the Simms Hospital, later to become Memorial Sloan-Kettering, was established. It was followed by other cancer institutions in the United States: Roswell Park Memorial Institute in 1911, Pondville in 1926, Ellis Fischel State Cancer Hospital in 1940, and The University of Texas M.D. Anderson Cancer Hospital in 1941.

Lest you think that cancer nursing was behind in oncologic knowledge and practice in those earlier days, let us look at some of the other disciplines. The staffs of the four cancer hospitals were exceptions because they had the knowledge and sophistication of current practice. The early professional care teams were composed of physicians, nurses, and usually medical social service workers.

The early treatment for cancer was surgery, often radical, and usually performed by general surgeons. Early radiotherapy was given by the radiologist, not usually a trained radiotherapist, and was done using 250-V machines, not the megavoltage apparatus and cyclotrons of today.

Medical oncologists arrived on the scene in the late 1960s and early 1970s when chemotherapy was in its infancy. The pharmacist has been the primary dispenser of medications until the advent of chemotherapy. The position of hospital chaplain in cancer centers was created around 1974 at M. D. Anderson. The early stoma therapist was often a patient with a stoma who helped provide support and equipment to patients.

What were the nursing implications in the early 1950s and 1960s? The majority of patients were treated surgically, often without benefit of the sophisticated anesthesia, blood component therapy, and antibiotic therapy used today. The concept of post-operative recovery rooms and surgical intensive care units did not exist. Actually, at M. D. Anderson, when the new building opened in 1954, no provision had been made for recovery rooms and we quickly converted two adjacent rooms, with four beds each, for this purpose, followed by a surgical intensive care unit. As patient needs changed, particularly with chemotherapy treatment, a medical intensive care unit was planned and opened.

Cancer was a dreaded disease in the 1940s and 1950s. Patients and families viewed this as a death sentence. Patients at the cancer hospitals generally were given their diagnosis and told their treatment and prognosis. But this wasn't true everywhere because some physicians felt patients would not accept treatment if they knew that the result of treatment was a stoma or the loss of a limb. Some people believed cancer was contagious, particularly if there was an open lesion or drainage from an orifice. Patients could often accept the words *tumor* or *growth* but not *cancer*.

Nurses too had a fear of cancer. Many times, when I was out speaking to nurses, I would ask them to take a piece of paper and write the words that came to mind when I said "cancer." Overwhelmingly, they responded with "death and pain." You really couldn't blame them for this attitude because they really didn't see that many survivors.

There has been a marked change in providing information to the public and patients. The Cancer Information Service (CIS), a nationwide telephone information service, was initiated and founded by the National Cancer Institute in 1976 because they felt a need for patients and the public to be informed. M. D. Anderson established the first one.

Organized, coordinated patient information services in cancer centers provide reliable and timely information to patients and families. I was responsible at M.D. Anderson for getting the patient education program established, and recruited staff in 1979. The department of patient education, with a director and health educator, started the program. It has been very successful. I believe that the initial concept of having interdisciplinary staff work together planning and executing programs and developing patient education programs and materials made it possible for physicians and those in other disciplines to make their contributions. Systems were also established for documenting patient education on the patients' medical records.

The long-term, chronic nature of cancer afforded us the opportunity to know patients better and to establish special relationships. Realistically, nurses do become emotionally involved and have long-term friendships. Actually, in those early days the concept of the nurse–patient relationship did not provide for such friendships, but many of us visited in patients' homes, went out socially with them, and became friends with them and their families.

I began my career in cancer nursing by accident. I had worked for the Missouri Division of Health as a district public health nurse. In 1950 I received a call from the director of public health nursing asking me to take a job as a consultant and to set up a continuing education program for public health nurses using the Ellis Fischel State Cancer Hospital as the resource facility. I told the director that I lacked specific knowledge and experience of cancer nursing but accepted her challenge: "You're not too dumb to learn." And learn I did.

I had some excellent physician mentors at EFSCH, who spent much time helping me learn through new patient multidisciplinary conferences, patient rounds, follow-up clinics, time in surgery, and radiotherapy, where I could actually see what was going on. Then I could determine the nursing care needed. I learned from the nursing staff; some were practical nurses. They often looked at me askance, even though I explained why I was there and that eventually public health nurses would be coming for education programs. My approach was to determine what I needed to know, then go to the unit and hospital nursing staff and say, "May I help you do this today?"

For example, at Ellis Fischel, radiotherapy was administered by low dose 120KV 250 KV machines—the only ones available at that time. This low dosage was not skin-sparing. Cervix patients were usually treated twice a day and sites were rotated front and back, plus many had transvaginal radiotherapy as well. These patients had very red, moist reactions with desquamation. Prevention of infection was most important. It was a real nursing challenge to apply dressings to the treated area which included breaking the blister formations, properly cleaning the area with ether and air spray, and applying lanolin and dressing at least three times daily. We received our reward when the patient returned to the clinic several months later, healed.

The whole treatment program changed with the development of the cobalt 60 unit by Drs. Gilbert Fletcher and Leonard Grimmet in the 1950s. This equipment also led to the first combined treatment modality: surgery plus radiotherapy.

Surgery was frequently the treatment of choice. Radical surgery began in 1900. Support services in the 1950s with anesthesia, blood component therapy, antibiotics, and rehabilitation were minimal. Radical head and neck surgery often made it necessary to tube feed patients. There were no disposable units or catheters, but the old red rubber tubes. There were no local facilities at EFSCH for learning esophageal speech post total laryngectomy. I talked the Missouri Division of the American Cancer Society into paying for two men who had had laryngectomies to do an educational program for two of our patients and our medical and nursing staff. We were as excited as the patients who learned the basic skills that evening. I set up a program with funding from the Missouri Division of ACS to help our patients learn esophageal speech in their home towns.

Not only did surgical patients have to deal with the physical and psychosocial aspects, but they also were frequently very uncomfortable and a real challenge to the nurses. There were no disposable supplies such as needles, syringes, intravenous fluid containers, and bags holding blood units. There were no disposable or permanent supplies for patients with colostomies or urinary diversions such as irrigating equipment, disposable or pemanent bags, skin barriers, etc. At Ellis Fischel, surgeons performing pelvic exenteration in the early 1950s had no temporary appliances. Patients were constantly wet. We used dressings with pads covered by large rubber dams; zinc oxide was placed about the stoma/pelvic area in an effort to prevent excoriation. One manufacturer (the Rutzen Company) designed a temporary and permanent urinary diversion bag. Patients' measurements were sent off but it was usually a week or two before the appliance arrived. Initial policies established at both Ellis Fischel and M. D. Anderson were: (1) patients remained in the hospital until the nurses could teach them to apply, remove, and reapply the appliance; (2) any necessary supplies or equipment were obtained for the patient, who would be taught their proper use prior to discharge; (3) anything the patient needed subsequent to discharge would also be supplied since local resources were not available in those days.

If we were assigned to care for a colostomy patient we would prepare to do the irrigation while teaching the patient. Equipment would consist of an enema can for the tap water for irrigation, tubing, and a red rubber catheter. I always used a large baby nipple; I cut off the tip and put it in the stoma backward to help keep water in while irrigating. The only thing I had for a return flow was a bed pan. Patients were taught to dilate the stoma daily to keep it patent. After the patient was regulated, only four-by-four gauze pads were placed over the stoma. Again, we had to be sure the patient had been adequately taught before being sent home with written instructions.

Most patients with breast cancer had radical mastectomies. Heavy pressure dressings covering the chest area, including the arm on the surgery side, were applied. These dressings were to take care of drainage and to promote healing by getting skin flaps to stick to the chest wall. There were no catheters and suction available as there are for mastectomy patients today. Surgical nursing care was pretty simple compared with today's complex care.

Physicians' orders for postsurgery would usually include provisions for early ambulation, maintenance of fluid balance, medications for pain relief, antibiotic therapy, treatments, and dressings, depending upon the site involved. Nurses also gave psychological support to patients and families, and did the patient teaching. We had preprinted instructions for specific aspects of care. When feasible, we referred patients to the public health nurse in the community.

Cancer was a hush-hush disease. Rarely would you find an obituary identifying cancer as the cause of death—it was usually called "a lingering illness." Cancer nursing was an undesirable field in the early 1950s, actually rated by student nurses at the bottom of the list for entry position.

At EFSCH I set up orientation and continuing education programs, then termed "inservice education" programs. I developed policies and procedures and a manual for the nursing care of patients. When this was accomplished I was then ready to set up the educational program for public health nurses—the ultimate goal.

The continuing education five-day program was used as a model. It was so popular because so few cancer nursing experiences were available. I quickly expanded it to include other hospital nurses, faculty from schools of nursing, and visiting nurses from other cities and states.

One day I had a call from the regional public health services officer inquiring about the program and wanting to visit. Rosalie Peterson, R.N., M.S., Ph.D., director of the nursing section field investigation and demonstration branch of the National Cancer Institute came. She quickly became my mentor and officially appointed me a consultant to her section branch in 1952. She sent her nurses to take my program. She involved me in a number of nursing- and cancer-related activities at the national level. She recommended me to R. Lee Clark, M.D., for the position of director of nursing at M. D. Anderson.

When I went to interview, I had to request to meet with nurses. When Dr. Clark offered me the position, I told him I was interested if I had the authority as well as the responsibility. "They're yours," he said and helped me over many a rough spot. In those early days, the nurses, including directors of nursing, were not too high in the echelon. I had to ask to be placed on, and have nurses placed on, various hospital committees and Dr. Clark's weekly department-head meetings. These committees were established through the formal organization and structures of the medical staff and institution. It didn't take me long to realize that if I brought something up I had better be well prepared. Many times I would go to see the chair before the meeting to go over items. My staff were excellent in helping me prepare. We had many special committees and task forces set up for specific aspects.

When I came to M.D. Anderson as director of nursing at the new hospital in 1955, there were approximately 170 nursing personnel. Only one-third were registered nurses. I quickly requested staffing changes and funds for a staff that consisted of 75 percent RNs and 25 percent other staff in order to provide quality care. When I moved from the director's position in 1977, there were 1,200 nursing staff members in the department.

The salary for a staff RN was $252 per month regardless of hours worked or duties assigned. I advocated (and received the necessary support from the hospital administration) for providing adequate salaries and numbers of qualified staff to improve patient care. It was very difficult to recruit nurses. They felt working in a cancer hospital was too depressing.

My experience at Ellis Fischel Hospital proved invaluable because M.D. Anderson had the same needs in organizing the department of nursing. Nurses at M.D. Anderson were in the forefront, developing new, expanded roles and innovative approaches to the care of cancer patients in collaboration with physicians and members of other disciplines. Nurses at M.D. Anderson also shared these developments freely with other nurses. Charges for educational services were unheard of; it was an expectation for us.

We had many visitors—both nurses and physicians. Pat Burns, R.N., Roswell Park, came for help in organizing her nursing department. Robert Tiffany, from the Royal Marsden in London, spent time with my education director and myself because he needed help to set up a cancer nursing education program at his hospital.

Early nurse practice legislation in Texas made no provision for expanded roles. It was not until 1970 that an amendment to the nurse practice act for practitioners was passed.

I remember the first nitrogen mustard given at EFSCH in the early 1950s. Only a physician could administer the drug. There was a specific technique. The drug was unstable. It was made clear to the patient that this drug was palliative, not curative. Chemotherapy was given as a single agent and used until no longer effective, then another single agent, if available, was used. Combination chemotherapy was not developed until 1966 when we had a better understanding of cell kinetics and research.

In October 1968 I began to discuss with assistant directors, supervisors, and head nurses the possibility of registered nurses assuming responsibility for the administration of investigational drugs, most of which were used in IV therapy, provided specific criteria and guidelines could be developed. I contacted the directors of nursing at the other three major cancer centers and the National Cancer Institute clinical center to see what their nurses were doing. None were giving any of these drugs and they expressed concern that I was even contemplating such a practice. I had been president of the Texas Nurses Association from 1962 to 1964 and had established a liaison committee with the Texas Medical Association. One of the committee's primary purposes was to look at the "gray areas" of practice and try to develop joint policy statements regarding medical and nursing practice. At the Texas Nurses Association we developed a policy statement on nursing practice relating to investigational drugs in 1967. This statement read: "It is agreed that it is appropriate practice for a registered nurse licensed in Texas to participate in research involving the use of investigational drugs provided the following conditions are filled: (a) the principal investigator, a licensed physician, is responsible for securing the necessary patient consent, (b) the nurse must have adequate information concerning the investigational drugs he is expected to administer in order that he may fulfill his professional nursing responsibilities, (c) investigational drugs should be made available through the agency pharmacy, whose responsibility it is to provide proper labeling and dispense in accord with the investigator's written order."

The Texas Medical Association would not issue this as a joint policy statement because they believed giving investigational drugs was strictly a medical function. At M.D. Anderson I met with the executive committee and requested that nurses be permitted to give chemotherapy drugs. The following key policies were established: (1) all investigational drugs are stored in the pharmacy and issued, properly labeled, upon written order of the physician investigator, (2) administration by any route is prohibited until adequate information concerning action, dosage, toxicity, precautions, and side effects are available on the nursing unit. This medical function was delegated to qualified registered nurses.

In January 1970 Catherine Herrington, R.N., assistant director of clinics, and Anita Mahaffey, R.N., B.S., set up a teaching program for the nurses in the clinic area where chemotherapy would be given. The first classes were taught by a physician because the nurses did not have adequate chemotherapy and investigational drug information. Drug data sheets were developed and given out freely to staff all over the states. I had so many calls to explain how this program was established and what the legal aspects for nurses were. Many visitors—both physicians and nurses—came to see the program. Our nurses believed this was a major improvement in the quality of patient care. Nurses who passed the course satisfactorily were permitted to give chemotherapy, including investigational drugs, per the approved guideline. This approval was also noted in their personnel record.

In the 1950s and 1960s it was common practice for drugs to be stocked on the units, and for nurses to calculate dosages and prepare the admixtures under less than desirable conditions. I actually took some of the chemotherapy preparations to the pharmacy and therapeutics committee.

In the 1950s M. D. Anderson had a very active pharmacy and therapeutics committee under the executive committee of the medical staff. I was a member. In the early 1960s dramatic changes in cancer therapy, which profoundly affected the practice of infusion therapy, included (1) the use of chemotherapy as a primary treatment modality for cancer patients, (2) the use of investigational antibiotic therapy, (3) the use of commercially available drugs in research protocols, and (4) questions of drug compatibility and information on stability.

Early problems with the preparation of chemotherapy agents, questions of compatibility and stability, and the fact that these functions rightly belonged to the pharmacist, resulted in two major recommendations being made in 1968: (1) all IV preparations were to be done in the pharmacy in a separate section using laminar air flow hoods; and (2) all IV solutions with additives were prepared in the pharmacy and delivered ready to be administered to the patient by the nurse. Thus the pharmacist rightfully assumed his or her responsibility, and the nurse contributed to IV therapy administration. The greatest gain was for the patient, who could be assured of safety and quality care.

M.D. Anderson Cancer Center today continues to provide a complete IV additive service which is in charge of preparing all IV admixtures and irrigation fluids and distributing IV fluids without medications. In the late 1960s and early 1970s no one could have projected the sheer volume, and changes in methods of administration, of today's infusion therapy. Approximately 2,000 patients are now examined daily in the clinic and 70 beds are designated for the ambulatory treatment center, where phase I and phase II drugs are given for outpatient therapy.

Nurses at M.D. Anderson Hospital became actively involved in the conduct of clinical trials with investigational chemotherapeutic agents.

We collaborated with principal investigators in reviewing protocols, developing drug data sheets, establishing policies and procedures for the administration of the drugs, observing patients for possible known and unknown side effects, teaching patients and families and preparing educational materials for them, and assisting in data collection and analysis. Nurses also had a major role in continued communication with, and providing emotional support for, patients and families.

Scalp vein or butterfly infusion sets were introduced in the late 1950s. These sets had plastic flexible wings attached to the needle which provided a better finger grip for more accurate insertion. At this time disposable Abbott® Venopaks were also available. There were some real problems with these systems particularly as they related to the cancer patient. The frequent venipuncture required by the scalp vein needles and the shortness of the catheters (1.5 inches) often damaged the superficial veins so that they could no longer be used for IV infusion, and the infusion sets often remained in place only a couple of hours. In addition, accidental extravasation from some of the drugs seriously harmed surrounding tissues. Also, cancer patients often had long-term and extensive IV therapy. Because of these special needs and problems, research was directed at alternate methods for IV access beginning in 1976. This was a collaborative effort between the department of developmental therapeutics and the department of nursing, with Millie Lawson, R.N., B.S., and Kenneth McCredie, M.D., as the primary investigators. Significant developments resulted from these investigations, which revolutionized infusion therapy for the cancer patient and resulted in safer, more reliable methods. These were (1) the use of a peripherally inserted (long-line) central venous catheter made of elastomeric silicone material, (2) the use of a fibrinolytic drug (urokinase) for declotting catheters, and (3) the use of portable pumps for the delivery of IV drugs. The catheter and pump programs made it possible for patients to be treated on an outpatient basis rather than being hospitalized during courses of drug therapy.

The first major improvement was the development of the long-line indwelling silicone elastomeric central venous catheter (CVC). This peripheral catheter was inserted by Millie Lawson, R.N., B.S., a specially trained research nurse in the department of developmental therapeutics, and later by nurses she trained on the infusion therapy team she supervised. The catheter was inserted by percutaneous venipuncture in either the right or left basilic or cephalic vein under specific sterile procedures. The position of the catheter tip in the superior vena cava was verified by a chest roentgenogram checked by the nurse. The nurse then sutured the catheter in place. Neither checking the X-ray nor suturing the catheter were generally done by nurses. The catheters were generally well tolerated by patients. Based on the results of more than

2,500 insertions performed and an average catheter indwelling time of 67 days, these catheters were considered reliable for IV infusions and relatively safe for long periods of indwelling.

In just a decade the infusion therapy program expanded to the present number of 4,500 patients with indwelling central venous catheters and 500 peripheral inserted catheters (PIC) per month. Catheters have remained in place as long as two and a half years. When the CVC program was initiated, a specific maintenance program was established. The IV team performed sterile dressing procedures twice a week to reduce the risk of bacterial infections. Providone iodine ointment was used and covered with permeable waterproof transparent tape. Between courses of chemotherapy, or when the patient with an indwelling CVC was discharged to home, patency of the catheter was maintained by placing a resealable heparin injection cap with a Leur-Lok® connector in the catheter tubing. A daily injection of 1 ml of normal saline with 100 U of heparin was made through the center of the cap. Patients and a family member were taught to care for the catheters, and to be able to identify any problems which needed to be reported to the physician.

When I started in cancer nursing in 1950 I was privileged to have some very good colleagues and friends. Since there was no organization, we frequently used the phone to call each other for information or help. My colleagues included Rosalie Peterson R.N., M.S., Ph.D., director of the nursing section field investigations and demonstration branch of the National Cancer Institute (I served as consultant to her section staff and she was my mentor); Katharine Nelson, R.N., M.S., Teacher's College, Columbia University; Dorris Diller, R.N., M.S., Skidmore College; Edith Wolfe, R.N., M.S., Memorial Sloan-Kettering Cancer Center; Norma Owens, R.N., Ph.D., New York University; and Jean Quint Benoliel, R.N., M.S., Ph.D., University of Washington. Also there were the directors of nursing at the other two major cancer hospitals, the director of nursing at the clinical center of the National Institutes of Health; and the consultants at the American Cancer Society, beginning with Marjorie Schlotterbach, R.N., M.S., in 1948.

In 1951 the first American Cancer Society nursing advisory committee was appointed with Katharine Nelson as chairman. Initially its purpose was to advise on educational programs and materials. I was appointed to the committee from 1954 to 1960, and from 1964 to 1980, together with serving on the professional nurse education committee and subcommittee on films. Virginia Barckley, R.N., M.S., was employed as ACS nursing consultant in 1962. Virginia's background in mental health was a definite advantage.

I believed it was extremely important to actually tell nurses about cancer nursing challenges, rewards, and problems. I was invited to speak at local, state, national, and international meetings. Topics varied, depending on the interest of the group. One of the more interesting presentations I gave was the keynote address entitled, "Cancer Nursing, the State of the Art," for the first National Cancer Nursing conference, sponsored by ACS in 1973. We were amazed that 2,500 nurses attended. The proceedings were published and widely distributed, as were subsequent conferences in 1977 and 1981. The state divisions of the American Cancer Society sponsored many conferences for nurses. I spoke at many of them.

As temporary advisors, Virginia Barckley and I were invited by the World Health Organization to go to Peru and conduct the first cancer nursing course for nurses in Peru. There were 400 who attended; we had expected 100. When we arrived we learned the nurses couldn't speak English and we couldn't speak Spanish—some fun to do the program! An OB nurse translated our talks.

Robert Tiffany of the Royal Marsden Hospital in London planned the first international cancer nursing conference in 1978. I chaired the morning session and gave the introductory remarks. In 1981 I was invited to present a paper at the second nursing conference.

After the first conference, a group of us spent the weekend at a castle for a retreat. The major item on the agenda was to determine how the American nurses and organizations could help nurses in other countries who desperately needed even basic cancer nursing training. Virginia was a respresentative for the International Union Against Cancer, but progress for nursing had not occurred. All of us felt cancer nursing needed more visibility and physicians' support.

When I learned that the 13th International Union Against Cancer Congress would be held in Seattle in 1982, I talked with Dr. Lee Clark and also with Diane Fink, M.D., of the National Cancer Institute to see if nurses could be represented on the joint programs as speakers, as well as to set up our own oncology nursing sessions, which had not been done previously. It took a lot of time to work with Dr. Fink in selecting the topics and speakers. One session had all nurse speakers; other sessions had medical and oncology nurse speakers. This participation provided excellent visibility for oncology nursing. In addition, all proceedings, including nursing sessions and presentations, were published as part of the official proceedings.

Virginia Barckley came to the American Cancer Society as the nursing consultant in January 1962. She had many ideas and concerns related to service to patients as well as nursing education. She was responsible for initiating the first work–study program for senior student nurses in cancer nursing with the idea of their gaining knowledge and skills as well as interest in the field of cancer nursing. This program provided the opportunity for students to spend the summer in a comprehensive cancer center or a clinical cancer center. Some financial support was provided to students from the state divisions of ACS. Funds for instructors' support came from the American Cancer Society. We participated at M.D. Anderson, taking senior students from many states. Many went back home and were good ambassadors for cancer nursing. All of us who participated in this program felt it was extremely worthwhile, and in my estimation, it was good for recruitment. Subsequently, a program was initiated to provide scholarships for faculty members who wished to attend a summer program in which we also participated at M.D. Anderson.

In 1958 those of us on the nursing advisory committee recommended the need for scholarships for graduate nurses to attend short-term courses in cancer nursing, and also for advanced educational preparation for nurses in the field of cancer. This was approved in principle, though funds were not allocated. Also in 1958 the nursing advisory committee recommended that nurses become members of all professional education and service committees at the division and local levels of the American Cancer Society. I chaired the committee on professorships and scholarships and Trish Greene was a member. She later became ACS vice president of nursing and patient care services.

In 1980, based on a recommendation of the nursing advisory committee, the American Cancer Society initiated a new scholarship program for nurses to be prepared at a master's level in oncology nursing. In 1981 there were 10 recipients of these scholarships. The next year ACS awarded 20 and continues to do so. Scholarships provide a maximum of $16,000 for two years. A report on the program is in the May 1994 issue of the *Oncology Nursing Forum*. From 1981 until 1992, 281 nurses had received scholarships.

We requested that the scholarships be set at $8,000 with a maximum of two years to obtain the master's. Arthur Holleb, M.D., vice president of medical affairs, was very supportive and obtained the funding. I talked with Dr. Holleb about providing sufficient funds in a scholarship so nurses could do full-time study.

I chaired a working group of the professional education committee of the American Cancer Society to develop a proposal for clinical professors in oncology nursing to be centered in nursing education programs meeting the criteria. This program was approved in 1980. Divisions of ACS provided the funding of $35,000 per year for three years. To date, there have been 12 professorships awarded in oncology nursing.

Members of the subcommittee on scholarships and professorships were concerned about the dearth of doctorally prepared nurses in oncology nursing. I was chairing this subcommittee when we decided to try for approval from the professional education committee of scholarships for doctoral education. We requested four the first year. I really worked hard to line up arguments for this proposal and it passed. These scholarships provide $8,000 per year for a maximum of four years.

Oncology nurses owe a real debt of gratitude to the ACS and state divisions of the ACS for support of all programs. The primary focus in all programs is improving care to cancer patients through more qualified staff. Members of this committee meet once a year, review all applications, make site visits, discuss, score, and make final recommendations for all scholarship awards and programs. In addition, the committee develops criteria to be met for the program and has a system for recipients to report back to the committee, which monitors progress based on the original goals.

The values of clinical research projects, both in the hospital and in the ambulatory care setting, increased dramatically with the use of chemotherapy in the early 1960s, followed by immunotherapy, blood component therapy, and various other procedures. In the early 1960s, M.D. Anderson clinics were open until 5 P.M. five days a week. In planning for the new ambulatory care facilities in the new hospital, physicians and nurses programmed two and a half times the number of patients and space needed, based on that data base. This was not even sufficient, and today 2,000 patients are seen daily in clinic. None of us could have predicted the dramatic increase in the number of ambulatory care patients.

It was exciting to be a part of the clinical research projects, and to see the positive results in caring for patients. There was a multidisciplinary collaborative approach to planning and problem solving. I believe the reason we succeeded was that we needed each other's contributions. We were willing to give and take, keeping in mind what was best for the patient. We had to break down barriers, be positive in what we could do, and not do what could not be done.

I'd like to give you some examples of how I was able to obtain some financial help for staffing and equipment.

In 1967 Emil Frei, III, M.D., who had worked with the germ-free environment concepts at the National Cancer Institute clinical center, planned to initiate such a program at M.D. Anderson. I met with him. As a proposal was being prepared to be sent to the National Institutes of Health at the National Cancer Institute, I submitted and justified a proposal, with a budget, for nursing staff and nursing care hours needed beyond the requirements for a usual medical/surgical cancer unit. Funds were also requested to augment central sterile supply staff for increased preparation and sterilized supplies and equipment. These funds were requested from National Cancer Institute grant competitive bids. I received funds for nursing staff, and supplies and equipment for patients as well as for central supply. I believe these may have been the first such nursing funds in a clinical research NCI grant.

We were able to use some of the concepts initiated for patient care in the "Bubble-Isolator" and had a good data base of our own. However, when Gerald Bodey, M.D., decided to do research using the concept of laminar flow, this was a totally new concept not previously used for patients anywhere.

Weekly multidisciplinary conferences were held with departmental representatives who were involved regularly in the research and patient care. Nursing representatives included the head nurse, supervisor, assistant director (medical), and myself. These conferences were working sessions for protocol review, planning, coordinating, problem solving, evaluating, and being kept up to date on further research planned and/or the results of current research efforts. Experience gained in the pilot project aided in the development of a 20-bed laminar flow unit for the clinical research center which opened in 1977.

I again prepared a budget proposal which was submitted with the grant request for NCI funding. In the 1973 competitive grant, I received funds for nursing staff, both on the patient unit and in central supply, for the preparation of huge volumes of supplies and equipment. Part of my grant proposal justification was pertinent patient needs and various approaches to the expanded role of the nurse.

The team led by Gerald Bodey, M.D., was focused on the patient and cognizant of the fact that such a program could improve survival rates of, for example, acute leukemia patients who would be using laminar flow rooms. In planning the unit, Dr. Bodey brought up the fact that visitors could not be in the unit. All of the nurses immediately said, "You can't keep patients away from families and friends." We proposed a solution which received administrative approval. An outside enclosed corridor that could be entered by a separate elevator outside the unit was built. The corridor was glassed in so patients could see out. Then we added individual phones at each bed and each room in the hallway so patients and family members could see and talk with privacy. I was so proud of all the nursing staff involved. All concepts, procedures, and care had to be researched, determined, tried out, and evaluated to see if it met germ-free standards.

When Edward Copeland, M.D., the physician investigator for intravenous hyperalimentation, sought grant support from the National Cancer Institute, I met with him and prepared a job description for the position. I prepared a budget request to be submitted with his request. Initially I received funds for one nurse and later for a second nurse as the program grew. Since I had been successful on a couple of requests, this continued to be my approach on other research projects. I would never have had enough staff on my regular department budget to provide for so many new research areas.

In the early 1950s and 1960s, and even with the advent of chemotherapy, patients had to be admitted to the hospital, maybe for a week or a month, for treatment. In 1980, Kenneth McCredie, M.D., worked with the Alza Corporation in California to develop a prototype portable infusion pump which we pilot-tested at M.D. Anderson. The pump could be worn on the upper arm and weighed 1.05 pounds. An elastomeric reservoir held 25 ml of fluid, about a 24-hour dose. We had the first patient come to clinic and return so we could check him. We were all excited because of the benefit to patients in terms of management, cost, mobility, and quality of life. It meant detailed teaching of patients and families in changing reservoirs. What a tremendous approach to infusion therapy! Think what it would be like if today's volume of such patients had to be hospitalized for treatment. Today there are a variety of pumps, depending on patients' needs and medications.

In 1970, when the institution decided that all facilities—hospital, ambulatory, operating rooms, recovery, and intensive care units—would be built, a medical planning firm was employed. At the first meeting all department heads were given a document with information to be prepared. I took it seriously and involved all administrative and educational nursing staff, and many staff at the hospital unit level, as the ward clerks. I set up teams for study areas: unit size, rooms, equipment, bathrooms, lighting, and others. Some suggestions we made were: (1) no more than 30 beds per unit; and (2) no more long halls—we wanted patients close to nursing staff. This concept was hard to sell to the architects. I wanted triangular nursing units with beds set around a central core. And I wanted completely open units. After much arguing with the architects, Dr. Clark okayed my plan. Again, we had statistics on why single, rather that multiple, units were needed. We had also asked for many clinic changes to expedite care.

I would like to point out that nurses and physicians in respective service areas planned together both for the hospital unit and clinic to provide the best facilities for care. I remember when we were talking about remodeled and new space for surgical intensive care, the head nurse was concerned because the layout would not provide any outdoor window space for patients to see out. I argued her point and the space was changed to provide what she felt was adequate for patients. We had an excellent data base on our needs for nursing education and office space. We received all we asked for, including different size meeting rooms and a patient unit demonstration model.

A valuable decision made was to use a mock-up patient room in which concepts and ideas could be tried. We built, tried, and evaluated four room changes before we decided what we wanted. All staff were encouraged to work in the mock-up room. Special days were scheduled for the staff assigned to this area, as well as others, to come and try out the placement of the bed and bedside equipment.

We wanted to continue providing cots for parents who wanted to remain with a child on pediatrics. Although we wanted "pull down" Murphy beds for the whole new hospital, Dr. Clark would not approve that much space, so our search for a comfortable bed/chair continued.

The National Cancer Act of 1971, revised in 1974, established a broad-based intensive program to reduce morbidity and mortality of cancer in human beings. The act provided for cancer control programs, educational programs, and research efforts. The act established the three major cancer hospitals as the first three comprehensive cancer centers.

I was fortunate to be appointed to committees that were going to plan programs as a result of the National Cancer Act legislation. At first I didn't know why I was appointed, because generally physicians, not nurses, were given such appointments. I had two new mentors: Diane Fink, M.D., director of the division of cancer control and rehabilitation, and Veronica Conley, R.N., Ph.D., chief officer of committee review, whose background was also in cancer. I learned I was appointed because I had a good clinical and cancer nursing background, and I was not afraid to speak out. I had no background in NCI grants (except when I applied for nursing funds), contracts, RFPs (requests for proposals), site visits, committee review activities, and recommendations.

Appointments

1973–1977 Appointment to National Institutes of Health, National Cancer Institute; Division of Cancer Control and Rehabilitation, Department of Health, Education, and Welfare

1973–1974 Member, Cancer Control Education Review Committee, National Cancer Institute

1975–1977 Chair, Intervention Program Review Committee, NCI; Division of Cancer Control and Rehabilitation, Department of Health, Education, and Welfare

I was the first nurse to chair an NCI Committee. This had been unheard of.

Some of us in nursing were concerned that there were no NCI funds for cancer nursing education. In 1972 John Bailer, M.D., the associate director for cancer control at the National Cancer Institute, visited M.D. Anderson Hospital to discuss medical education in cancer. As usual, R. Lee Clark, our director, always let individuals know that someone was coming. I wanted to see him about cancer nursing education and requested time to do this. The only time available was late in the day on the way to the airport, so on the busy freeway traffic between 5 and 7 P.M. I tried to convince him that there was a need for education for nurses in cancer. I also indicated that I believed established cancer centers could provide leadership in the preparation of personnel to staff future cancer centers and other programs. This was a surprise to him; he did not realize that there was any additional information nurses needed when taking care of cancer patients as compared to any other patients. However, he asked me to send him "a brief" of what I thought needed to be done. He would see what could be done. I prepared a simple brief including the need for continuing education programs for nurses and programs for faculty and students. Subsequently, I received a note from Dr. Bailer indicating that the proposal had been submitted to the cancer control advisory committee in January of 1973.

The committee deferred acceptance to have the program staff further investigate the current status of oncology nursing. Undergraduate and graduate programs and continuing education for nursing were studied since the cancer control program was looking for a nationwide approach for nurses in oncology. A request to submit a proposal was issued in 1974 and 15 contracts were awarded by the division of cancer control and rehabilitation of the Department of Health, Education, and Welfare for oncology nursing programs in cancer centers, community hospitals, and schools of nursing. I received a contract.

I also voiced my concern about the lack of enterostomal therapy programs for training persons in the care of those patients. In 1974 the National Cancer Institute division of cancer control and rehabilitation issued a request for response to a proposal for the establishment of an enterostomal therapy education program. I received a three-year contract as did Boston and Emory Universities. I asked Dr. Clark to establish a task force with physicians, nurses, and the central supply supervisor. We made many changes in our program for the care of stoma patients.

This program had its inception in 1984 and this year celebrates its 10th anniversary; 343 nurses from 37 states and 8 foreign countries have attended the program and been certified as enterostomal therapists. There have only been two program directors, Dot Smith, R.N., M.S.N.E.T., and Beverly Hampton, R.N., M.S., E.T. This program has made tremendous contributions to the care of stoma and other patients. From the inception of the program, all trainees received help with their own programs and problems. From the beginning the ET director and I worked closely with the International Association of Enterostomal Therapy to help promote and accredit programs.

Nurses have been represented on the National Cancer Institute's cancer control grant review committee since the 1970s, beginning with Eleanor Lambertson, Ph.D. and Ida Martinson, R.N. Ph.D. Ruth McCorkle, R.N. Ph.D. and I were appointed from 1979 to 1983 as members. I served at times as chair and/or member on site visit teams for the National Institutes of Health of the National Cancer Institute.

There were always excellent committee members—physicians, scientists, educators, ethicists, and others. Ruth and I educated them in cancer nursing. At the same time, there was much to learn from them. At times I chaired the grants review committee. This was an invaluable experience. I believe we established the visibility and the credibility of oncology nurses in nursing research and clinical care. We paved the way and made it possible for future appointments and for the recognition of true peer status.

Publications and Films

I have contributed 30 publications to journals. Some of these are classics, since there was nothing in the early literature. In 1970, with assistance from the M.D. Anderson medical communications department, I made a film, *To Take a Hand*, which depicted the psychological aspects of working with patients and nurses.

In 1986 I served as a consultant to the American Cancer Society in cooperation with the special projects staff of the biomedical communication department of M.D. Anderson for the development and production of a videotape entitled *Cancer Nursing—the Critical Difference*. The videotape received first prize at the American Nurses Association film festival.

Professional Awards and Honors

I received many honors and awards for my contributions to cancer nursing and oncology nursing. These also reflect the work, cooperation, and support of my staff, for without their help I could not have done many of these things. Also, I believe some awards recognize the change in status of oncology nursing.

1966 Professor of Oncology Nursing, The University of Texas, M.D. Anderson Hospital. There was provision for conferring professor status for clinical achievement.

1981 I was the first nurse recipient of the American Cancer Society's Distinguished Service Award "as an internationally recognized pioneer whose sensitivity and extraordinary effort helped to create the specialty of cancer nursing. She trained many of today's leaders in the field, stimulating them to pursue their individual areas of interest. During thirty years as Director of Nursing at M.D. Anderson, she infused her work with a caring concern, always making time to visit patients."

1983 National Cancer Program, Cancer Control Grant Review Committee, "for Outstanding Contributions to Programs of Division of Extramural Activities of the National Cancer Institute 1979–1983," Washington, D.C.

1986 First recipient of Distinguished Merit Award for national and international contributions from the International Society of Nurses in Cancer Care at the Fourth International Conference on Cancer Nursing. Virginia Barckley, R.N., ACS nursing consultant, and I were both honored with this award because the society could not determine who had done the most for its first award.

1988 Ph.D. Honorary, Doctor of Public Service, conferred by St. Louis University, St. Louis, Missouri for splendid contributions in oncology nursing. This is my alma mater. This was the first honorary doctorate awarded to a nurse and a woman.

1989 Received the first National Nursing Leadership Award from the American Cancer Society for national and international contributions in cancer nursing.

1991 Received Honorary Membership Award from the Oncology Nursing Society for contributions nationally and internationally in oncology nursing.

I rarely had time on the job, with a very large, active department of nursing, to do any of the extra committee work and other activities, such as reviewing, writing recommendations for both NCI and ACS applications, contributing to the literature, or preparing numerous speeches. These were my evening and weekend jobs, or I did them on the airplane to or from a meeting or early or late in a hotel room.

After my father died, my mother came to Houston to live with me. She had her own activities while able, but developed congestive heart failure and other problems such as small strokes. I often had to be called out of a meeting to go home and change a portable oxygen tank. There were no home health services as there are today. I was blessed with a good part-time maid. If I left town I had to see that nurse coverage was available. My mother would fuss about all my running around, but I would hear her proudly telling her friends what I was up to. I guess one of the best trips she took with me was to an ACS conference in Orlando, Florida, when she got to see the Gardens. She had a keen mind, enjoyed traveling, and we got to be extremely good at traveling with a wheelchair.

One of my young nephews from Missouri once came for the Christmas holiday. I took him with me to the hospital to make rounds and left him at one of the nursing stations while I went to check on something. When I came back, the nurses were having a great laugh. He had asked the nurses what I did, but their responses didn't mean much to him. So when he got home he said, "Grandma, you know all Aunt Renilda does is just stand around and talk."

I'm sure the nurses in oncology nursing today will continue to add to the rich traditions of the past. Each decade will have its own challenges and contributions—which can be added to the legacy.

Notes

Abbott Venopaks is a registered trademark of Abbott Laboratories.

Leur-Lok is a registered trademark of Becton Dickinson.

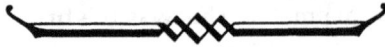

22

Ryan Iwamoto

I vividly remember an intense experience I had when I was about four years old. An accident occurred in which my arm was caught in the engine compartment as the hood of the car was shut. I am sure time "stopped". . . for me, my parents, and the neighborhood as I was yelling at the top of my lungs. I remember being taken to the hospital but refusing to leave the car, much less go into the ER department. I was more frightened of what would happen in that department than of what had just happened to my arm. I distinctly remember curling up and hiding on the floor of the front passenger seat, making myself as small as possible so that no one could find me, much less extricate me from the car.

Since I would not go into the ER, the nurse came out to the car and gently examined my arm as I huddled in that little space. When she found no damage, she allowed me to return home with my parents. The nurse respected my need for protection and security, she allowed me to be where I was, and she met me there. I believe that was my first lesson in nursing.

When I was in high school, I had aspirations to become a doctor. Family members had medical problems and medicine intrigued me.

In college I soon found the math and science courses uninspiring. It was actually a third-year calculus course which was my Waterloo. I decided to reevaluate my career goals. I went to see a career guidance counselor at the University of Hawaii and took the Strong Interest Inventory. What I remember is that I had interests which were compatible with librarians and YMCA directors! Although those are wonderful careers for others, I could not see myself pursuing those jobs. Recently I had the opportunity to participate in the Strong Interest Inventory when they were updating their data banks. Interestingly enough, I continue to have similar interests as librarians and YMCA directors.

Having an interest in art, I decided to enter the school of architecture. As there was a moratorium on admission to the school, I took prerequisite classes in art, urban planning, and environmental sciences. I found those courses very enjoyable and effortless. I began to apply to other schools of architecture, at the University of California, Berkeley and the University of Southern California, both well known for their schools. I was accepted to both and received a very generous scholarship from USC.

At that time in my life, I was very involved with the InterVarsity Christian Fellowship at the University of Hawaii. Each summer, Bible study camps were held in California for students on the West Coast and Hawaii. The summer before entering architecture school, I attended this camp and met several nursing students, both men and women. A seed was planted for I had never even considered nursing as a career, much less thought that there were men in nursing. These students talked about how they enjoyed their classes and the interactions they had with patients. When I returned home, I began calling the local hospitals and asked to speak with nurses, physical therapists, social workers, physicians, pharmacists, and others to learn what they enjoyed about their careers and their thoughts about the future of their professions. What impressed me at the time was that the nurses were working in a variety of settings, seemed to feel that there were many possibilities for someone with a nursing background (very key for one who was having a difficult time making a decision), and seemed truly satisfied with their work. To the consternation of my parents, I decided to turn down the offer to enter architecture school and began preparing to enter nursing school.

The interviews for nursing school at the University of Hawaii were held in groups of five candidates with about four faculty members. When asked why I wanted to become a nurse, I believe I said that I saw nursing as a steppingstone to eventually becoming a physician! It is hard for me to believe today that if I had said such a thing I would have been admitted to the school. If I didn't say it, I certainly thought it. Again, my difficulty in making a choice was evident.

It was soon after I began working as a nurse that I started to appreciate nursing for the profession it is, offering its unique contribution to and perspective of patient care. I no longer saw my career in nursing as a "steppingstone" toward becoming a physician. I discovered that the "carative" philosophy of nursing fit well with who I was and with what I felt I had to offer others.

In nursing school I had an opportunity to participate in a summer colloquium on miltidisciplinary cancer care. Teams consisting of a medical student, a social work student, a graduate nursing student, and an undergraduate nursing student worked together to evaluate and participate in the care of cancer patients in local hospitals. The facilitator of the program, Joanne Itano, orchestrated a program which allowed me to meet many of the cancer nursing leaders in Hawaii, many of whom are friends and colleagues to this day. It was through this program that I met Grace Ann Ehlke, a faculty member at the University of Hawaii School of Nursing, who shared with us her personal experiences with cancer. My team was assigned to St. Francis Hospital in Honolulu. This hospital had started the multidisciplinary CARES (CAncer REhabilitation Services) program which provided outreach to the local community as well as to the outer islands. At this hospital, Doris Ahana and Phyllis Lum (then Tanabe), the clinical nurse specialists, provided guidance and knowledge about cancer care as well as a little hand-holding as our very novice team ventured into the fray. It was at that point that I thought that if I ever got out of nursing school, I would eventually like to become a clinical nurse specialist. As I look back I am amazed at the solid foundation of mentoring I received early in my career.

My senior clinical experience in nursing school was on a neurological/orthopedic floor. This floor was a demanding floor for in addition to having patients who were on respirators, comatose after multiple traumas (e.g., automobile accidents, falls, etc.), the floor also had patients with chronic problems such as multiple sclerosis. The "aha" moment came to me as I was caring for a particularly "difficult" patient. Nursing students were frequently assigned to this patient because she was experiencing an exacerbation of her multiple sclerosis, could not provide her own self-care, and needed bed baths, frequent turnings, and transfers to the commode. The care she required was exhausting to provide and she was not a particularly grateful patient; in fact she was usually unhappy about her care or food. Her call light was frequently turned on for help. In retrospect I can better understand the fears and anger she probably was experiencing which were manifested by her behavior.

One morning as I was giving her a bed bath, I began thinking about a Scripture passage that has ever since been the inspiration for what I do.

> "For I was hungry, and you gave Me something to eat; I was thirsty, and you gave Me drink; I was a stranger, and you invited Me in; naked, and you clothed Me; I was sick, and you visited Me; I was in prison, and you came to Me." Then the righteous will answer Him, saying, "Lord, when did we see You hungry, and feed You, or thirsty, and give You drink? and when did we see You a stranger, and invite You in, or naked, and clothe You? and when did we see You sick, or in prison, and come to You?" And the King will answer and say to them, "Truly I say to you, to the extent that you did it to one of these brothers of Mine, even the least of them, you did it to Me." (Matthew 25:35–40).

That was the point in my life at which I began to see a glimmer of the holiness in each person. It gave me a new perspective about honoring and respecting each person.

Upon graduating from nursing school, I was hired to work at St. Francis Hospital, the same hospital where I had participated in the multidisciplinary cancer program. As there were no openings on the oncology unit, I worked on an orthopedic and surgical unit. As is the case in any hospital, there were many cancer patients on that unit. For a novice nurse, it was a whole new world, meeting people in the most extreme of situations. I remember caring for a Hawaiian woman who was a hula teacher. The surgical wound for her gastric cancer was not healing, probably because the cancer was continuing to progress. All nursing resources were gathered to care for her. What I remember was her dignity in the face of death. As a hula dancer, she had long black hair. When chemotherapy caused alopecia to occur, her hair was carefully taped to her scalp. It was so important not to lose that part of her. Her family was with her constantly, guarding and caring for her. I learned the importance of caring for the patient and family as a unit. They could not be separated from her.

I eventually was able to transfer to the oncology unit. I had grown particularly fond of an elderly Chinese woman and her husband. Her husband came to the hospital each day to spend time sitting at her bedside, helping with her needs. One evening when I was on duty, she began to have extreme difficulty with breathing and choking. With the flurry of activity, I became so involved in attending to her physical care that I didn't notice that her husband had left the room. He may have even been asked to leave the room because of the code team suctioning her airway, monitoring her condition, and because of how upsetting the situation may have seemed to him. She quickly died. I went to look for her husband and found him sitting alone in the small recreation room we had on the floor which has a wonderful view down to the city and the ocean. He was sitting in a recliner, intently watching the setting sun, the orange-red glow illuminating his face. Cautiously I approached him and told him that his wife had just died. "I know," is all that he said, tears slowly welling up in his eyes. We slowly walked back to her room. I spent a few minutes in silence as he sat next to her.

The pastor of the church I attended, Ted Ogoshi, was very active in hospital ministry and especially involved in cancer care. We had some interesting discussions about the spiritual aspects of caring for others. Each year he would send a letter to each member of the congregation on his or her birthday. The letter he sent me included a haiku that he had written:

The medaka[1] seeks
The short clear stream instead of
The dirty river.

In 12 words he had captured the essence of the choices one makes in life and death.

I attended graduate school at the University of Washington where Betty Gallucci and Doris Molbo were professors. Graduate school was a wonderful time of being able to focus educational energies and pursue my interest in cancer care. Doris Molbo introduced me to the American Cancer Society as a volunteer. Her own work with the society and eventual appointment as the first ACS professor of oncology nursing in the nation was an inspiration. I remember how Doris challenged me to scrutinize an issue from all perspectives yet to continually be open to all possibilities. Betty was my thesis advisor and gently yet firmly guided me through the process. Her encouragement and enthusiasm buoyed me through graduate school. It was during graduate school that I joined the Oncology Nursing Society, attending the Congress that was held in San Diego in 1980.

Before graduating from the master's program, I began the process of looking for a job. I was torn between looking for a job in Seattle or returning to Hawaii. A friend from Hawaii who is a school counselor gave me wonderful advice. She suggested that I needed to find a job that I looked forward to going to at least 50 percent of the mornings. Another friend said that I should choose where I wanted to live and that within five years the "job of my dreams" would probably become available. If not, it would be time to move on. I chose to stay in Seattle. There were no clinical nurse specialist jobs in Seattle at the time and so I began looking for staff nursing positions. I sent my letter everywhere and began hitting the pavement with resume in hand.

One of the hospitals I went to was Virginia Mason Hospital. The personnel department secretary called the nursing supervisor, Dagny Rolph, who immediately came over to see me. Dagny will forever be the "face" of Virginia Mason for me. Here was a petite woman in her starched white uniform walking with me to meet with Ann Reiner, then the head nurse of the Peter Canlis Cancer Unit. As we walked through the halls, we came upon a visitor to the hospital who appeared lost. Dagny stopped, her kind smile radiating, and escorted this person to the place he needed to go to. I remember thinking, "This place takes care of people!"

I worked as an assistant head nurse on the oncology unit. Working with Ann Reiner was a wonderful experience. Her sensitivity and clarity challenged me to grow and develop professionally and personally. Ann's

---

[1]A small river fish.

integrity to self and others continues to inspire me. When an opportunity to develop a clinical nurse specialist position in the radiation therapy department occurred, Ann encouraged me to apply.

One of the radiation oncologists at Virginia Mason Clinic read an article that appeared in *Seminars in Clinical Oncology*. It was written by Laura Hilderley and addressed the role of the nurse in radiation oncology. After reading the article, this physician approached the director of nursing to discuss his interest in having a nurse in the radiation therapy department. Ann suggested to the director of nursing that I help write the job description and clinical responsibilities. Using Laura's article and the American Nursing Association's definition of clinical nurse specialists, I wrote the job description with Ann's guidance. One of the radiation oncologists I worked with was Willis Taylor, who at the time was the national president of the American Cancer Society. Dr. Taylor's deep commitment to ACS was inspirational and cemented my dedication to volunteerism.

A few years later I met Laura Hilderley. We were both rushing to a special interest group planning meeting at the annual ONS Congress. This was the first year that groups were being formed around specialties such as radiation therapy. I introduced myself to her and thanked her for her article which was the impetus for my job. As usual, Laura was gracious and very interested in learning more about me, and how I was faring as a novice radiation oncology nurse. Here was this well-known leader at the forefront of cancer nursing truly interested in my professional development! Her response was immediate and warm-hearted. I remember thinking that her interest in and commitment to others were qualities I would try to develop in myself. Later, Laura asked me to write my first manuscript for publication in a radiation oncology nursing textbook that she and Karen Hassey Dow were working on. As my editor, Laura provided guidance and encouragement every step of the way.

Brenda Nevidjon had moved to the Seattle area and we met through mutual friends. Brenda helped me to make contacts and negotiate my involvement at the national level of the Oncology Nursing Society. Her encouragement and persistence in spite of my hesitation helped me overcome insecurities I had about involvement on the national level. I eventually served as a reviewer and then associate editor for the *Oncology Nursing Forum*. Under the editorship of Sue Baird and then Rosemary Carroll Johnson, I learned about the inner workings in the field of publications. I am now serving on the editorial board of *Cancer Practice*, working with Genevieve Foley, editor. It has been an exciting endeavor to be a part of a journal in its early development.

Brenda also coordinated my nomination for the ACS Lane Adams Award. Receiving the award was a humbling experience for I felt I did not have the qualifications to merit the award. However, the award ceremony filled me with pride for my chosen profession as I heard the wonderful stories of the other awardees. In the nomination, Brenda crystallized for me my philosophy of care when she used the image of a shepherd in describing the care I provide. As a clinical nurse specialist in radiation oncology, I have the opportunity to work with patients and families experiencing cancer. It is truly "shepherding" in that I help the patient and family negotiate the system, walking with them, helping the patient and family through the experience of receiving radiation therapy. Providing symptom management, education, counseling, and resources are daily experiences.

I also appreciate the humbling times when defeats occur, when there are problems I can't untangle, and meanings elude my understanding. I cared for a middle-aged woman who was dying from an especially aggressive breast cancer. Within a year of diagnosis and definitive therapy, she began coming to our radiation therapy department for multiple courses of palliative radiation therapy. With each successive course of therapy she appeared more and more weakened yet determined to do all possible. She spoke anxiously about her only daughter's upcoming wedding and her strong desire to be there to walk her daughter down the aisle. The wedding was about two months away and it didn't seem that she would be alive for the wedding. A few days into the radiation treatment, I received a call from this woman's daughter. I could hear the fear in her voice as she talked about her mother's deteriorating condition. Her mother was very lethargic, staring off into the distance and talking about seeing people who were not actually there. This was frightening and upsetting to her. When I asked how she thought her mother was doing, it was revealed that her parents did not talk much about her cancer or the treatments she was receiving. She felt that her mother would soon be well again as she had always done in the past. Since she wanted her mother to feel well during her wedding, she had thought of postponing the wedding for a later time so that her mother could recuperate. In my heart I felt that she should move the wedding up because I thought that her mother was hanging on until the wedding. I found it difficult to help this woman and her family face the future, to help them maintain hope, to not take away from the wedding, and yet to assure that the time the family spent together was cherished. I felt intense pain and sadness in talking with this young woman who was preparing for a very happy moment in her life yet beginning to have an awareness of the gravity of her mother's illness.

Another woman who was being simulated for palliative therapy for a large fungating recurrent breast lesion had decreased arm mobility because of contracture of her chest wall and shoulder. She had difficulty lying flat on the treatment table, much less raising her arm out of the treatment field. She lived about a hundred miles away from the treatment center. Three separate appointments were used to attempt to simulate her treatment. Each time her pain was so intense that pain control efforts, including IV sedation, were futile. What I remember most clearly was her chanting in pain. It was a repetitive moaning. For me, it was the moment I realized that this treatment for this woman was far worse than the disease itself. I found myself becoming numb to her pain in order to concentrate and administer the IV sedatives. This realization was a moment of grace for I then was able to refocus my attention to the woman laboring in pain. I realized that the medicines were getting in the way of my caring for her.

As sometimes happens, people wander into our department looking for help. One day I happened to be at the front desk when a distraught woman appeared at the front desk asking to see a doctor. The receptionist looked at me to triage this situation. I asked the woman to come back to an exam room to talk. Within a minute I realized that this woman was mentally disturbed. She talked incessantly with tangential thinking and was obviously upset by an encounter she had had with a physician in our general internal medicine department. She talked in a paranoid manner and clung to me, sobbing about events which occurred years ago. My first reaction was to get out of there, call the security guard, and in general flee the situation. It was a busy clinic day and I really did not have the time to attend to this woman. An immediate second thought was that I needed to respond to this person and the pain and fear she was experiencing. I realized that I could not assuage, much less heal, her mental anguish, but I could help her through the system.

I called the physician's office where she was last seen, and they told me to direct her back to that physician for he was making arrangements for her care. One of the fears she had was that she was going to be involuntarily committed to the state mental institution and feared that the stigma would stick to her for the rest of her life. I went with her to the physician's office to give her reassurance and make sure that she got the help she needed. Unfortunately, the office staff, obviously frustrated and tired from trying to work with her earlier in the day, appeared callous and abrupt, scolding and cajoling her as with a child. Since an exam room was not available for her to wait in, we sat in the hall outside the doctor's office. In the midst of the busy clinic, with the office assistants trying to make arrangements for her to receive psychiatric care, she suddenly looked at me and said, "I don't need to stay here if I don't want to, do I?" My heart went out to her. She was frightened, being pushed around in the medical center, and any fragment of control that she had was being taken away. This was her way to maintain that control. I said, "Yes, you don't need to stay." She stood up and left the department, with me in tow. I tried again to get her to see the physician, assuring her that he would not do anything against her wishes, but was unsuccessful. She asked directions to the exit. When I returned to my department, I realized that perhaps there was a better response. I could have said, "Yes, you don't need to stay, but I think it would be better if you did." She had trusted me and I could have provided her the reassurance that she would be taken care of. These moments happen so quickly; in a flash, the opportunity to make a difference is gone.

One patient I cared for was a young teenaged boy about 15 years old who received chemotherapy for testicular cancer. He seemed studious, regularly receiving his chemotherapy beginning on Friday so that he would not miss too much school. He was quiet and reserved, bringing his homework into the hospital to get whatever he could completed before the antiemetics took effect and he fell asleep. Needless to say I don't think he got much done. Since I was his primary nurse, I usually took care of him when he came in for his therapy.

A few years ago, this young boy, now in his 20s, came to my department to thank me for the care I gave him. I didn't recognize him at first but immediately recognized his name. We spent time catching up on what had happened in the intervening years. He spoke about his family, various jobs he had held, and he shared that he wanted to become a nurse. He said that it was because of the care that I provided him that he wanted to become a nurse. I cannot describe the intensity and wonderfulness of that moment. I have heard it said that the happiest moment in a man's life is when his child is born. For me, this was like having a child born—to feel that what I did made such a difference, that what I did resulted in some good. The fact that it was so unexpected made it all the more intense. I felt at that moment that I could die and be happy that my life had been worthwhile.

As a nurse I consider it a privilege to walk with a patient through his or her experience. I feel honored when patients allow me to enter that very private and sacred area of their lives—their fears, hopes and dreams—at a time of great vulnerability and strength. Connecting with another human being is the basis for the care that I provide. I especially enjoy the creative aspects of being a nurse, using innovative resources and approaches to help solve a problem. I cherish the ability to make a difference, to show a helpless person that her or his life is respected, that she or he has dignity. By trusting my heart, listening to the small quiet inner voice, and responding to the needs of others, I have been able to care for others. But I have also been given the precious gift of lessons for living and appreciating life. I am so grateful for these lessons: not to take things for granted; to truly stop and appreciate each moment and to go on.

Lessons Patients Have Taught Me

Live each day, each moment to the fullest. Value the preciousness of time. Life is a gift; regrets in life are rarely for what was done, but for those things left undone, untried, unsaid. Enjoy life. Carefully make choices about the activities you commit to. Life is too short to spend time in endeavors that are unfulfilling or constantly frustrating. Cherish relationships. Don't take people for granted. Listen with your heart. Be present. Healing occurs in common things, not necessarily magical moments: reconciliation between family members, a telephone call, preparation of a favorite food. Death is not the enemy, the enemies are: broken relationships, not being true to oneself, hardness of heart, abandonment, fear, unwillingness to forgive, and pride. At times the only gift we have left is love.

In the introduction to his book *Meetings at the Edge*, Stephen Levine writes, "The process of growth is, it seems, the art of falling down. Growth is measured by the gentleness and awareness with which we once again pick ourselves up, the lightness with which we dust ourselves off, the openness with which we continue and take the next unknown step, beyond our edge, beyond our holding, into the remarkable mystery of being." Throughout my career as a cancer nurse, my encounters with patients and families experiencing cancer have enriched my life. It is never easy and always challenging as I try to listen sensitively to the needs of the person I am caring for. With each encounter I believe I am affected, am changed, experience growth, and am enriched. As I walk with people in their journey through extreme situations, on the edge of life, it is a powerful, life-changing experience. My journey so far has been scary, exhilarating, mundane, sacred, and deeply joyful.

References

Levine, S. *Meetings at the Edge.* (Garden City, NY: Anchor Press, 1984), xiv.

23

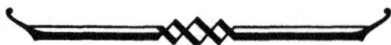

Judith Johnson

To accomplish great things,
  we must not only act,
  but also dream,
  not only plan,
  but also believe.

—Anatole France

Living with cancer . . . most people in the medical establishment 20 years ago considered such a concept unique. Cancer was something you died from. Or cancer was something you cured. But it wasn't an illness that people lived with.

About 20 years ago, however, I had two very good friends diagnosed with cancer. Their illnesses were serious. They understood they would probably die from the cancer. But in the meantime, they realized that they also had to live with that cancer. And as I watched both of these women, I realized how difficult a time they were having—not just because of the illness, but because of their lack of information and resources. They didn't understand what was going on. Their families weren't prepared to deal with the cancer. And no one knew how to talk about it. Support groups were almost nonexistent at that time, and I couldn't help but wonder what could be done to help my friends and their families deal with this situation.

My friends' experiences piqued my interest in this subject. I conducted an exhaustive search and found no type of existing educational program for them, even though they felt strongly that, had there been some type of education or support available, their cancer experience would have been made easier.

The Gap in Cancer Education Becomes Apparent

At the time, I was a nursing instructor teaching pathophysiology at Mounds-Midway School of Nursing and working with students in the cardiac intensive care unit. I was quite focused on cardiac care and had intended to pursue that nursing specialty. I was also beginning graduate work at the University of Minnesota with the intent of someday getting a master's degree in public health nursing. This was in the early 1970s, and the topic of death and dying was coming to the forefront. Everyone had read Kübler-Ross's material, including me, and most were thinking about cancer from a death-and-dying perspective. But I had two friends who were still living, and they were struggling to find the tools that would help them live more successfully during that time. Their experiences provided the incentive to send me in the direction of cancer care.

Thanks to more and better treatment options, people were living longer with cancer. They needed concrete information and support to help them adapt to a life with cancer. An independent study that addressed the sexual concerns of cancer patients and their spouses, a research study that proposed teaching nursing students specific aspects of cancer nursing, and the opportunity to work with a cancer support group at the University of Minnesota Hospital were all experiences that helped me gain further insights into the problems and concerns of cancer patients.

By 1976 I was considering potential doctoral thesis topics, having completed my master's degree and the major portion of my doctoral studies. I needed a topic that combined my major field of study in adult education with my minor in community health. It seemed logical to pursue my interest in cancer and try to design a health education course for people who needed to learn to live with a chronic illness.

To prepare myself, I began studying the role of patient education in other chronic diseases, specifically diabetes. I soon learned that diabetic patient education was a well-established discipline where people attended a series of classes to learn about their illness. Studies showed that educated patients felt more in control and were more compliant because they had a better understanding of their disease. I wondered: why couldn't this same philosophy be transferred and applied toward living with other chronic illnesses?

My intent was to develop a course that could be adapted to any chronic illness, but because I needed a definitive population for my research, I chose cancer patients as my subjects. My two friends had planted "the seed of need" in my brain, and I felt compelled to follow that path. I was already connected to the American Cancer Society in a volunteer capacity, serving on various committees and boards.

Gathering People and Resources to Research the Concept

One of the principles of adult education is that an advisory board of users should always be integral to the development of any program. I couldn't just arbitrarily decide what cancer patients needed to know. I needed a group of experts in the field to help me assess the educational needs. In this case, those experts were cancer patients themselves. So my first step was to contact North Memorial Medical Center, since they had one of the few established cancer support groups. Not only did this group exist, but I soon learned that they were a very strong and active group. Once I discovered this, my hope was to solicit their help by asking them to become my advisory board.

Pat Norby, cofounder of I CAN COPE, was one of the people who facilitated the Share and Care support group. She also was the nurse responsible for administering most of the chemotherapy at that hospital. She knew this group of people well, and I enlisted her help. Pat was instantly excited about the potential for such an educational program. We developed a partnership, she as a member inside the institution, and me operating as a graduate student on the outside. Together we sketched out an outline of what would be included in the course. We took the idea before the physician group, administration, and other hospital personnel to garner support.

What DO People with Cancer Need to Know?

We were on our way! But our next step was a critical one: determining exactly what people with cancer wanted and needed to know. To accomplish this, I conducted a large needs assessment, a series of questions that I asked a diverse group of people—those who were newly diagnosed, those who were living with cancer, those who were considered cured, and friends and/or relatives of people who had recently died from cancer. After questioning more than 100 people, some patterns started to develop, which were compiled into 15 general topical areas. I presented these topics to the advisory board of patients and asked them to prioritize the topics so I would know how to organize the course content.

Communication: The Number One Area of Interest

Interestingly enough, their number one topic was "how to talk to my doctor and/or family." Communication. To this day, communication is still a primary concern and one of the most difficult areas to cover in I CAN COPE classes. People didn't understand what their doctors were saying, and they were too intimidated by the doctors to admit their lack of understanding and learn how to ask intelligent questions. With friends and family, patients became emotional and tongue-tied. They were afraid and found it difficult to talk honestly about frightening topics such as pain, fear, abandonment, and death.

Thanks to the important input of the advisory board, communication became a key factor in the design of I CAN COPE. We attempted to weave some aspect of communication into every course session. For instance, the terminology matching sheet in session 1 is designed to acquaint patients with medical terms frequently used by their doctors. By using these terms throughout the classes, people become familiar with the words and their meanings.

Class Design: Factual Information
Before Emotional Issues

As I approached the design of the class format, one key element seemed very important. I needed to get people comfortable with one another before moving into sensitive issues that involved group sharing of feelings and emotions. For this reason, most of the factual information about cancer and its treatment was built into the first three classes: what is cancer? what treatments are available? what are the potential side effects? and what can you do about them? I hoped that within this nonthreatening educational framework, class participants would slowly become comfortable with one another and would be ready for the more emotional issues like intimacy and self-esteem.

In most cases, history has shown this philosophy to be sound. By the fifth or sixth class, most participants are able to discuss topics that are more emotional and don't necessarily center on black or white issues.

As course content began to take shape, I realized that very little resource material existed for use in cancer patient education. I spent a lot of time exploring libraries, bookstores, film libraries, and any other places where I could get ideas for visual aids to supplement the teaching materials. I didn't want this course to be a series of lectures. I wanted to get people interacting, both with one another and with their environment. As materials were developed, the advisory board of patients gave their input as to appropriateness and readability.

Guest Speakers Become a Key Course Component

I felt strongly that the teaching of the course, for the most part, should be conducted by experts in the field. For this reason, I enlisted the help of physicians, nurses, and other specialists as resource people. In most cases, the resource people responsible for developing class content became the original instructors. Today, the newly revised I CAN COPE materials continue to recommend using professionals as course instructors: physicians to teach medical facts, nurses and nutritionists to teach side effects and symptom management, therapists to teach communication and sexuality, and a wide variety of resource people (lawyers, estate planners) to teach ancillary living skills.

The demonstration project was really taking shape now, and Pat and I were getting excited about actually testing it out with patients. In November of 1976 I approached the board of directors of the American Cancer Society, Minnesota division, and asked if they would provide funding for AV equipment and materials to support the project. Everett Schmidt, M.D., then president of the board, chose my concept as his "president's project," and provided $3,175 to fund a demonstration project in cancer patient education. By January of 1977 the pilot program was designed, funded, and ready to launch as a research study.

Learning to Live with Cancer: Is the Topic Significant Enough to Earn a Ph.D.?

Just as my dream was about to be launched, my bubble was about to burst in the academic community. The review board responsible for approving my thesis proposal was not convinced that it was an appropriate research topic. It seemed they didn't believe it was a significant enough project to warrant a doctoral degree. Today I can smile about it in light of the tremendous success of the program. But at the time, I was devastated.

I tried to analyze why the committee rejected my proposal, and my hunch was that they perceived cancer patients as people who are dying, and they couldn't understand why I would want to design a course for living with cancer. The dominant view of people with cancer at that time was not at all positive. And this was a topic never before addressed in adult education. This committee was accustomed to looking at more global issues within formal educational structures such as academic institutions. This cancer education program was being held in a hospital, and it was a much more personal approach to education than they had experienced. I believe the committee was leery of approving a Ph.D. in such a new area. On a certain level, I could understand their thinking, even though the rejection was very frustrating.

Despite the rejection, this project had a life of its own, and I was committed to seeing it through regardless of where I ended up academically. But the fact that the committee had labeled it "not significant" kept eating at me. My advisor and I sat down and rewrote some of the material to make the statistical design tighter, then resubmitted it to the committee. Fortunately, they approved the proposal after the second submission, and I was elated. This was truly a day of celebration!

Designing the Research to Measure Course Effectiveness

In January of 1977 I started collecting the data. With Pat's help, we recruited 52 people to participate in the research. All of them were adult outpatients who had been diagnosed with or had had a recurrence of cancer within that year. They were invited to enroll in a course where they would learn about cancer and were told that this course was part of a research project (Johnson, 1982). A key factor in this research was the job of assessing changes in people's knowledge and attitudes—specifically, their general knowledge of cancer, anxiety level because of the cancer, and overall meaning in life. This was based on literature suggesting that if people are vulnerable and anxious, they lose a sense of the meaning and/or purpose in life.

After Pat and I completed the program content, I went through the materials and assembled a set of questions based on the course, called the Course Inquiry, which was intended to test the patients' knowledge of cancer and its ramifications. I chose a second instrument, the Purpose in Life (PIL) to measure the effect the course had on participants' meaning in life. Spielberger's State Anxiety Test was used to measure participants' anxiety levels. All the participants were given these three questionnaires in January–February and again after the treatment group had completed the course.

Using this precourse baseline data, the participants were then paired. In a paired design, two people are matched using the scores from their questionnaires. This creates a similarity between the two groups, which eliminates the possibility of one group being totally mellow and the other being overly anxious. After identifying 26 pairs, I flipped a coin, and one-half of the pair was randomly assigned either to a treatment group or to a control group.

In April the "treatment group" began attending eight classes of what was then titled, "What Will I Do? Learning to Live With Cancer." We kept close track of this group—what people were absent from class and when. Interestingly enough, we had one class member die during the class series. He was not someone who was expected to die; his prognosis for his type of cancer had been good. He was an artist, a relatively young man, who was really engaged in the process of living and learning about his cancer. But he had a sudden recurrence, and he died of complications. I was concerned that his death would heighten the anxiety level of the class.

What we learned, and continue to learn at I CAN COPE classes across the nation, is that the group can generally handle a death well. This group talked about it openly. One week after he died, his wife came to class and brought a recent piece of his artwork that showed a long road going off into the distance. You couldn't see the end of the road. It was very poignant and meaningful to all of us. It was as if he was giving the group his final message.

Comparing the "Treatment" Group to the "Control" Group

In the week between the April treatment group finishing class and the May control group starting class, all the study participants were retested using the same three questionnaires. Results showed that the persons attending the April class reported an increase in their knowledge of cancer, more meaning in life, and a decrease in their anxiety.

What I didn't anticipate was that the control group would also register changes. I assumed their retest scores would be basically the same as the scores from their original testing in January. To my amazement, their anxiety level had gone up a bit, their meaning in life had gone down, and their knowledge about cancer had stayed about the same.

The differences in the test scores between the treatment group and control group turned out to be highly significant. In fact, it was so significant that the committee questioned the validity of the results.

Is It the Course? Or Is It More Than That?

I can't claim that the results were totally due to the educational focus of the course. We know that the benefit of mutual support is hard to measure, and at this time, support groups were almost nonexistent. But I have to believe that much of the decreased anxiety and increased meaning in life was due to the camaraderie participants found in being with others engaged in a similar struggle. For whatever reason, the results did look suspect because across the board they were so strongly significant. To satisfy my own curiosity, over the next couple of years as the course was held, I continued testing people prior to starting the course and again after its completion. Results consistently showed a drop in anxiety along with an increase in both knowledge of cancer and meaning in life. That made me feel more comfortable about the verity of the original results. These differences in test scores provided significant evidence, to my mind, that an organized patient education course can help people acquire knowledge that facilitates their adaptation to living with a chronic illness, specifically cancer.

The Course Is Born—Now It Needed a Name

The original course title, "What Will I Do? Learning to Live with Cancer," seemed too long and cumbersome. We felt a short, descriptive title, something that would address the negative stigma assigned to the word *cancer*, was needed. Interestingly enough, COPE was the name of a deodorant at that time. Pat and I and one of our patients were on a long car trip traveling to a speaking engagement and started kicking around course title ideas. We felt the *can* in cancer could symbolize the powerful message within the word: you *can* make this illness manageable if you are willing to take a large problem and break it apart. What *can* you do? You *can* cope. And so the title was born.

I CAN COPE Grows and Expands

We knew I CAN COPE would work in a large, metropolitan setting. But what about small-town America? Marvyl Patton, a cancer survivor and social worker, assumed the challenge of piloting the program in Waseca, Minnesota, a small farming community with a 35-bed hospital. Together with her Make Today Count support group, Marvyl adapted the program to her environment. The tremendous response to the course showed that it could work equally well in a small-town setting.

In the summer of 1977, the Minnesota division of the American Cancer Society provided funding of $20,000 to assist in the total packaging of the course material for mass distribution. Pat and I worked with Gene Sylvester and Associates to put together a package which contained a teaching manual, participant handbooks, filmstrips, tapes, handout materials, and an evaluation packet. Representatives from 184 Minnesota hospitals were trained, and in 1978 I CAN COPE was launched statewide in Minnesota.

I CAN COPE Goes National
After a Minnesota Beginning

In May of 1978 Pat and I traveled to the 14th annual meeting of the American Society of Clinical Oncology (ASCO) and the 5th annual meeting of the Oncology Nursing Society (ONS). This was the first national presentation made after the initiation of the pilot project. To our delight, the response to the program was overwhelming. Nurses in particular immediately starting asking to see course materials. The persistence of this nationwide body of professionals was truly the driving force behind the American Cancer Society's recognition that I CAN COPE had nationwide applicability. In 1979 the national office of ACS officially adopted the program, to be distributed by the service and rehabilitation department. Pat and I worked with the regional offices of ACS to train facilitators throughout the country.

Traveling Nationally and Internationally for
I CAN COPE

From the program's inception, I have always believed that the cancer patient is the best person to describe the benefits of I CAN COPE from a personal perspective. For that reason, wherever Pat and I went, we insisted that a patient travel with us. In most cases, the patients' stories ended up being the highlight of our presentations. Much thanks goes to Boehringer-Ingelheim, Inc., a drug company that also believed in this concept and frequently covered our expenses as we traveled around the country to teach others about I CAN COPE.

By the time the program was 15 years old, more than a half million people had been served in more than 50 ACS divisions nationwide. When the package was displayed as part of the American Cancer Society exhibit at the International Cancer Congress in Buenos Aires, Argentina, I CAN COPE had officially gone international. Since then, the program has been audited by people from several other countries and is being presented or talked about in Canada, England, Ireland, Israel, the Netherlands, Australia, Sweden, Norway, Switzerland, and Japan. South Africa has put the entire course on videotape. A physician from the area of the Soviet Union where the Chernobyl accident took place has been visiting Minnesota and attending training sessions so she can adapt I CAN COPE for use in her country.

The Program Premieres in Book Form

In 1983 Linda Klein came to me with the idea of writing a book about I CAN COPE. I could see this as a natural vehicle for taking the message of I CAN COPE out of the classroom and into people's homes. After several years of working closely with patients and studying course material, we finally had the first book ready, and it was published in 1988. Five years later, Linda and I once again worked with patients and updated the book using more current material. The second edition of *I Can Cope: Staying Healthy With Cancer,* published by Chronimed Publishing, was released in February 1994.

I CAN COPE Stands the Test of Time

In 1991, the American Cancer Society conducted a large national evaluative study of I CAN COPE (McMillan, 1993). The findings showed that the goals, objectives, and basic overall framework of the program had stood the test of time. A large national revision work group then completely dissected the program, taking out elements that were outdated, bringing audiovisual materials up to date, and adding components that involved more individual patient participation and self-care strategies. We even inserted relaxation and imagery exercises, complete with an audiotape of relaxation music. I CAN COPE was now updated to fit a 1990s lifestyle!

I CAN COPE—The Concepts

Cancer as a Chronic Illness

Up until this time, cancer was something you died from, not something you lived with. I believe I CAN COPE opened the doors for a more open discussion. By giving people an opportunity to get together and learn, we also gave them hope—hope that they could go on with their lives in a productive manner, regardless of time constraints.

Knowledge Is Power

An overriding aspect of learning you have cancer is a feeling of powerlessness. The medical establishment assumes control of your treatment plan. The disease assumes control of your body. What is left to the patient's control? By giving the patient a thorough understanding of the illness, I CAN COPE leads people toward self-care skills: proper nutrition; honest communication with doctors, family, and friends; stress management; pain control; relaxation skills; and survival strategies. Armed with this knowledge, and the supportive environment of other cancer survivors, quality of life naturally should follow—and in most cases, it does.

No Two People Are Alike; No Two Cancers Are Alike—Cancer Is More Than One Disease

In the beginning, doctors were sometimes hesitant to send patients to I CAN COPE because they felt it would be damaging for patients to compare stories. They were worried that someone with a good prognosis might leave the class depressed because someone with a similar diagnosis was doing poorly.

In the classes, we stress that cancer is actually more than 100 different diseases, and even the exact same type of cancer affects individuals in totally different ways. Sometimes I don't think we give cancer patients enough credit for the wisdom, strength, and determination they exhibit after their diagnoses. Most people are anxious for knowledge and are capable of assimilating the bad with the good.

I CAN COPE—The People

Nothing in the whole experience has been more gratifying than watching the various players who participated in the growth of this program, starting with the original advisory board. I truly believe that the reason the course design has worked so successfully through the years is because this board was constantly involved during the evolution process. This group of eight individuals was very committed and took great ownership. As a representative sample of the various types of cancer—breast, testicular, melanoma, myeloma, lung—they realistically voiced the needs of all cancer patients.

The first group of graduates from the pilot program also became strong advocates and lobbied vocally for increased funding and support for I CAN COPE. One of the patients owned an audio-visual company. He often expressed appreciation for what he learned from the program, and when he died, his family donated a very expensive video machine to be used in pictorially documenting I CAN COPE. This kind of support contributed greatly to its success.

And finally, every person who has been through the course represents a success for Pat and me—success in that we have made a difference in that person's life by giving them tools to go forward and live a life of high quality, despite their chronic illness. Probably my ultimate joy was helping to take care of former Senator Hubert Humphrey prior to his death. We had many conversations about I CAN COPE, and although he was too ill to attend the course at the time, he did make contact with the National Cancer Institute to suggest that they pursue a similar path in terms of patient education.

In 1978, after Humphrey's death, Pat and I met with his wife, then-Senator Muriel Humphrey, at her office in Washington, D.C. In the Congressional Record of May 15, 1978, she inserted the following words supportive of I CAN COPE: "We must remember that these types of beginnings need nurturing, so that in time they may come to fruition for all of our people."

The growth of I CAN COPE—from infancy to an internationally-recognized program—is undoubtedly the experience that gives me the most pride when I look back on my years in the field of oncology nursing, and one which I believe has enhanced the lives of thousands of cancer patients.

References

Johnson, Judi. "The Effect of a Patient Education Course on Persons with a Chronic Illness," *Cancer Nursing*, Vol. 5 (April, 1982):117–123.

McMillan, Susan C., Mary B. Tittle, and Dawn Hill. "A Systematic Evaluation of the I CAN COPE Program Using a National Sample." *Oncology Nursing Forum*, Vol. 20, No. 3 (1993), pp. 455–461.

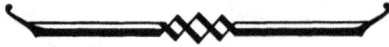

24

Susan A. Leigh

The year was 1960 and Sister Mary Elizabeth assigned the students in my eighth grade class to look into the future and write their autobiographies. An added challenge was that the final page had to have a physical shape to it, one that would illustrate our chosen profession. For me, this would be easy. After years of pre-adolescent research and introspection, I had already decided by the age of 13 what direction my life would take. And it even had a shape—a nurse's cap.

My "years of research" started in the fifth grade as I scoured the library for every Cherry Ames and Sue Barton novel I could find. Their lives were so exciting! Each story found these untiring young women in different exotic locations doing different kinds of nursing. They were nurses on horseback or skis, in jeeps or boats. They worked medical miracles, solved crimes, traveled to foreign countries, and could always get a job. The title of *nurse* was equated with heroism, romance, and mystery, and the world was at their disposal. That's what I wanted to be. Being a nurse would be my ticket to adventure. So off to nursing school I went, and an adventure it has been.

My nursing career started at the University of Arizona in Tucson. It was the mid-1960s, and I left a protected family environment and a tiny Catholic high school to attend a college that had a larger population than my entire hometown. I no longer felt like a big fish in a small pond but rather like a tadpole in an ocean, and I was often overwhelmed. Not only were the school and city full of challenges and distractions, but our country was then in the midst of a controversial war that personally affected many in my age group. The social situation was impossible to ignore.

While nursing school challenged me both academically and socially, I also found myself challenged financially. It was during my junior year that I was introduced to the army student nurse program, and it seemed like an interesting alternative to more student loans. Within a week of merely sending away for information, I found an army recruiter on the doorstep of my dormitory with some very appealing offers.

As the war in Vietnam had been a major strain on the army nurse corps, the military was desperate for new recruits. Graduate nurses fresh out of school were targeted to fill many open slots both stateside and overseas. With my limited experiences at that point in my life, I figured that no matter where I was sent, I wouldn't have been there before. Thus, it would be an adventure. And I could always hope for an assignment other than Vietnam. While many nurses joined the army with the singular intent to go to Vietnam, I readily admit that I was not one of those individuals. So after many months of deliberation, I signed up.

Getting through my senior year was then much easier. Not only were my school expenses covered by the army, but I also had medical benefits and privileges at the local air force base. I had a monthly paycheck, money to pay for a car, and a job after graduation. I had no aspirations to specialize in any aspect of nursing at that point, and coming from a baccalaureate program, I felt I needed a good deal of general, practical, on-the-job training. That was exactly what I got.

After basic training in San Antonio, I was sent to Letterman Army Hospital in San Francisco—a dream assignment as long as I stayed away from the antimilitary Haight-Ashbury district. As a second lieutenant, affectionately known as "butter bars," my first duty as a graduate nurse was caring for patients on the neuromedical/neurosurgical ward. Many of these young men had spinal cord injuries from the war or from stateside accidents, and were para- and quadraplegics on Cir-O-Lectic® beds. With my limited clinical experience, I found myself in the capable hands of veteran corpsmen who helped me learn how to draw blood, insert IVs, and master the mechanical devices on this particular unit. Dealing with the psychological trauma was even more of a challenge than the physical. Yet I flourished in my new profession as I learned the technical and interpersonal skills that helped me to feel like a real nurse. Looking out at the Golden Gate Bridge every morning from the eighth floor solarium, I wondered how long my luck could hold out. I really enjoyed this assignment, and loved living in the Bay Area and working in this hospital. But my luck ended after eight months.

My orders to Vietnam came in May of 1970, and within a month I was on my way to Southeast Asia. I was so socially naive and inexperienced that my initial fear was not necessarily of the war, but rather of surviving the incredibly unbalanced male–female ratio! While some nurses felt like it was a dream come true, I considered it a nightmare. And with a name like Lieutenant Leigh (pronounced *lay!*), what I really needed was a sense of humor.

The year that I spent in the Mekong Delta at the 3rd surgical hospital is a story unto itself. I don't think anyone or anything can prepare a person for a war zone, and many of us were so young that we had limited life experiences to help us cope. Needless to say, it was the major challenge of my life up to that point, professionally and personally. It was a year of extremes—exhausting, exhilarating, frustrating, and challenging. I can't say that I wish I had never gone to Vietnam. I can say, though, that I wish the war had never happened, and that our politicians and military should learn how to deal with conflict in a different way.

No one returned unchanged. By the time I came home a year later and had completed my obligation to the army, I had serious doubts about whether or not I even wanted to be a nurse anymore. The reality of war had stripped me of my innocence and idealism, and military priorities were the antithesis of my hopes and beliefs. I needed time to regain some energy, heal my spirit, and do some major decision making. So I sold my 1965 red Mustang (what I wouldn't give for that car today!) and bought a Volkswagen bus. I was thinking that I wanted to slow down, smell the roses, savor the sights and sounds, and bask in the beauty of the world around me. I couldn't rush past anything in a Volkswagen. So I packed up the family dog and headed out for mini-adventures. I traveled around the western United States, camped, took photographs, visited friends and relatives, and felt a sense of freedom unlike anything I had experienced before. I had paid my dues, so I thought, and I was cruising.

Emotionally, I felt better every day. But physically was a different story. I seemed to get more tired and short of breath, was pale, and had a constant, irritating cough. To satisfy my mother, I went to the local veteran's hospital in my hometown for a check-up where they drew some blood and suggested I go to physical therapy for the knots in my shoulders. I downplayed my symptoms and attributed them to exhaustion from the past year, and the outpatient doctor agreed with me that nothing was wrong that rest couldn't cure. Of course, that's what I wanted to hear. So I continued cruising until I ran out of money and had to start thinking about working again. Meanwhile, the love of my life had returned from Vietnam, and I went to visit him at an army post down south. This was February of 1972.

While dancing into the wee hours of the morning to the newly released album *American Pie*, I noticed that it was extremely hard for me to breathe. I felt so out of shape as I stuggled for air and coughed. And then out came a small amount of blood-tinged mucous. A repeated incident prompted a chest X-ray at the local army hospital which showed a large mediastinal mass and left hilar adenopathy with left pulmonary parenchymal involvement. One look at that X-ray had my physician boyfriend convinced that I was in big trouble, and he had me on a plane home that night. I was immediately sent to the veteran's hospital in

Tucson, and after three long weeks of tests and multiple examinations, I was finally diagnosed with nodular sclerosing Hodgkin's disease.

During these three weeks of work-up, the chest X-rays from my discharge physical seven months prior were retrieved from the army. They had been read as negative, yet showed obvious disease. I thus had grounds to petition for a retroactive medical discharge, and to receive all care through government hospitals. So I was transferred from Tucson to the Palo Alto VA which was affiliated with Stanford University Hospital, and I began a journey that would impact my life even more than Vietnam had.

Having survived an external war, I was then thrust into an internal one. I wasn't ready for this. My nursing textbooks said Hodgkin's disease was terminal, and in fact my maternal grandfather had died from Hodgkin's disease at the age of 36. The patients with cancer for whom I cared as a student had all died. Yet one of my best friends in Vietnam was diagnosed with this very same disease right after I had returned stateside. Could we have caught the disease from each other? Was there something in the environment? No one seemed to know or even care to speculate. Anyway, he had received a new form of treatment called chemotherapy. Even though it was too early to tell how he would do, there was at least a spark of hope for me.

Fortunately, the physicians who were in this war with me were some of the leading experts in the treatment of this form of cancer. Remember, this was 1972. Hodgkin's disease was one of the first malignancies to be treated with potentially curative high-energy radiation therapy and multidrug chemotherapy. So, under the circumstances, I was in the right place at the right time. There was, though, disagreement as to the stage of my disease. While no disease was discovered below the diaphragm, the majority of the oncologists decided to treat me as a stage IV because of the extranodal disease in the lung. Yet I was probably a II-a-e. I then underwent six cycles of MOPP (mechlorethamine, vincristine, procarbazine, prednisone) and total nodal radiation to shrink the large masses before beginning X-ray therapy. The mantle radiation that followed totalled 4,400 rads with 2,000 rads given to the left lung due to the parenchymal involvement. Suboptimal treatment was delivered to the remaining "inverted Y" fields (para-aortic, splenic, and pelvic) due to thrombocytopenia and leukopenia from the prior chemotherapy. It was a long and difficult year, and besides losing half my hair, a lot of weight, my ovarian function, and most of my self-esteem, I also lost my boyfriend. After therapy was discontinued, I felt and appeared much sicker, both physically and psychologically, than I had when I was diagnosed. As the multiple losses had taken their toll on both my body and my spirit, I began the period of "watchful waiting" and anticipated recovery. This is when I really started to learn what it was like to be a survivor. As I could write a separate story about my year in Vietnam, so too could I write a separate story about my year undergoing treatment for my cancer.

Oncology fellowships at the time were brand new, and this special training for physicians was as much trial-and-error as was my survival journey. The doctors gave me my chemotherapy (what a scary thought!) at the VA, and radiation technicians treated me at Stanford. Nurses cared for me on the wards, but generally did not have a clue as to how to support me, medically or emotionally. There were two nurses in Tucson who spent time with me and prodded me to talk about my cancer, but that was it. I think it was especially difficult for most of the nurses since I was a young female in a hospital system primarily for older males, and on top of that, someone who had a disease that was historically terminal. There were no specially trained social workers either, so support was hit-and-miss, if at all, and I remember feeling tremendously isolated. My main contact was with physicians, and they were so optimistic and hopeful about my potential cure that I found it difficult to express my fears or concerns. When I cried after I found out I would be sterile after therapy, a physician said to me, "We're going to cure you. What more do you want?" There was little understanding of the need to grieve, to deal with physical and emotional changes, or to live with anxiety, fear, and uncertainty. The only measure of success at that time was longevity and cure, and it took me years to understand the complexity of recovery. What I did realize after all those months was that this new specialty, the treatment of cancer, had a tremendous need for nurses who were willing to listen and who would attempt to understand the issues beyond medical treatment. I decided that this was where I belonged profession-ally—eventually.

My physical recovery took over a year once treatment stopped. My blood counts stayed below normal for a couple of years, and I never completed the abdominal radiation therapy. But my emotional recovery was an ongoing process. Days of sheer joy were interspersed with days of depression. As my priorities had so drastically changed, it was often difficult to relate to my old friends or feel comfortable socially with new ones. At times I felt old beyond my years, yet there was also a childlike feeling of wonderment and exhilaration for every new day. Life was miraculous, but often very confusing.

Around this time, my friends from nursing school were pursuing graduate degrees, so I thought I would give it a try and utilize the GI bill. I was disappointed that there was no advanced degree in oncology, and I was disinterested in the general med/surg course work. While I was struggling with school, I had a real scare which hospitalized me for a possible recurrence of my Hodgkin's disease. When I found out that my abdominal pain was not liver involvement but a false alarm, I once again reevaluated my priorities and decided that graduate school was not worth the aggravation. That is when I received an offer that seemed too good to be true.

My oncologist at that time, Dr. Stephen Jones, was assistant director of the new hematology/oncology program at the University of Arizona Medical Center. Two nurses had been working with this new group over the past year, and they needed another part-time RN to help with research protocols and to give chemotherapy. I was offered the position and I grabbed it. This is exactly what I wanted to do professionally, and I felt that my personal experiences could do nothing but enhance my on-the-job training. My heart and soul went into my work. Contrary to everything I had been taught in nursing school, I established close bonds with many of my patients, many that turned into friendships. Life seemed to have meaning again, and I made myself available to anyone who needed to talk. After all, we could "swap war stories," as Dr. Jones would often say. Meanwhile, a lot of energy was going out of me, but not enough was being returned. In less than three years, I burned out.

Looking back upon those early years in oncology nursing, I realized that I was as needy as many of my patients. They gave to me just as much as I gave to them, and that was probably my first peer support network. I had difficulty understanding how the other nurses could be so strong, and many of the physicians felt I was hypochondriacal when it came to my own health and overemotional when it came to my patients. Yet it was beyond me how people could *not* be emotional working in an area such as this. On the one hand our society was just starting to talk about death and dying, while on the other hand we were developing entirely different expectations for survival. Death was seen as failure.

The death of a young single mother from recurrent Hodgkin's disease was the "straw that broke the camel's back" for me. Leticia was extremely needle-phobic. I worked hard using relaxation techniques to calm her so that I could get a needle threaded into her damaged veins in order to deliver chemotherapy. Then she recurred for yet a third time, and eventually died leaving behind a five-year-old daughter. I was not only sad, but I was also scared to see someone so young die of the same disease that I had had. No one knew what to say to me. Since I had cried after being with Leticia when she heard the news, rumor had it that I couldn't control my emotions, and that I should be kept away from patients. I decided it was time to leave.

Healing happens on many different levels and can last for months, years, or even a lifetime. It was good for me to be away from oncology altogether at that point because I still had so many issues to deal with myself. One psychologist suggested that there were counterphobic elements to my working with cancer patients, and that maybe I should pursue another specialty area. Yet after some psychotherapy, a lot of serious thought, and a year away from hospitals, I seemed to be drawn back to oncology. But my role would be somewhat different this time.

I spent the next five and a half years doing pharmacokinetic research studies, and spent anywhere from 24 to 72 hours with patients and their families. The time spent with my study subjects was intense but brief, so I was better able to limit my involvement and I saw less death. Then something happened that shook my foundation again.

Two of my former Hodgkin's disease patients became ill with leukemia and died very suddenly. We had all received combination chemotherapy and radiation therapy, and knew that leukemia was a risk factor. But when it actually happened to two of my favorite patients, I was terrified. Even though I knew that their diseases had been more extensive and aggressive than mine, and that they had both received more treatment than I had, it was still very difficult to separate their situations from mine. So I lost two more wonderful friends and a little bit more security. Feeling so vulnerable, I left oncology nursing once again.

Perhaps I should have learned a lesson through all this and stayed away from this particular nursing specialty. I did take some more time for myself, a year to be exact, to travel and think and heal and read Richard Bolles' *What Color Is My Parachute* to help me figure out what to do. But all my searching led me back to oncology. As I made the determination that this was where my heart and soul resided, another job offer came from the cancer center. This time it was in the division of cancer prevention and control (CPC), and I would set up and monitor prevention studies. My friend and colleague Lois Loescher not only offered me the job, but would be my supervisor. This was the beginning of an extraordinary chapter for me, both personally and professionally.

My working life was somewhat synchronized with my survival journey. I started out in a very acute care setting surrounded by illness and therapy, and then gradually made the transition to more relaxed and less emotionally intense work. While my cancer history would always be a part of me, I was continually learning how to incorporate it into my life and benefit from my experiences, especially where work was concerned. While CPC studies allowed me flexibility and occupied my time, I never quite felt passionate about this area of oncology, and I missed interacting with cancer patients. When Debi McCaffrey (Boyle) called to see if I would like to attend a meeting in New Mexico to explore issues concerning cancer survivors, I excitedly jumped at the opportunity.

Debi was not only an oncology clinical nurse specialist in Phoenix, but she was (and is) a renowned public speaker who was in great demand. Due to her hectic schedule and prior engagements, she was unable to attend this meeting, and asked if I would be interested in going in her place. I remember wanting to scream, "Cancer survivors! Someone is seriously interested in cancer survivors?" I could hardly contain myself. You bet I wanted to go. And off I went to Albuquerque in October 1986.

There were about 22 of us from all walks of life and from all age groups sitting around a table. Many represented national or grassroots organizations, and about half of us were actually cancer survivors. Over the weekend we found ourselves discussing a vast array of issues pertaining to life after cancer and the diverse experiences and interests we brought to the meeting. We celebrated the increasing numbers of people living beyond their diagnosis and treatment, and yet were concerned about problems that continued for years after going off therapy. Besides biomedical complications, we identified issues such as limited psychosocial support, lack of information, uninformed consumerism, insurance problems, employment discrimination, living with chronic anxiety, limited access to state-of-the-art treatment, health maintenance, and the lack of survivorship-related research. It was felt that the medical profession was not concerned enough with quality of life issues for adults with cancer, and specifically for long-term survivors. Also, limited resources were being wasted in duplicating efforts to develop supportive programs, publications, and networks around the country, and there was no specific organization that was coordinating these efforts and advocating for adults with cancer. We thus identified the need for a national organization, and the National Coalition for Cancer Survivorship (NCCS) was born.

At that first meeting I sat among some really incredible people: Cathy Logan who started Living Through Cancer, a community-based support organization in Albuquerque, and who was responsible for pulling this meeting together; Fitzhugh Mullan who had authored a book about his cancer journey entitled *Vital Signs,* had published a wonderful article in the *New England Journal of Medicine* entitled "Seasons of Survival," and was the co-host of this gathering; Michael Lerner who ran Commonweal, a week-long support program in Northern California, and was a leading proponent for integrating alternative and conventional modalities; Harold Benjamin who started the Wellness Center in Santa Monica and had just published *From Victim to Victor;* Neil Fiore, a psychologist and survivor who authored the book *The Road Back to Health;* Dr. Paticia Ganz who was a pioneer in the area of oncology rehabilitation; and many others who had started their own community hotlines and organizations, along with representatives from a number of national organizations, including ONS. I sat there in awe, and in silence.

I concentrated on every discussion, and was overwhelmed with the energy, enthusiasm, and expertise in the room. These people were talking a language that I thought only went on in my own head. Over the years as I had mentioned some of my concerns to physicians and nurses, I had often found myself patronized, ignored, or labeled a hypochondriac. But here was a roomful of people validating these thoughts that I had learned to keep to myself, and I really got excited. But what would I now do with this information?

When I returned to work and talked so enthusiastically about my weekend, Lois could not have been a better ally. She sensed the importance of this issue and set up a meeting with the CPC leadership. Dr. Frank Meyskens willingly gave us free rein to study the issues and develop some sort of program. With a small grant, we went to work reviewing the literature on long-term and late effects of therapy, and developed an instrument to assess the impact that cancer had on survivors. Debi McCaffrey and others worked on these projects with us, and both were published, one in the *Annals of Internal Medicine* and the other in the *Oncology Nursing Forum*. After two years of pulling the necessary information together, an adult long-term follow-up clinic was proposed with both physiological and psychosocial components, much like pediatric survivor clinics. It was an idea whose time had come, so we thought. But we were ahead of our time, and the proposal was not accepted. As my funding ran out, I suddenly found myself without a job.

It continually amazes me how disappointments can lead to challenges and opportunities. Before I found myself jobless, I had been introduced to another aspect of career development, once again via the mentorship of Debi McCaffrey. At the 1987 ONS Congress in Denver, Debi pulled together an instructional session on a topic new to the society. You guessed it: cancer survivors! What an experience for someone who had never spoken before a large crowd. The panel consisted of Debi as moderator; Fitzhugh Mullan, president of NCCS and a cancer survivor; LaMarr Bomaretto, a survivor of three separate cancers and leader in the Denver cancer community; and me. As I looked out over the crowd of approximately 2,000 nurses who came to our session, I was so nervous that I honestly thought I would lose bowel and bladder control. But I kept telling myself, "You can't be wrong, you can't be wrong. This is your own personal experience." After an emotional and tearful introduction by Debi, and a few moments of knocking knees, dry mouth, and quivering voice, I made it through the 20-minute presentation with flying colors and actually enjoyed the experience.

That presentation was the beginning of a new direction for me. I had discovered the power of the spoken word, and the usual shrinking violet blossomed on stage. I might have been nervous, but I covered it up and enjoyed the speaking and the response I received. My voice was heard, my self-confidence improved, and I was proud to speak on behalf of cancer survivors. After that, the invitations to speak snowballed, and I have been busy ever since. So when I realized that I would no longer have a job at the cancer center, it was Lois who believed in me and who encouraged me to do more speaking.

Another special mentor, colleague, and good friend has been Judi Johnson, the creator of the I CAN COPE program. Her intelligence, creativity, and generosity have made her a leader among leaders, and I have been fortunate to work with her and learn from her. As I delivered the Ciba-Geigy Quality of Life lecture at the 1992 fall institute—which, by the way, was the most incredible honor I have ever experienced professionally—I was thrilled to have Judi in the front of the audience. As she had been such an inspiration to me over the years, I felt stronger in her presence. As Judi was recovering from a stroke, I reminded her of the inspiring message shared by Karen Hassey Dow in her "Enduring Seasons of Survival" presentation: that we should not only aspire to survive, but to thrive.

Survivorship has been a topic at ONS ever since that 1987 session. After meeting informally for a number of years, we now have a focus group for nurse survivors and a special interest group (SIG) on survivorship. Every major meeting has sessions on survivorship-related topics, and much of the research in this important area will come from oncology nursing. Survivorship is not just about long-term survival. As Barbara Carter and others have written, it is about the process of living with, through, and beyond cancer. As such, it is an integral part of all oncology nursing.

With many new doors opening, I have become a consultant, lecturer, and writer with a very specific focus: survivorship. My good friend Lois has not only introduced me to computers, but she has encouraged me to write and to continue speaking. And NCCS has become a major part of my professional life as I have served three years as secretary, have chaired the speakers bureau, and am currently president. I find myself challenged on multiple levels, and am constantly learning from my survivor peers and colleagues.

An area that has been a major concern of mine over the past decade is the issue of late effects and the importance of systematic follow-up for long-term survivors of adult cancer. This type of follow-up is terribly inadequate in our current health care system, and may be an even greater challenge with impending changes. The voices of survivors themselves must be raised in unison to advocate for continued access to care, for choice in physicians, for continued funding for research and clinical trials, and for funding psychosocial support. I remain committed to the idea of continued follow-up now more than ever since I was diagnosed with cancer for a second time in December 1990.

No one can say for sure whether or not my prior therapy, specifically the radiation, played a part in the development of my recent breast cancer. But I am mightily suspicious since the single tumor was in the field that received an extra radiation boost due to parenchymal involvement. A number of articles have recently been published about the increased incidence of breast cancer in long-term survivors of Hodgkin's disease, and this strengthens the case for survivor clinics or programs, and continued, systematic follow-up. Our choices are also different because of our prior therapy, and each case must be assessed individually. There are no automatic formulas or answers for survivors with recurrences or multiple cancers. Because radiation was not an option for this second malignancy, and because the risk for contralateral disease was unknown, and because all the physicians conferring on my case agreed not to give me any more chemotherapy, and because I was node negative and not the best candidate for Tamoxifen (at least during the week this decision was made!), I decided—after *much* deliberation—to have bilateral mastectomies with immediate reconstruction.

Even though this was my second time around with cancer, and I have been an oncology nurse and patient advocate for many years, nothing about this experience was easy. I was more afraid than ever before. But once I got over the initial paralysis, I was able first to find the internal strength, and then the information and support that I needed to start making decisions. I knew most of the doctors that I needed. I called nurses who specialized in breast care. My family and friends were more experienced at being supportive this time. I sought out other breast cancer survivors and those who had experienced multiple cancers. I really understood the need to connect with others who "had been there." The only real glitch—and it was a distasteful one—was a major incompatibility with the plastic surgeon. My decision to have reconstruction piggybacked the silicone implant controversy, and my surgeon was somewhat less than pleased about me questioning his judgment, to say the least. But I did not feel comfortable with any decision at that point, and our relationship went from lukewarm to painfully frigid. I felt his interactions were verbally abusive, and I finally could not bring myself to return to his clinic. What began as a tantalizing option turned into a nightmare.

This is yet another story that could embellish this central one. But to make a long story short, it took me a year to figure out what to do so that I could feel comfortable with my decision. I refinanced my house, pulled out some extra cash, and found another plastic surgeon whom I adore. Without criticism or sarcasm my new doctor helped me review my options and supported my choice. He congratulated me for asking questions and being informed, and hugged me when we had the plan figured out. His kindness and compassion blended with his technical and artistic skills, and our continued relationship is mutually satisfying to us both. Meanwhile, my experiences with breast cancer have been an inconvenience—mind you, a major one. I have hardly skipped a beat though, and I have felt support from family, friends, colleagues, and fellow survivors unlike anything I ever imagined. Practice makes perfect, so they say. If nothing else, prior experience can surely be helpful.

The area of oncology is an exciting and satisfying place to be in our current society. I am continually struck by the ingenious ways we nurses create niches for ourselves so that we can be most effective in our work. We now have a whole cadre of enthusiastic cancer survivors who are ready and willing to advocate for themselves and for the health care community. I am proud to be an oncology nurse, and I am forever grateful 'or the opportunity to "give back" in whatever way I can.

Note

Cir-O-Lectric is a registered trademark of Stryker Corporation.

25

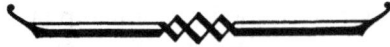

Jean Nelson Lonergan

My career in oncology started in 1981. As a new graduate I began working on a medical unit with overflow oncology patients. I was continuing my work toward a bachelor's degree and was working part time while I finished school. What was different about this unit was the sense of compassion and level of sincerity among my coworkers, but it was the patients themselves that sold me on oncology. My expectation was that this unit, and oncology in general, treated a primarily geriatric population and I had little experience being around the elderly; my grandparents had died while I was a youngster. What I found was an untapped source of strength, knowledge, and energy. The oncology patients' ability and struggle to deal with today, and their appreciation for life, invigorated me and actually gave me strength.

My first summer in nursing was indeed a challenge. Just being a "new graduate" and learning the necessary skills needed to be a nurse took most of my energy. I had wanted to be a nurse since I was a little girl, although no one in my family had been a nurse and I had had no exposure to the field. I just had this sense that nursing was the right field for me. (Growing up in a family of educators, many family friends told me I was destined to be a teacher. That part was certainly correct.) So each morning that summer I jumped out of bed and was so excited to put on my white uniform and cap.

There were a number of obstacles the unit faced that first summer. In this small community hospital, the word *oncology* had yet to be understood or defined. The unit was developing and trying to identify itself as a specialty area while justifying its value in a small community hospital. The challenges were numerous. Being identified as the "death unit" certainly brought comments from the unit staff and retention was a concern. Physicians other than oncologists were routinely ordering chemotherapy. Chemotherapy certification for nurses was just being initiated. And telling a patient he or she had cancer, or educating a patient and family regarding the disease, was definitely *not* considered a nursing function. While my friends and coworkers were supportive, many questioned my choice in specialties. Even my family couldn't quite understand my desire to work with "people who are dying." "How depressing," I heard over and over. But I found that the rewards easily outweighed the negatives. And I was just beginning.

Perhaps one of my incentives for working in oncology was the newness of this specialty. Or, it certainly may have been the challenge given to me by my college dean upon hearing I was transferring out of nursing to continue work on my bachelor's degree in another field. "This is a huge mistake. You'll never make a good nurse," she said. I was inspired to prove her wrong. I would become not only a good nurse, but a quality oncology nurse.

That first summer, I had the opportunity to meet Mark. He was young, in his 30s, with two small children and he was dying of lung cancer. He was the first patient I actually watched deteriorate before my eyes. At that time, all I thought I could offer him was morphine.

I became quite attached to both him and his family. They had an unbelievable inner strength. Toward the end it was really tough. I remember him saying that he could "see the light" and his wife encouraging him to "walk to that light." I was so touched by their love. I remember crying and his wife coming up to me and putting her arm around me telling me "it was going to be all right." Here she was comforting me! It wasn't until later that I realized the difference between sympathy and empathy. At that point in time, she was comforting me and I was little support to them. I knew I had overstepped the boundaries. But I learned to walk that thin line many times over. Despite many people telling me that I shouldn't get involved, I knew myself and I knew that I couldn't do my job well unless I did get involved. Soon I learned that there was more to oncology nursing than just administering morphine. Over the years, I've kept a list of all those I've known with cancer. Mark is number one.

I really loved being at the bedside, identifying ways to make someone more comfortable, to lend support to a family member when death was near, and to cheer a "clean" X-ray. The patients' toughness and their energy for life was so overwhelming. They inspired me. I am a firm believer that we cannot know our own strength until we are given the opportunity to use that strength.

Within two years my career changed directions and I became the unit manager, or "head nurse" as we were called then, for our 19-bed unit. I was 24 years old, scared, and overwhelmed! There was a lot I didn't know yet, but I had a great staff and found an excellent oncologist who loved to teach. It was a challenge moving from being a friend and colleague of the staff to all of a sudden being their manager, especially at such a young age. But I think I won their respect and their confidence as I still maintained my bedside skills, working right along with the staff, day in and day out. We laughed, we cried, we struggled at times, but we won many battles too.

Mary was another special patient I learned from. She was in her late 50s and also had lung cancer. She had been a "fraternity mom," and could out-smoke, out-drink, and out-cuss most of us. Her philosophy of life was simply to "get the most out of each day as possible." Mary came in routinely for her chemotherapy, accompanied by her daughter. And then she came into the hospital to die. It was Mother's Day weekend. I remember that Sunday vividly. She asked to speak to me. She felt today was "the day" and did not want her daughter to come in. Her daughter was exhausted from keeping a vigil at her bedside and so I called her and expressed Mary's wishes. She understood. Around 2 P.M. Mary was in significant pain and so we placed her on a morphine drip. My staff and I sat on her bed and held her hand. I remember my family stopped by so I could wish my mom a happy Mother's Day. Mom saw the tears in my eyes and knew it was a tough day. All I could say to her was that I loved her. I didn't have to ask the staff to stay. They wanted to be there with Mary. She died around 5 P.M. surrounded by her friends. I'm not sure why Mary sticks out in my mind as we certainly faced death on more than one occasion. I guess it was the trust that we had established with Mary. She knew we would not let her die alone and that we would make her as comfortable as possible. We lived up to her trust in us.

Not all scenarios, however, turned out the way we wanted. I remember Steve. He was in his 30s and had colon cancer. He had married his high school sweetheart and had two young children. Steve became a frequent visitor to our unit. When Steve became terminal, his wife came to me one day and said, "Jean, whatever you do, please make sure that I'm here when Steve dies. We've been together through everything and I won't be able to go on if he dies without me here." I promised I would do everything possible to see that she was there.

One week later I came in around 5 A.M. to see my night shift staff. Steve was awake and we had a nice chat. He expressed his thanks to all of the staff for their great care throughout the past year. He was alert and very talkative. When I came out of morning report, I was told by one of the night nurses that she had just gone in to say good-bye to Steve and found that he had died. They had not yet called his wife. That was one of the toughest phone calls I ever had to make.

For about a year, I had a utopia. My staff was excellent. The support of the oncologists was tremendous and I was learning the challenge of management. We were just beginning to become involved in clinical research. "4 Southwest" was now known as the oncology unit, not the "death unit." Nursing had advanced enough to be able to talk openly about cancer and its effects and we were beginning to see a number of educational resources being developed. My challenge was educating the staff and sharing my commitment. I attended my first Oncology Nursing Society (ONS) Congress and was overwhelmed at the amount of support available through my peers. This enthusiasm led me to attend numerous other conferences, at my own expense, in an attempt to learn this new and exciting specialty. Once we developed our educational program, it was time to share our knowledge with our colleagues in rural Nebraska.

We took our program on the road and presented over 40 programs in one summer on chemotherapy administration and caring for the oncology patient. It was my philosophy—and still continues to be today—that we must share with each other the knowledge and experiences we have gained. By sharing, we can only enhance the quality of patient care. I indeed had become a teacher.

Designing a patient classification system that would capture the physical, emotional, and psychosocial challenges in dealing with these patients on a daily basis was one of my biggest headaches. It was a daily struggle to balance staffing requirements with sound, quality patient care. I think that's a battle we continue today, in all settings.

As our unit developed, so too did the physicians' confidence level in treating challenging oncology patients on our unit. I owe a great deal of thanks to Dr. Scot Sorensen who challenged me and my staff. He set very high standards and expectations and then took the time to work with us to meet those challenges. He taught me to expect the best and to only offer the best oncology care. I still maintain that expectation.

My next challenge was to develop a bone marrow transplant (BMT) unit. These complex and challenging patients were being referred to the academic center 50 miles away. My instructions were to assess, develop, and implement a plan for including transplant patients on our unit. I spent the next year traveling and educating myself and my staff, as well as designing a 2-bed BMT unit. Unfortunately, after developing the unit, because of administrative and political issues, the unit was never opened. This was a major disappointment for all of us dedicated to this project.

Shortly after that decision was made, I began to assess how oncology nursing had impacted my life. Working 65 hours a week certainly had taken its toll. I lived my life on that unit. Being single was certainly an asset for working those hours, but my personal life was certainly affected. I realized that my life was very one-dimensional and in fact I was suffering from burnout. I took a long look at what I was doing and where I was headed and decided to use the knowledge I had just gained regarding BMT to pursue an opportunity in transplantation. This meant leaving my secure unit and moving on. It was a very emotional and tough decision.

Today, as I look back on that time, I realize what a great opportunity my first few years in oncology nursing were. I worked with many talented and supportive people. And while I'm not at the bedside today, I try never to forget the faces and the smiles of those I was able to touch.

I began working in the BMT unit at the University of Nebraska Medical Center in the summer of 1987. It was as overwhelming and as exciting as I had expected. I quickly adapted to the new challenges of BMT nursing. Working in BMT is so different because things are so intense for a significant period of time. Length of stays of 60 days in an isolation room were not unusual at that time, so we, as oncology nurses, had to be very creative and highly motivated in keeping both the patient and family members responsive to their daily tasks as well as physically and emotionally healthy. Thus it was very easy to develop long-term relationships with these patients. It was a nice opportunity to be involved at the bedside and a nice reprieve from management for me.

I did have an opportunity to be a mentor to several new graduates on our floor and to share my knowledge of oncology nursing with them. On more than one occasion on the night shift, I remember sitting patiently while IVs were being placed in my hands and arms by new graduates learning IV techniques. I also got to share a lot of my prior oncology experiences with them. One of the other things I hope I was able to mentor was the commitment to sharing our knowledge with each other via attendance at ONS Congress, writing articles and abstracts, and doing public and professional speaking. Today I think we take a great deal of these resources for granted.

Following a year on the BMT unit, a new nursing position was being created in the BMT coordinator's office, which was currently staffed by three physician assistants. They were introducing a nursing position to make the team multidisciplinary. It was a position working with lymphoma patients throughout the process of transplantation. I decided to "go for it" and accepted this new position.

For the next five years I had the opportunity to teach myself and many of my peers what a "coordinator" was. Today, the title and role of a BMT coordinator has become fairly established. I consider myself a leader in helping to develop that position. I was lucky to have had the opportunity to define my own job. And it didn't take long. My definition, "anything and everything that nobody else wants to do, doesn't do, or won't do" pretty much summed up the job. It was a challenging position and I had an opportunity to work with a great team. This position afforded me even more responsibility than being a manager, and I was given a significant amount of independence and flexibility. I owe significant thanks to Dr. Jim Armitage, Dr. Julie Vose, and particularly Dr. Philip Bierman, who took me under their wings, allowed me to design the coordinator role, and showed me what teamwork and striving for excellence was all about.

One of the greatest parts of my job was to meet with visitors from hospitals across the world, who had come to observe our BMT program and see about setting up their own program. I got to meet nurses, physicians, and administrators from a variety of settings and to hear and learn so many diverse ideas and plans. It was an opportunity of a lifetime. In addition, my team allowed me the necessary time for such activities as developing and presenting clinical lectures, patient education materials, and other teaching materials which I was later able to share with a significant number of my colleagues through pharmaceutical speaking bureaus, national and international conferences, and my activities within our BMT special interest group. I owe a great many thanks to these colleagues for covering in my absence so I could share what I had learned and developed.

As a coordinator, I worked at the bedside, both inpatient and outpatient, watching these patients "give it their all" for that one shot at curing their disease. At times we were successful, and at other times we were not. But I was always inspired by the dedication and the resilience of these patients and family members. They were accepting and gracious in the attempt.

Being a coordinator also expanded my vision of oncology and the team members and components necessary to make a successful program work. I could not merely focus on my eight-hour shift or the care requirements necessary for that day, but rather I had to interface with a significant number of different departments setting up pretransplant evaluations and posttransplant follow-ups. I had to rely on my colleagues constantly, in all settings. I dealt with the business side of nursing and experienced firsthand the harshness in telling a patient he could not be transplanted as his insurance company felt this therapy was "experimental." I dealt daily with staffing issues, both inpatient and outpatient, in attempting to get a patient admitted or seen in the outpatient clinic for an urgent platelet transfusion. And then I was responsible for keeping myself and my team updated on the 100 patients I managed across the country in all different phases of the transplant process. The word *challenge* does not even begin to describe this role. Today, in my opinion, the coordinator position is still the least recognized and rewarded in BMT nursing (except to those talented and energetic individuals who serve in that position).

A number of people have given me the strength over the years to keep the pace and have served as my mentors. Barbara Morton, R.N., June Eilers, R.N., and Susan Stensland, M.S.W., who kept me motivated to do more than just meet the requirements of the eight-hour-a-day job will always have my gratitude. Doing more than expected certainly made the days lengthier, but also more rewarding.

Through BMT, I was privileged to meet some outstanding people.

It was in 1989 that I had the opportunity to meet Carmen. Carmen had Hodgkin's disease and was seeking a transplant. I remember receiving the urgent phone call at 6:30 P.M. on a Friday evening. I had just gotten home from work when I received a call from one of the physicians. "Jean," he said, "you have to call this lady and get her down here. She needs a transplant now."

Carmen did receive a transplant but we were not able to cure her disease. We had the opportunity over the next four years to get to know each other well. She was a challenge and inspiration. She truly loved and lived life. She had a lengthy history of this disease and was a very informed and intelligent patient. Carmen was to have been a part of my wedding plans, but unfortunately she died two months prior. She and I remained friends until the day she died in 1993.

One of the moments I am most proud of in my professional career happened prior to my leaving the university. We spent two years putting together an international BMT nursing symposium and as cochair I spent a significant amount of my personal time dedicated to that goal. We were rewarded by having over 400 attendees, both national and international BMT and oncology nurses. Trying to explain to my colleagues where the heck Nebraska is, was in itself a learning experience! So these oncology nurses descended upon Omaha, Nebraska, in August of 1992. It was a huge success and I'm very proud of that accomplishment. For me and my colleagues, it was an experience of taking an idea, watching it develop, and seeing it come to life.

A trend I started to identify prior to my leaving Nebraska was the expanded utilization of ambulatory and home care for the BMT patient population. Improvements in supportive care techniques such as the utilization of the colony stimulating factors, began to have a positive influence on patients' length of stay. Discharge was occurring in less than a month, rather than two or three months. Thus I was spending more of my time in the outpatient clinic and following up with home care. Another career change was in the making!

I was offered a position in Chicago, a city I had always wanted to live in. Chicago offered a metropolis of transplant opportunities in regards to both employment and continuing my education. My decision was to make the move. A number of colleagues could not believe I would give up such a wonderful position, and to be honest it was a very difficult decision. But I knew I had done all I could at the university, had reached my goals, and it was now time to set new goals and to meet new challenges.

I accepted a position working as a national transplant specialist with a home care company. My job would be primarily nursing program development, but also sales support. Specifically I would be developing and educating home care nurses throughout the country. What I saw as a new and exciting opportunity for educating and sharing my knowledge base with home care nurses, was seen by many of my colleagues as leaving the field. More than one colleague confronted me with the message that I had "sold out." It was a personal and professional risk that I was willing to take. And it couldn't have turned out better.

Today my career continues to focus on transplant patients in a new setting, the home. My days of wearing white are over, but my admiration for those who do so remains. On the outside I may wear a business suit, but the inside of me still deals with the issues of pain, nausea and vomiting, lack of appropriate patient teaching materials, and even the lack of knowledge about our own specialty. I see in our specialty the need for further knowledge by many of our colleagues who do not have the opportunities, the support systems, or the teachers I was exposed to. Today I work to see that this lack of knowledge does not impede patient care.

I have the opportunity to educate not only my fellow clinical nursing colleagues, but many nurses in a variety of settings, including case managers. If we don't take the time to educate the ambulatory nurse in the referring physician's office, or the case manager who is responsible for the continued reimbursement, or the home care nurse who is responsible for the monthly IGIV infusion, then we are not offering the best in quality to our patients. Am I still contributing to cancer patients and their care? My answer is a heartfelt yes! Yet I am doing so in a much different way than the young and naive nurse of 1981 ever dreamed.

My life changed rather drastically upon my moving to Chicago. I soon learned what it was like to come home for dinner at 5 P.M., to have a personal life, and not to be on a beeper 24 hours a day. Today I balance a life with my wonderful husband Greg, my job, and my career. I remain as dedicated as ever, but allow time for my happiness too. I'm fortunate to have a wonderfully supportive husband who helps me do my job even better. Greg didn't know me in my first 12 years of oncology practice, so today he can only share my new challenges.

A number of factors influenced my decision to practice in oncology care. Nevertheless, it's easy to identify what has kept me in oncology nursing: the patients. Whether I'm in my office, at the bedside, or in the patient's home, I continue to remember who I work for. Have I been successful? My answer would be a most definite yes. And I can honestly say I did prove my college dean wrong!

I now recognize that cancer affects the young and the old. Coming from a family with a significant and lengthy history of cancer, I am realistic in the knowledge that I may one day be personally affected by this disease. I am confident that oncology nurses will be there for me also.

It was and is a challenge being a "professional friend." I owe a lot of my inner strength to my family. My parents taught me to care and to give generously. Oncology nursing gave me the opportunity.

"I cannot give life nor take life, but I can challenge life." This thought is what I would share with my future colleagues and is what has carried me through my days of oncology nursing. Being a dedicated oncology nurse is tremendously rewarding, but it is accomplished by taking and giving a part of yourself. I have served in a number of positions and in a variety of roles during my 14 years in oncology. Each role, whether it be friend, social worker, physician, nurse, teacher, or educator has been a vivid learning experience. Each practice setting has added to my education and to my sensitivity of the numerous roles we all practice in oncology. One of the changes I have seen over the years in oncology and nursing in general, is how rapidly and easily we have all become so specialized. I would simply challenge future oncology nurses to be open to new settings and new roles and especially to be free to give of themselves. The rewards will be tenfold.

It's hard to define a "legacy." I just know I learned from the best and now I have the opportunity to work and teach among the best. In my eyes, sharing the rewards, the hope, the inspiration I've been given is not a choice. It's a privilege.

26

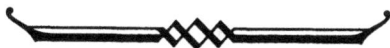

Deborah Mayer

In 1973 I graduated from Pennsylvania Hospital School of Nursing's diploma program at the age of 20. For the next two years, I worked in Philadelphia as a staff nurse in OB/GYN, predominantly in a neonatal intensive care unit. I had dreams of becoming a pediatric nurse practitioner or of working with pregnant teenagers in the Philadelphia school system. I was thwarted from some job opportunities because I did not have my B.S.N. I was looking for a nursing job that did not include shift work when I heard about a medical oncologist, Dr. Richard Smalley, who was looking for a chemotherapy nurse. I had just completed an IV course but knew nothing about chemotherapy or cancer. I naively thought that helping people enter and exit the world were two ends of the same spectrum and required a lot of similar nursing skills. I got the job!

Little did I know that job would start me on a career path that continues to be rewarding and stimulating almost 20 years later. My first patients taught me what became my foundation for cancer nursing. Ms. S., a young woman with advanced abdominal sarcoma, told me that she expected us to do the best we could in controlling her tumor but that if she couldn't sleep, or move her bowels, or was in pain, then whatever the amount of time didn't matter to her. She taught me the importance of symptom management and that quality of life was as important as quantity of life. Mr. B. taught me my real venipuncture skills. He required chemotherapy twice a day for a week as an outpatient (before all the venous access devices of today were available). He guided me with patience and understanding ("Let me get comfortable," "This is my better arm," "Relax and take a deep breath"). I learned early on to listen to my patients since they inevitably knew best. I had cared for Mr. C, who had head and neck cancer, for a long time. I said good-bye before leaving for a month-long oncology nursing program at Roswell Park Memorial Hospital because he was deteriorating. When I returned I was surprised to find he was still alive but I decided not to visit him until my second day back at work. He died that night and I regretted not having visited one more time. He, like so many cancer patients, taught me the immediacy of the moment.

I have learned many valuable lessons from the people I have cared for. My philosophy about life and nursing have been shaped by these experiences. In many ways, it created a developmental dissonance for me. Not many 23-year-olds were seeing and being affected by the things that I saw. As a result, I participated in things that I might not have (for example, a hot air balloon ride) or extricated myself from things that weren't important or weren't working for me (for example, my marriage) since I am all too aware of how finite our lives are.

Throughout my career I have been impressed with the combination of hopefulness and altruism felt by cancer patients as they enter treatment. I learned to do the best I could for the individual I was working with but always sought to have future patients benefit from those lessons learned. That has been the underlying motivation for my extensive presenting and publishing—to have others gain from those experiences and to make a difference beyond the individual patient.

I remained at Temple University for six years and progressed from being a chemotherapy nurse to a primary care nurse practitioner, to the oncology coordinator. Dr. Smalley became my mentor in ways I continue to be grateful for. He encouraged me and supported my attendance at the Roswell Park oncology nursing program for a month. An outcome was an original study on factors affecting chemotherapy-induced nausea and vomiting which I presented at the 1977 Denver ONS Congress and published in the *American Journal of Nursing* in 1979. (I bought my first professional suit for the Denver conference and remember how excited I was when Tish Knobf, from Yale, called me to tell me my abstract had been accepted.) Many of the people I worked with attended my first presentation. Dr. Smalley supported my attending a primary care nurse practitioner certificate program at the University of Maryland as an interim step to obtaining my B.S.N. (requiring a four-month absence from work). I became an active participant in the Southeastern Cancer Study Group and helped establish, along with Connie Henke, the first cooperative group nursing committee. I also was one of the founders of the Delaware Valley Cancer Nurses Association which became one of the first ONS chapters. Oncology was a new field. I was learning a lot from my mentor, not only about cancer care but also about teamwork, collaborative practice, conducting clinical trials and nursing research, and presenting and publishing, as well as organizing and running committee meetings! Dr. Smalley and I truly had a collaborative practice and worked as an effective team; I have never been able to replicate that to this day. This experience became a gold standard which I continue to strive to attain in whatever practice I am in. He also taught me that physicians were my colleagues and coworkers so I gained confidence in interacting with them as peers. I gained confidence in myself as I gained competence in all of these areas. I also thought that all nurses had these opportunities and experiences and was surprised, later in my career, to realize otherwise.

Dr. Smalley supported my attendance at all ONS Congresses from the very first one in Toronto in 1976. After the Congress that Sue Baird chaired in 1978, I went up to compliment her on a job well done. She recruited me to be on the congress committee for 1979 in New Orleans and my career in ONS was launched. I have since developed many important friendships from my ONS colleagues which have lasted over the years and across life events. In fact, for a number of years, I saw many of my ONS colleagues more frequently than my family since we were meeting so often. My most treasured ONS friendship has been with Pearl Moore. We met on a Congress committee when she was ONS treasurer and our friendship has evolved over the years. I have learned about meeting planning from my Congress activities, about finances as treasurer, and about strategic planning and leadership from my time as ONS president.

In 1981 I was recruited to become the head nurse for the new NCI Biological Response Modifiers Program (BRMP) clinical oncology research unit that would be established in a small community hospital in Frederick, Maryland. The staff and I started and developed that unit with vision and the resources to make it a reality. We were able to institute primary nursing and the nurses became involved in clinical research from protocol development through publication and presentation. I remember fondly and greatly valued at the time the eagerness and enthusiasm with which the staff took on this task, and how they grew with the experience. In continuing to conduct phase I and II clinical trials at the BRMP, I was learning about biologic response modifiers and began sharing that knowledge about the burgeoning new "fourth modality" of cancer care. I was also learning to become a nurse manager—it was the first appointment I had in a nursing department (my position at Temple University was in the department of medicine). I developed more of my philosophies on participative management which later influenced my ONS presidency. My work in Frederick was an incredibly challenging and rewarding opportunity, but being single and living in a small town made me personally very unhappy. In considering other job opportunities, I was again turned down for not having enough formal education. I vowed that I would not leave my current job for a "lateral" move but would save enough money to support myself through graduate school. This took two years. In the meantime I had to get working on my B.S.N.! After ten years of sporadic course work, I finally completed my B.S.N. from the University of the State of New York Regents Program in Albany. Little did I know when Tish

Knobf called me in 1977 that I would be attending Yale on an American Cancer Society scholarship in 1983.

After running unsuccessfully for a board of directors position in 1980, I was elected as ONS treasurer in 1982, and again in 1984–86. When I first started as treasurer, the ONS budget was about $100,000 per year. It is now a multimillion dollar budget for a complex set of corporations, including the foundation, certification corporation, press, and society. One of the most distinctive memories I have of that time was being on the interviewing committee for the ONS executive director. Pearl Moore was one of three candidates, all of whom offered something unique to the organization. Hiring Pearl was one of the best decisions we ever made and one of the best things that ever happened to ONS!

Connie Henke Yarbro informed me right after the election that I had also just become a trustee of the Oncology Nursing Foundation. I asked, "What's the foundation?" The foundation was initiated by Connie as a mechanism to start the Mara Flaherty Lectureship with sponsorship from Mara's family, friends and her employer, Porter & Novelli Associates. The board of directors was also the foundation's trustees, usually meeting the night before an ONS board meeting. Since its inception in 1982, the foundation has grown and consistently supported oncology nurses with funding to conduct research, further their education, and conduct public education. Ellyn Bushkin later chaired the foundation and brought new energy and vision about our activities. She contributed greatly to the next phase of the foundation's development. I remember the impassioned plea for expanded support of the society for foundation activities—we all wanted to give her the shirts off our backs at the end of it! Colette Carson stepped in admirably to stay the course of the foundation as Ellyn's cancer made it exceedingly difficult for her to carry on. She assumed the chair when Ellyn resigned and is again helping the foundation grow financially and mature organizationally. Colette and I have worked closely over the years on the Congress committee, the ONS board, strategic planning, and the foundation. I have developed another very important and meaningful friendship with Colette through these experiences. I have been proud of and very committed to the mission of the foundation. In fact, I have made provisions in my will for a contribution to establish a research grant on cancer survivorship/rehabilitation.

I was particularly grateful for my friendship with Colette when we attended Ellyn's funeral together in April 1993 and when we listened to her husband Bernie movingly present her Mara Flaherty Lectureship in May 1993. Ellyn's death was a tremendous loss to many. During my career, many important oncology nursing colleagues have died of cancer, Bobbie Scofield, Linda Arenth, and Ellyn Bushkin, to name a few. It reminds us all of the relentlessness of this disease that we are so devoted to working with. It also reminds me that as our specialty matures, and many of us with it, cancer will not be uncommon amongst us. Our own mortality confronts us in many ways.

While in graduate school, and ten years after entering the specialty, my grandmother died of lung cancer, after successfully being treated for breast cancer. I was very close to her and she was an important person in my life. I remember the shock and anger I felt—after all, shouldn't the work I did protect those I cared about from developing this disease? I truly learned the benefits of hospice and bereavement care in caring for her. My other grandparents also died around this time, one from colon cancer, one from lung cancer, and one from complications after a hip fracture. I began to question the appropriateness of aggressive cancer treatment.

Another important change occurred for me during graduate school. I was exposed to nurses in other specialties in the medical/surgical clinical nurse specialist program. I learned more about and was struck by the comprehensive rehabilitation approaches used for patients with cardiac disease and others with chronic illnesses, and wondered about the lack of similar programs, on a uniform basis, for cancer patients. I stepped back from my previous treatment-oriented interests and began thinking more about the long-term issues of the cancer patient. That is when my interest in cancer rehabilitation truly began, an interest that would become realized later in utilizing my ONS president's grant, sponsored by Smith Kline, to develop the first ONS position statement on "Rehabilitation of the Person with Cancer" in 1989.

As I was completing graduate school, which was my first real full-time college experience, I saw Bobbie Scofield, another ONS colleague, at a New England regional oncology nursing conference. I was considering where I should move and what type of job I should take when she told me of a teaching opportunity at a new graduate program at the Massachusetts General Hospital Institute of Health Professions. I negotiated their first joint appointment as clinical nurse specialist and assistant professor. A joint appointment is always challenging—how to balance and manage clinical practice and academic expectations. Working with graduate students became another new and rewarding experience for me. It was a chance to indirectly effect cancer patient care through others. I tried to mentor these students as I had been mentored. It turned out that Judy Spross was also considering a position at the MGH IHP at the same time. We knew each other from ONS and a trip we had taken together to Asia and welcomed the opportunity to be colleagues on a day-to-day basis. We worked together at the institute for the next eight years. It was another valuable collegial experience for me. I also developed many wonderful friendships in Boston, including one with Karen Hassey Dow. We have since collaborated on health policy issues.

During my time in this position, I became ONS president. I never planned on being president. As ONS treasurer and board member from 1982 to 1986, I began to realize that we needed to look at how we decided which ONS activities should be conducted beyond the basic issue of whether we could afford it or not, and how the board, committees and staff worked. ONS was clearly at a crossroads—no longer a small business but in many ways still thinking and acting as if we still were. We hired a management consultant, Marguerite (Peg) Schaefer, to advise us. As a result, it became apparent that we needed to strategically plan for ONS's future. A small group of us were given the task to address; this group included board members Judi Johnson, Colette Carson, Barbara Holmes, Pearl Moore, and myself working with Peg. Over the next one to two years, we revisited the mission, did internal and external assessments, and struggled long and hard about who we were, what business we were in, and who our customers were. It was a tremendous learning experience from Peg, master of strategic planning.

It was my commitment to seeing this process through that led me to run for ONS president. The timing was right for me personally and professionally, and it seemed the next logical step to take. Barbara Holmes, my friend and colleague, also decided to run for president. I think it was the first time that the nominating committee had two volunteers come forth to run for president! We were proud of the way we handled the election and maintained our friendship, even kidding that the "winner" might be the "loser" and vice versa. I was the last of the two-year-term presidents from 1987–89 (it is now one year as president-elect and one year as president) which had its pluses (being in office long enough to see change through) and minuses (the personal and work compromises that occurred with a heavy travel schedule).

Many of the strategic planning recommendations could not be initiated until there were structural and procedural changes made within ONS. This was a tremendously challenging and difficult time for many within the ONS leadership. For example, we began including committee chairs at board meetings and having at least one of the two committee meetings held simultaneously to facilitate communication amongst them and to make them more a part of the whole organization. Another example was bringing our publishing activities "inhouse" with the development of and expansion of the Oncology Nursing Press. Minor changes to the mission were made but major changes to the bylaws were necessary. This strategic planning process has provided structure and direction, as well as flexibility, in addressing the needs of oncology nurses, ONS members, and ONS as an organization. I consider implementing the strategic planning recommendations and process as my major accomplishment and the legacy of my presidency.

In addition to a lot of travel and hard work, I had many wonderful opportunities and experiences as ONS president. My mother and sisters flew in to Pittsburgh to attend my first president's reception. They have supported me in many ways throughout my career and have physically been present for most major accomplishments. I had the luxury of a full day of consultation with a communications expert, provided by Smith Kline, on improving my public speaking abilities. I attended my first international cancer nursing meeting in London and attended a concert that Princess Diana also attended (she really is beautiful). I also attended the 50th anniversary celebration for NCI, a black tie dinner held at the Organization of American States in Washington, D.C. During my tenure, I met many ONS members and was impressed by their level of interest and commitment to our profession and to improving cancer care. It was a pleasure to see that the philosophies I had developed early in my career were mirrored in so many of my colleagues.

Completing my presidency created a personal and professional crisis for me. I did not enter the office as president but left it as one; I was a different, more mature person from these different experiences. My perspectives had broadened and deepened about many personal and professional issues. My focus of care was shifting from the individual with cancer to more policy-related issues that had the potential to influence care in broader ways. My job was not as satisfying as it had been and my personal life was quieter and emptier once the travel slowed down. During this period of adjustment, which lasted over six months, I saw a career counselor. After all, what could I aspire to now that I had been ONS president? I had been a nurse for over 15 years by then and thought it might be time for a second career. Maybe I should become a librarian or lighthouse keeper. . . . After some testing and counseling sessions it was clear that I was in the right field but that I needed some changes in the type of work I was doing to better fit my new interests and abilities. I transferred to a full-time teaching position within the same organization. I also enrolled in a health policy doctoral program at Brandeis University and started my coursework. During this time, I also became involved with and eventually married a very good friend of mine, Graeme Fisher.

Just when I thought there was little more for me to do in the larger professional picture, I was nominated for and presidentially appointed as the first nurse to a scientific seat to the National Cancer Advisory Board (NCAB). ONS had lobbied for a nurse to be appointed to this board for years. I had had the privilege of observing some of these discussions as ONS president. Although I thought it was important to have an oncology nurse on the NCAB, I didn't envy who it might be since the meetings were long and frequent, requiring at least four two- to three-day meetings at NIH in Bethesda, Maryland, annually. Little did I realize that it would be me a few years later for a six-year term, not expiring until 1996!

The NCAB is basically the board of directors for the National Cancer Institute and the National Cancer Program. The NCAB is comprised of 18 presidentially appointed individuals, 12 "scientific" seats, and 6 "lay" seats, along with a variety of ex-officio members representing a variety of governmental agencies. The original National Cancer Act of 1971 mandated that the National Cancer Advisory Board perform the second phase of research grant review (it must approve any grant, above $50,000, prior to funding disbursement), the annual review of the scientific activities of the National Cancer Institute programs, and provide the director of the NCI with recommendations on specific issues. During my term, I have again learned a great deal and influenced, in a small way, some cancer issues on a national level. Not long after my appointment, I was asked by the director, Dr. Sam Broder, to organize a minisymposium on "living with cancer," a distinctly different type of NCAB presentation, for the May 1992 meeting. This was a challenge since I had just had my daughter, Amelia, and was home on maternity leave. I was proud that two nurses, Betty Ferrell, R.N., Ph.D., and Diana Wilke, R.N., Ph.D., were among the presenters and did an admirable job. The minisymposium included the topics of cancer rehabilitation, pain, and the psychosocial and palliative aspects of cancer care and research. This was then published as a series of commentaries in the 1993 *Journal of the National Cancer Institute* (Volume 85, Nos. 10,13,14,15, and 16). I am also experiencing the politics of cancer in a new way. More attention and resources are slowly shifting to some of these areas.

Over the last few years, I have appreciated the honors bestowed upon me. In addition to my NCAB appointment, I was a recipient of an American Cancer Society scholarship. The Oncology Nursing Society selected me for the first ONS/Ciba-Geigy Pharmaceuticals Quality of Life Lectureship Award in 1991 and awarded me their Distinguished Service Award in 1992. In 1993 Judy Spross and Marcia Grant successfully nominated me for fellowship in the American Academy of Nursing. It was an added honor since Pearl Moore was also inducted into the academy in the same year. My family was again present for me at this important event.

In 1993 I relocated to Toronto, Canada, since my husband is completing a radiation oncology residency. I have assumed a clinical nurse specialist position at the Ontario Cancer Institute/Princess Margaret Hospital with a focus on breast cancer. I am learning to live in a different country and work in a different health care system. Many of the basic clinical issues, however, are the same. Needless to say, I have had to postpone my doctoral studies indefinitely. My challenge now is in balancing my family life with my professional life. Being very satisfied with all that I have accomplished, it is time to put my energy into my new family—which I really appreciate and value.

I am excited about the future of cancer nursing. It is "fraught with potential." With our evolving health care system, we can be in influential positions to help shape the future of cancer care. I am sure those changes will always remain grounded in how we can make a difference for the people experiencing cancer today and in the future.

Reflecting back on my career, I appreciate the richness and variety of my experiences and the many people who have touched my life. It has not always been easy, but I have been very fortunate in having had unique opportunities come my way, excellent mentoring to provide a solid foundation for my career, the development of meaningful friendships that have enriched my life, and the fulfillment of starting a family later in life. I am not sure where the next 25 years in cancer nursing will take me, or our profession, but I am sure it will be interesting. I have been very fortunate and successful according to a Ralph Waldo Emerson poem:

What Is Success?

To laugh often and much;
To win the respect of intelligent people and the affection of children;
To earn the appreciation of honest critics and endure the betrayal of false friends;
To appreciate beauty;
To find the best in others;
To leave the world a bit better, whether by a healthy child, a garden patch or a redeemed social condition;
To know even one life has breathed easier because you have lived;
This is to have succeeded.

27

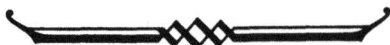

Ruth McCorkle

I graduated from Maryland General Hospital in Baltimore in 1961 and began my career as an operating room nurse. As a student, I loved my operating room rotation and had a clinical instructor who told me I had "the right stuff to be a great OR nurse." It meant a lot to me that someone thought I was good and wanted to keep me around. I saw the operating room as an environment where nurses and physicians talked with each other and the success of the surgery was dependent on teamwork. I felt like an essential member of a team where most of the surgeries were completed without mishaps; but the unsuccessful ones are still very vivid—the gunshot wounds to the head, the vascular anastomoses that wouldn't hold, the lack of skin to graft severe burns, the amputation of a small boy's leg as a result of a lawn mower accident, and the stillbirths of emergency C-sections. It was a time when I had little opportunity to talk about my feelings. I was a young woman in my early 20s with responsibilities far beyond my years. My salary was $220 a month, higher than most because I got extra pay for being on call.

As the Vietnam war escalated, I found myself wanting to do something; our president had been assassinated; the nightly news showed scenes of young men wounded on the battlefield. In 1964 I joined the Air Force Nurse Corps as a second lieutenant. I was stationed at Mather Air Force Base in Sacramento, California. The area was desertlike and I lived on base with two other nurses. We had rattlesnakes in our backyard. Midway into my tour of duty, I had to do air evacuation out of Vietnam. I received firsthand a view of the horrors of war.

There was little to comfort any of us as we felt so helpless in the face of the number of bodies and the men with parts of their bodies missing and the smells—the smell of blood. I thought I'd never get rid of the smell. I was overwhelmed with the number of losses we experienced. I was always exhausted so there was little time or energy to talk to anyone.

After I completed my 26 months in the military, I returned to my parents' house in Baltimore and continued to pursue my baccalaureate degree at the University of Maryland. I stayed in touch with a few of the nurses I met in the air force for a few years, but as we each married, we lost contact. One of my reserve coworkers at Andrew's AFB in Washington, D.C., was enrolled in graduate school at Maryland with me. She told me about an exciting new role in nursing called the clinical nurse specialist.

The GI bill was a blessing. After I completed my B.S.N., I applied to the University of Iowa to get my master's degree in medical/surgical nursing. I wanted to become a clinical nurse specialist and I wanted to work with a group of patients with whom I could form a relationship. I wanted to work with patients and know what happened to them. I knew that I could no longer continue to work on a person's body—to try to repair it—and not know if he or she lived or died.

In 1969 I took the pathophysiology course the summer before the fall semester started and worked nights in ICU at a community hospital. The hospital didn't have a physician in house at night, but one was available on call. There were two nurses who worked nights and if the unit was empty or had a low census, one nurse would be reassigned to a floor that had an increased demand. One particular night the unit was empty, my coworker had gone to the obstetrical unit to help with several women in labor, and I used the time to study for an exam scheduled the next day. About 2:00 in the morning, I got a telephone call telling me that a man with severe chest pain was being transported by ambulance and was expected to arrive in about ten minutes. I notified the supervisor to alert my coworker that I might need her. I called the physician on call so he could begin his trip to the hospital. He told me he would wait until the patient arrived and let us determine if he needed to come in. I had been alone in similar situations many times. It didn't seem like an unreasonable request, thinking my coworker would return before the patient arrived. Within minutes the patient was hurried into the bed, oxygen was attached, EKG leads were connected, and the IV was started. The man was diaphoretic, moaning, ash-colored, with labored breathing. I called the physician to report his status and his signs of cardiac distress as documented by the EKG and vital signs. There was no question the man needed morphine and he needed it immediately. The physician told me to wait until he arrived and he would evaluate the patient for pain. He lived 20 minutes from the hospital. It seemed like an eternity. My coworker was detained in the delivery room and the supervisor was attending to another emergency in the ER. I had completed all my tasks for this patient and I was alone with him. His moaning increased and I thought, "I'm not going to lose another one." I pulled up a chair, lowered the side rail, and started to stroke the man's hand. I looked him in the eye and told him, "I don't know if you're going to live or die, but I'm not going to leave you." I told him, "Breathe with me—nice and slow—take a breath—let it out." And before my eyes, the terror in the man's eyes left him. His normal color returned to his face, his moaning lessened, and he stopped perspiring. By the time the physician arrived, the man's appearance of distress had improved and I was concerned the patient wouldn't be medicated for his pain, but morphine was ordered as soon as the physician looked at the EKG. This was a powerful experience for me. I knew I had been present with many young men as they died and I had tried to comfort them. I told them that their lives had had meaning and that they had served their country. But this was the first time I confronted death with a patient and together we were able to divert it and postpone it. My presence, my touch, and my connection with this patient helped to keep him alive and it happened without medication.

Reading became my salvation. I had never read very much in school, only what was required. I never subscribed to a professional journal. I decided to go to school full time and I spent many days in the library looking at journals and books on nursing. By the second semester of our graduate program, we had to declare a specialty. I didn't have a preference for any one specialty and my classmates had selected all the other "more appealing" specialties: cardiac, renal, endocrine, pulmonary. I decided to major in cancer nursing.

There wasn't specific cancer content in our program, but there were some isolated articles that highlighted the special problems of patients diagnosed with cancer. Learning primarily occurred by tutorials and self-direction. One article that had a lasting effect on me was Jeanne Quint's 1963 article, "The Impact of Mastectomy" in the *American Journal of Nursing*. She stressed that women newly treated for breast cancer were concerned about their future and not about the surgery or cancer per se. I was fascinated with Jeanne's interest in these women after they were discharged from the hospital. It helped me to realize that what I had learned in the past could be used in a constructive way to make me a better nurse. My background in surgery could be used to help many of the women understand what to expect and to adapt to the experience in a positive way. The same year, Dr. Kübler-Ross published her first book entitled *Death and Dying*. I was able to have a few contacts with Dr. Kübler-Ross in Chicago because of the close proximity to Iowa. I traveled there and she was very receptive to coming to Iowa and talking with my graduate class several times about our experiences with dying patients.

At Iowa I had the opportunity to be exposed to the ideas of Ada Jacox (1969), Carol Lindeman, Myrtle Aydelotte, Rozella Schlotfeldt (1975), Kay Norris, and clinicians like Marian Johnson, Mary Wagner, and Ann Paulen. I took my first CNS job in oncology at the University of Iowa Hospital in 1971. Karen Bellars had just left the position and the administration and staff loved her. The first six months of the job all I heard was how wonderful she was and I feared I would not be able to be as effective. The biggest challenge of the job was working with so many patients with metastatic disease. Many had multiple problems such as bone mestatases, ascites, pulmonary effusions, brain metastasis, and constant pain. Physicians were extremely reluctant to medicate patients with narcotics and when they did, proper dosages and schedules were not used.

As Dr. Kübler-Ross shared her experiences with dying children, it gave me a new courage to approach dying patients, and energy to sit with them and to listen to their stories. I found the library my retreat. The authors seemed to be writing directly to me. Another wonderful article in *AJN* described "Christmas at St. Christopher's" by Cicely Saunders (1965). Dr. Saunders made me want to visit St. Christopher's Hospice outside London and to see firsthand the miracles of pain management and compassionate care. I was able to train there in 1972. My experience was unbelievable. The weekly support meetings with Dr. Collin Murray-Parkes talking about loss helped me on the road to recovery from my own losses.

It was a place where staff met regularly to share their own pain and suffering. Each of us had experiences that had affected us that needed to be shared in an environment of love, concern, and safety. As a result of the group work, I was able to sit with many patients who were dying and felt that I was able to make a difference in the way they died. The night before I left St. Christopher's, Dr. Saunders made me promise that I wouldn't initiate changes in practice about hospice until six months after I returned to Iowa. In retrospect, it was one of the most important promises I've ever made. The principles of hospice care were so progressive that my enthusiasm for improving practice would have initiated a negative reaction, potentially bringing about little or no reception to the need for change. Gradually, as clinical situations occurred where the outcomes were extremely grim, I was able to introduce suggestions for changing our approaches to patients with progressive cancer. These experiences led me to begin my own contributions to the literature and helped me to clarify my own philosophical basis for practice.

At St. Christopher's, Dr. Parkes (1971) and Dr. Twycross (1972) steered me in the direction of exciting research opportunities in symptom management. I soon realized that through research it was possible to find ways of managing challenging and often impossible clinical problems. There were a number of other authors in the literature who I felt were writing directly to me: John Hinton (1963), Avery Wiseman (1973), and Barbara McNulty (1971). With each clinical experience I had with patients, I made detailed notes on cards, summarizing the problems and what I had tried to do about them. Gradually I had a data base that helped me to see commonalties among clinical problems and helped me to realize that my patients were my best teachers. Each situation was reviewed and gradually I found I was able to improve the situation for the next patient; I continued to improve my nursing care so that many of the early problems experienced by so many patients were avoided. Eventually, a knowledge base for effective symptom management has evolved in the United States. I am very proud to have been a part of instituting change in clinical practice.

In 1975, after completing my doctorate, I moved from Iowa to Seattle, Washington, to work with Jeanne Quint Benoliel. In that year, the Fred Hutchinson Cancer Center was instituted. A small group of us founded Hospice of Seattle and we helped John Bonica expand the University of Washington Pain Clinic to treat the cancer patient as a part of its routine services rather than as a consultative service. All of these professional activities were happening in the mid-1970s after the Cancer Act was passed; ONS was founded; and one of the first cancer nursing texts was published. We had a common purpose: to improve care on behalf of our patients.

My first teaching responsibilities included supervising undergraduate students. Senior nursing students selected the clinical areas where they hoped to work and I had a group who wanted to learn to care for adult patients with cancer. They were very bright, highly motivated, and eager to learn. Within my first month of clinical supervision, I had an experience that had a profound impact on the way I relate to physicians and other health professionals. One special student was assigned to a woman with metastatic breast cancer who was scheduled for a bilateral adrenalectomy. The woman was in her late 40s, was married, and had two sons. She talked frankly about her cancer and her fears of dying—dying in pain and dying before her sons were old enough to be without a mother. The student was reluctant to respond to the woman, but our evening clinical provided her an opportunity to sit with the woman and develop her confidence in talking about sensitive issues with patients. The student was terrific; she listened and told the patient that if she were her daughter she would want to know what was happening to her mother. The student charted her assessment of the situation and noted that she had talked with the patient about dying. The next morning the student returned to the unit only to be confronted by the surgeon, informing her that she was never to be assigned to another patient of his and if he had any influence he would see to it that she would not graduate. The surgeon told the student that the success of his surgery was dependent on his patient having a positive mental attitude and complete belief that the surgery would be a success. He did not want the patient to have the slightest doubt of its potential success.

He asked the student the name of her instructor and he immediately called the dean's office, who in turn notified Jeanne Benoliel about the incident. The student paged me and as soon as I completed a procedure with another student, I arrived to talk with and comfort the student about the encounter. We reviewed what had happened and how it could have been different. I tried to find the surgeon, but he had left the unit for the operating room.

Within the hour, Jeanne Benoliel paged me and asked if we could meet. I reviewed for her what had happened and underscored how neither of us had done anything wrong. And yet I wondered why I was feeling we had done something wrong. She said quietly and firmly, "You and the surgeon have different goals for this patient and you both are focusing in on your areas of expertise. You recognize the surgeon for his expertise and contribution, but the surgeon doesn't know who you are or what you know. You have to educate him and it may take time." She went on to tell me that I had to meet with him as soon as possible. I told her he was in the operating room until the end of the day. She said "Perfect! You want to get him alone, at the end of the day, and after he's been on his feet all day. You need to apologize, but also tell him that you've been recruited to the school for your expertise and that you very much would like to work with him. Ask him if he has any advice and how he would recommend you supervise students in the future. Tell him you need his help."

This experience taught me the importance of directly confronting conflict as soon as it occurs and the importance of clarifying roles, especially when there is an overlap of responsibilities. Within the next year, Jeanne and I developed our community-based graduate program, "Oncology Transition Services" (Tornberg, McGrath, and Benoliel, 1984), and the surgeon became one of our most trusted colleagues. The patient who had the adrenalectomy became our founding lay board member for Hospice of Seattle. She worked with us for three years and taught us early on the need for ongoing care throughout the cancer trajectory and the need to include the family as an integral part of that care.

What a lucky break for me that no one wanted to specialize in oncology nursing when I studied for my master's. I remain very grateful that I've had so many wonderful opportunities. My advice to nurses who are struggling with clinical problems where there are no easy answers or no solutions:

- Search the literature for creative answers.
- Let the authors in the scientific and clinical literature befriend you.

• Enlarge your world of professional colleagues. Write authors or telephone them, dialogue with them about what they've written, meet them at conferences, search them out.
• Keep systematic notes on common problems.
• Always remember that our patients are our best teachers.

References

Hinton, J. M. "The Physical and Mental Distress of Dying," *Quarterly Journal of Medicine* 125 (1963):1–20.

Jacox, A. "Who Defines and Controls Nursing Practice?" *American Journal of Nursing* (1969).

Kübler-Ross, E. *On Death and Dying*. (New York: Macmillan, 1969).

McNulty, B. J. "Partners in Patient Care," *Royal College of Nursing/British Medical Association Conference Proceedings* (1971).

Parkes, C. M. "Psycho-Social Transitions: A Field of Study," *Social Science and Medicine* 5 (1971):101–115.

Quint, J. C. "The Impact of Mastectomy," *American Journal of Nursing* 63 (1963):88–91.

Saunders, C. "The Last Stages of Life," *American Journal of Nursing* 65 (1965):3.

Schlotfeldt, R. M. "Research in Nursing and Research Training for Nurses," *Nursing Research* 24 (1975):177–183.

Tornberg, M., B. McGrath, and J. Q. Benoliel. "Oncology Transition Services: Partnerships of Nurses and Families," *Cancer Nursing* (April 1984):131–137.

Twycross, R. G. "Principles and Practice of Relief of Pain in Terminal Cancer," *Update* (1972).

Wiseman, A. D. "Coping with Untimely Death," *Psychiatry* 36 (1973):366–378.

28

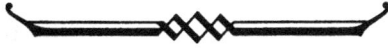

Christine Miaskowski

Caring for children was my goal as I completed my baccalaureate program. However, there were no openings in pediatrics when I started my first nursing job. I started working as a staff nurse on an acute medical unit in a university teaching hospital in New York. The majority of the patients cared for on my unit had a cancer diagnosis. There were no organized staff development programs nor any orientation programs to prepare a new nurse to provide care for oncology patients with so many complex problems.

Working for two years on this unit, almost always on the evening shift, allowed me to develop lasting relationships and numerous memories of patients with cancer. In addition, what appealed to me about working evenings was getting to know and understand the problems and experiences of family caregivers.

In 1976, I became the assistant head nurse on the unit. In that capacity I had the opportunity to influence the selection of patients admitted to our unit. Perhaps unconsciously, we began to care for a larger percentage of oncology patients compared to other medical conditions. As I accepted my promotion, I realized that I needed to return to school for a master's degree. At that time in the New York area there was no master's program in oncology nursing. I pursued a master's degree in medical/surgical nursing at Adelphi University.

My master's program was wonderful! During the years 1976–1979, several things happened in my life that, upon reflection, charted the course of my professional career in oncology nursing. The first significant experience was attending an oncology nursing continuing education program at Boston University. This program, sponsored by the National Cancer Institute, provided me with a wealth of knowledge on the pathophysiology of cancer, the treatment of cancer, and most important, nursing's role in managing the complex problems cancer patients experience as a result of the disease or treatment. An aside that might be meaningful is how I negotiated attending the Boston meeting. I went to my director of nursing and told her about the program. The program was free, but she needed to provide me with the time to attend the meeting and transportation to the meeting. I offered to teach a staff development program when I returned from the conference. My director of nursing agreed and I am very grateful and truly indebted to her to this day.

The old adage that knowledge is power is certainly true. The information I obtained at the Boston program and my experiences in the master's program synergized. I did return to Albert Einstein Hospital in the Bronx and taught the staff development course in oncology nursing. But that was only the beginning. My exposure to the experts opened ways to improve nursing practice on my unit as well as in the rest of the hospital. With my colleagues at Einstein, we developed policies and procedures related to chemotherapy, radiation therapy, and venous access devices. At this point I began to develop a keen interest in the management of pain.

During this period of time, the hospice movement was flourishing. Again, I was fortunate to be able to attend a palliative care medicine conference at the Royal Victoria Hospital in Montreal. There I got to hear presentations from Balfour Mount, Cicely Saunders, and Kathleen Foley. The early work of these wonderful professionals was an inspiration to me. I realized that most patients did not have to die in intractable pain as a result of cancer or cancer treatment. I came back to my unit after the Montreal conference truly inspired to begin to effect changes in pain management. However, changing physicians' and nurses' behaviors about pain management was and still is extremely difficult. The time was 1976, sustained-release morphine preparations were not available, and I remember that one of my greatest struggles was trying to get night nurses to wake the patients up to give them their pain medications around the clock.

In addition to working on my master's degree and attending continuing education courses, several other things happened in my life in 1976 that solidified my commitment to oncology nursing in general and pain management in particular. First of all, my father was diagnosed with laryngeal carcinoma. His treatment course involved radiation therapy, followed by a laryngectomy, subsequent recurrence of disease, and more radiation therapy. My father's illness spanned two years. My most vivid memories include walking into the intensive care unit the night of his surgery and being overwhelmed by the tubes, drains, and incisions, and not being able to hear his voice. More vivid in my mind, however, is the memory of my father dying in intractable pain. Dad received large doses of morphine while at home. I taught my mom how to give him injections. However, what I know now, but didn't know then, was that my dad was suffering from a neuropathic-type pain that was most probably a result of the surgery and radiation therapy he had received. Opioids are not as effective for neuropathic pain, but I didn't know, nor did the physicians, that he most probably would have benefited from a tricyclic antidepressant. What this experience did for me was solidify my commitment to cancer pain management.

Another event that facilitated my growth and development in oncology nursing also occurred between 1976 and 1977. It was during that time that I met Dr. Beverly Nielsen. Beverly was on the faculty of Adelphi University and was coordinating a continuing education program in oncology nursing. Again, more education; that seems to be a recurrent theme of my career. I attended the program and the next year Beverly invited me to become a faculty member in the program. Accepting that invitation was the beginning of a lifelong friendship and facilitated my involvement in the Oncology Nursing Society.

Beverly was a wonderful mentor. I think this is an important area for each of us to consider in our career development. We need to seek out and develop relationships with good mentors. Beverly supported me in achieving many of my professional goals. I remember going to my first ONS Congress with her. She helped me get oriented to the meeting but more important she introduced me to her friends and colleagues in ONS. I remember feeling so overwhelmed as I met many of my "heroes" in nursing.

Completing my master's degree in 1979 allowed me to change positions within the hospital. I spent two years as a staff development instructor. Part of my responsibility was developing an oncology nursing orientation program for the hospital. At the same time, I was still teaching in the continuing education program at Adelphi University and helping to establish an oncology master's program at the university.

The year 1982 brought new challenges and excitement in the workplace. At this time I became the clinical nurse specialist for the oncology and critical care units at Albert Einstein Hospital. In my new role, I began to get more involved in symptom management, particularly pain management, with the oncology patients. However, it was very difficult trying to do all of the pain management care as a single individual. And then a miracle happened! A neuro-oncologist, Dr. Ronald Kanner, was hired by the hospital. Ron had done a pain fellowship with Dr. Kathy Foley at Memorial Sloan-Kettering Cancer Center and had been hired by the hospital to develop a pain service.

The director of nursing at the hospital suggested that Ron call me when he came to ask her for nursing support for a pain management service. That was the beginning of one of the most, if not the most, rewarding professional relationships I have ever known. We worked together to develop both an inpatient and an outpatient pain service. Ron taught me a great deal about the management of pain from a medical perspective, and I taught him a great deal about the management of pain from a nursing perspective. Ron also served as a mentor by introducing me to key people in the American Pain Society.

The years 1985–1987 were very eventful and fulfilling for me as well. During those years, again with Beverly Nielsen's assistance, I became actively involved at the national level in the Oncology Nursing Society. I served as a member of the clinical practice committee, then became chair of that committee, and was subsequently elected a member of the board of directors of ONS. All of my contacts and experiences in ONS were extremely rewarding. I was able to network and develop long-lasting friendships with oncology nurses from around the country. I also learned a great deal about how professional organizations function. This knowledge has served me extremely well in my subsequent involvement with other professional organizations. The ONS devotes a lot of its time and resources to mentoring people. It fosters the growth of professional nurses. Being actively involved in my professional organization was a milestone in my career.

The recurring theme in my professional career surfaced again in 1983, namely education. I decided to pursue a doctoral degree. Serendipity and mentorship were involved in my choice of programs. As part of my master's program in nursing, I had heard a lecture by Dr. Barbara Hansen. Dr. Hansen is a nurse physiologist who did work on tube feeding-induced diarrhea. She did her original experiments on monkeys and subsequent studies on humans and determined that it was a lactose-intolerance that produced the diarrhea associated with tube feedings. I remember going up to Dr. Hansen at the end of the lecture and telling her I wanted to be just like her. She became a role model for me.

When I decided to pursue a doctoral degree, I decided to study physiology. That decision necessitated my obtaining a second master's degree in biology (more schooling). I then spent three years in an animal laboratory completing the requirements for my doctoral degree. Mentorship again played a major role in my professional development. As I was ready to choose a dissertation advisor, Dr. Jaya Haldar, a neuroscientist, was hired at St. John's University. I met with her and decided she would be an excellent role model, a wonderful advisor, and a wonderful mentor. Every one of my expectations were realized by this wonderful woman.

After completing my doctoral degree in 1987, I had to decide what to do next. Serendipity continued to be a major influence in my life. I had heard about a postdoctoral fellowship program called the Clinical Nurse Scholars Program sponsored by the Robert Wood Johnson Foundation. The week after I defended my dissertation, I flew to Washington, D.C., to present some of the findings from my dissertation at a meeting of over 14,000 people. My poster was in the neurology section and as I glanced at the program brochure, I realized that the next group of posters related to nutrition. I happened to look over the titles and authors and saw a poster being presented by B. Hansen on nutrition using a monkey model. I remember walking down the aisle of posters trying to remember what Barbara Hansen looked like. I remember walking up to her poster and asking her whether she was the nurse who had done the tube feeding research. She was the person. I shared with her that I had received my Ph.D. in physiology and that she was one of my heroines in nursing. She asked me what I was planning to do, now that I had completed the dissertation. I told her about my desire to apply for the Clinical Nurse Scholars Program. She smiled and shared with me that she was on the board that reviewed the applications. Sometimes I just sit and wonder what the odds were of my meeting her in a crowd of 14,000 people!

I applied for the fellowship program and was selected, another milestone in my career. Accepting the fellowship necessitated that I move to San Francisco. I wanted to go to San Francisco to do postdoctoral research in pain with Dr. Howard Fields. However, no decision in life is ever easy. The day I found out that I was accepted into the Clinical Nurse Scholars Program, I also found out that my mother had uterine cancer. With support from my physician and nurse colleagues in oncology, I was able to make the decision to accept the fellowship and also help my mother through her surgery and radiation therapy prior to moving to San Francisco in 1988.

Mentorship, a recurring theme in my professional career, also had a prominent role in my life at the University of California, San Francisco. I was very fortunate to have both a nurse/scientist mentor, Dr. Marylin Dodd, and a physician/neuroscientist mentor, Dr. Jon Levine. My postdoctoral experience provided me with an opportunity to get back into the field of pain. Doing my doctoral degree required that I devote a substantial amount of time and effort to my work. Being actively involved in the Oncology Nursing Society (I was chair of the clinical practice committee at the time) was a sufficient amount of professional activity.

Doing the postdoctoral fellowship provided me with numerous new experiences and challenges. I had to move clear across the country, make new friends, find a place to live, and begin a new job. People whom I had met through the Oncology Nursing Society were living in and around San Francisco and provided me with advice and support through the first few months of a difficult transition.

Life in a research laboratory is very much like life and work on a nursing unit. I guess group dynamics are group dynamics wherever a group is assembled. The time I spent in Jon Levine's lab (1988–1990) was probably one of the most exciting times in my professional career. I began to learn a tremendous amount about what was required to become a successful researcher and scholar in an academic setting. These ideas were reinforced from a nursing perspective by Marylin Dodd.

Success in any setting, but particularly in an academic setting, is not easy to achieve. I think one of the major attributes that contributes to success is having a clear vision of what you want. Planning a five-year trajectory that is carefully thought out, yet with enough flexibility for "pitfalls" is no easy task. But an organized plan helps to keep one on track. It helps one make choices (something I've never been very good at) and allows one to mark progress and celebrate achievements.

Having said that, I found that trying to establish a five-year plan following my postdoctoral fellowship was one of the most difficult things I had to do in my professional career. Making choices, as I said earlier, was not easy for me. Now I was being forced to choose between an academic research career and a clinical research career. In addition, I had to choose where I wanted to live as well as work. Several important factors entered into helping me make my ultimate decision as I traveled around the country interviewing for both academic and clinical positions. The central factor that influenced my choice of position was the "gestalt," so to speak, of the environment where I would live and work. From a purely physical perspective, the San Francisco Bay Area has one of the most optimal climates in the country, if you don't mind the fog and earthquakes.

However, a more important factor in making a choice about where one wants to live and work is the professional environment and who you will be able to "talk to" as you do your work. Mentorship became a prominent theme in planning my future professional life.

I chose an academic research career, partly because that was what I had been trained to do, partly because I had never done that before, but most importantly because it would allow me to do the things I wanted to do and hopefully benefit patients and oncology nurses as well. Looking back now after three years, I know that I made the right choice for me.

Pausing to examine my professional career has allowed me to meditate on and thank God for the wonderful people who have been part of my personal as well as professional life. My career has been blessed with rich and fruitful experiences. I am grateful that I had both the strength and the insight and perhaps the courage to say "yes" to certain things without always seeing the bigger picture. I'm deeply grateful to the patients in my life who provided me with so much inspiration to continue my research in pain management. I was blessed with two wonderful parents who taught me to value and respect life and to do all that I can to benefit the human condition. Their love has sustained me through some very difficult times. Finally, I am deeply indebted to all of my professional mentors and friends who provided me with inspiration and guided my professional development. No words can express the gratitude I feel toward each and every one of them. One way I try to repay the debt to each of my mentors is to be a mentor to other nurses who come into my life.

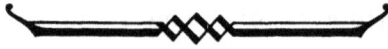

29

Pearl Moore

In 1969 while I was working as the director of a hospital school of nursing, my mother was diagnosed with cancer of the stomach. Even today I can still feel the devastation, the fear, and the hopeless feeling when the surgeon spoke with my brother and me in the hospital waiting room. The surgeon and oncologists, with our permission, felt my mother must not be told the truth for she would "never handle it." Instead she was told she had a severe stomach inflammation requiring removal of the stomach and drug therapy for the inflammation in the liver (not referred to as metastases). Thus began a year of evasions, half truths, and outright lies. Added to this were the ravages of the illness such as weight loss, fatigue, and pain; the difficulty of intra-arterial hepatic infusions; and the nausea and vomiting and hair loss from the chemotherapy. One wonders how could an intelligent person not know she had cancer? How could intelligent children allow this deception? How could doctors and family members be such cowards? Well, we were all afraid of talking about what was happening. Talking about it acknowledged the inevitable. Besides, in the 1960s few people were told they had cancer.

The other thing that was sad was that almost all of the caregivers would stand in the doorway of my mother's room—How are you? they would ask and then run before she really answered. Why? I wondered. Was it because she might ask the questions we were all avoiding, or might staying in the room mean a slip-up and the truth would be revealed?

For all of us it was a sad year. In the meantime my mother took care of all of her affairs, talked about the things she needed to talk about, and generally came to terms with her last days—always protecting us.

After this experience, a master's program started at the University of Pittsburgh in which you could study to be a clinical nurse specialist in oncology, neurology, nephrology, or cardiac nursing. I knew that I must enter this program. I had seen firsthand what devastation cancer brought physically and emotionally to all it touched. I had seen caring people unable to give real care. In 1972 I entered the program and thus I entered the second stage of my career.

I loved the program, the theory, and the clinical. I was a sponge, absorbing everything. I moved from a responsible job to the student role with ease. My preceptor was an oncology clinical nurse specialist, Eileen DePastino, in an OB/GYN hospital working with patients with gynecological malignancies. I observed her with awe—this nurse who had previously been on my faculty. This compassionate, bright, skillful nurse taught patients, she taught staff, she planned 24-hour care, she gave support to patients and families, and mostly she talked about what the patients wanted to talk about or listened for as long as they needed to have her listen. This is what I wanted to do. It was why I had gone into nursing many years earlier. It was the care I wished my mother had received. Too late for my mother, but I at least could learn to help others.

While in school I learned about a new organization, the Oncology Nursing Society (ONS), which was to become my third career. But we will get to that later.

I graduated in 1974 and then I had to convince someone that they needed to have a cancer clinical specialist. Most of my classmates went into "inservice" departments or schools of nursing. But I wanted to do what I had been educated to do. I went to Montefiore Hospital where I was a known entity and convinced them to establish the role. No one was as uncertain as I as to how this new role would be accepted. But I plunged in. I asked head nurses and staff nurses to refer patients to me. I asked physicians to refer to me. I asked social workers to collaborate with me. I asked inservice instructors to let me give some classes and help in orientation. I asked the home care nurses to let me help. But most of all, I just walked in and started talking to patients. My one belief was that no one owned the patients, and if the patient or family wanted to talk with me, I had the right to be there. Well, before long my problem was not what to do, but how to do it all.

I had many referrals from many sources. I taught patients and their families. I taught nurses. I helped staff develop nursing care guidelines. I gave direct nursing care. I became a patient advocate and care coordinator. I loved it.

Toward the end of my first year, I attended a program given on pain by a neurosurgeon, Dr. Robert Selker. I answered some questions about physiology and I guess he thought I was smart. After the program he asked me to help with a National Cancer Institute site visit for a proposal the hospital had submitted to become a part of a National Cancer Institute cooperative study, the brain tumor study group. I agreed to help but I remember saying, "I'm not really interested in neurosurgery or neuro nursing." While preparing for the site visit, I learned a lot about malignant brain tumors; and when the hospital got the grant and I was asked officially to be the coordinator, I felt differently and wanted to join the group. Here was the opportunity to follow patients and families from the time of diagnosis to the time of recurrence. Patients who not only had all the problems related to cancer and cancer treatment, but also all the problems accompanying major neurological deficits. Also, I could see patients in the hospital setting, in the outpatient setting, and in their homes.

I took this new job and began an eight-year odyssey into what was the most demanding nursing I had ever done. I was caring for persons with cancer and severe neurological deficits who received experimental treatment. This challenge was often overwhelming for patients and families and for me. But it was also the most satisfying work I had ever done. I met patients a few days after the diagnosis was confirmed and was with them to their death; sadly, almost every patient died within a year. I was caregiver, teacher, advisor, counselor, charge agent, advocate, and friend. I will never forget these brave people and their families.

At the same time, I was learning about experimental treatments including intra-arterial chemotherapy, hyperthermia, and hyperfractionation of radiation. For many years I gave our patients chemotherapy, preparing the medication in a tiny cubicle (without a hood) and administering it without even wearing gloves. Long before OSHA guidelines, at an ONS conference, I heard about potential dangers. I began wearing gloves and asked others to do so too. This usually evoked much laughter. Today we know better.

Dr. Selker, a neurosurgeon, was the principal investigator of our program and was the best colleague a nurse could ever have. We respected each other and our respective contributions. In addition, he made certain that I received credit for my contributions. I remember well the day he asked me to give a lecture to the residents and interns about our protocols (not a usual event in our setting). He gave me credit in a *New England Journal of Medicine* report on the toxicity we were seeing in our patients on a particular chemotherapy regimen. Meanwhile, he was supporting me in becoming more and more active in the still fledgling ONS.

Eight years later, I began to burn out. I wasn't quite as patient and I was dreaming about patients all the time. I left this wonderful but draining job in 1982 and started my third career—executive director of ONS.

My first contact with ONS came when I was in graduate school. Several of us attended an American Cancer Society conference in Chicago in 1974 at which time a small group of nurses met to discuss forming ONS. I joined this group of a few hundred whose goal was to help each other, to share ideas, and to network. When I went to work later that year, as one of just a few clinical specialists, I realized how important this new organization was to me. The ONS newsletter wrote about things that I needed in my practice. It wasn't written anywhere else. At the ONS Congress (I never missed one, even to this day) I again was getting the information I needed so desperately.

In 1975 Lisa Begg, ONS president, moved to Pittsburgh and asked me to be the ONS bylaws committee chair, a job she assured me would not be difficult. Anyone who attended the Congress in Toronto in 1976 will remember that the bylaws caused such an uproar at the business meeting that they were tabled for an entire year. Perhaps the problem was that three of us drove to Toronto in my 1969 Volkswagen "Bug" and drove for two hours in the wrong direction (singing all the way). I arrived only in time to walk on to the stage for the presentation of the bylaws!

After that fiasco, Lisa still had faith in me and asked me to run for treasurer. On winning the election, I served as treasurer for two years. My dining room table became the first ONS finance department. I still remember the auditor sitting at my dining room table to do the ONS 1978 and 1979 audits.

What an exciting time to be on the board. Lisa and I with board approval hired our first staffperson in 1978—Nancy Berkowitz as an administrative assistant. Fifteen years later Nancy still remembers those early days when ONS got its mail at a post office box, when the office was in her spare room, and when she and I would meet in my brain tumor study group treatment room. Our second employee, Layla Ballon, was hired in 1980 to be the ONS bookkeeper. I remember telling Layla she would only work a maximum of "several hours a week." Today, Layla often puts in a 50-hour week and she looks at me and laughingly says, "just a few hours a week."

Other exciting things were happening, including the big decision to rent space for the first real office. Believe it or not this vote failed when first brought to the table. We were so afraid of not being able to pay rent; we were not ready for this big step. Finally, the board approved renting a small "cubbyhole" and the first office came into being in 1979—and we have been able to pay the monthly rent ever since!

Due to an illness I didn't run for a second term as ONS treasurer, but a few years later I did agree to chair the certification task force. Through an ONS membership survey, the task force found that ONS members overwhelmingly wanted certification. But the path to certification was frightening for ONS because it would involve over $100 thousand for costs related to forming a new corporation and for test development including testing company costs. But ONS persevered and formed a second task force charged with determining how to implement certification. A grant from the American Cancer Society helped us to start. These task force meetings, as most ONS meetings in those days, were held in our lawyer's office—because he was the only one with a real conference room. Edwin Grinberg was ONS's first lawyer and remains in that position today. He took this small group on as a client as a favor to a friend in Chicago and I don't believe he has ever regretted his decision.

In 1982 ONS was ready for a full-time executive director and the search team went to work. Because I loved ONS, because I was ready for a change, and because I would not have to move, I put my hat in the ring and I got the job.

I started as an ONS staff member on Valentine's Day in 1983 in our second office on Banksville Road—two rooms with three part-time staff. My first days and weeks were terrible. I would pace up and down, I missed patients, I missed nursing, I felt suffocated by the four walls. I was used to traveling to different hospitals, to offices, to homes. Most of all I wasn't sure what my job was supposed to be. What did the executive director do? Well, within a few months I became too busy to remember what I missed at the hospital. I had entered the business world without leaving oncology totally. I knew what our members were all about. Membership grew, chapters grew, and SIGs came into being. We formed the Oncology Nursing Foundation, the Oncology Nursing Certification Corporation (ONCC), and we formed a subsidiary to ONS—the Oncology Nursing Press, Inc. We grew to a staff of 52, with staff departments such as meeting services, finance, education, membership and public relations, office automation, government relations, and recently archives and research. We were becoming a large organization but one with heart—one that cared about people with cancer and one that was influencing cancer care.

We joined other organizations in liaison relationships including the American College of Surgeons (ACOS), the National Federation for Specialty Nursing Organizations (NFSNO), the National Organization Liaison Forum (NOLF), and the International Union Against Cancer (UICC), to name a few. With UICC, ONS reached out to what I believe was important to ONS—a global connection and an obligation to help others less fortunate than we in the United States. I came to sit on the UICC nursing project committee that Trish Greene chaired and eventually I became the chair. In recent years, UICC nursing courses have been given in many countries including Thailand, Indonesia, Hungary, Venezuela, Brazil, and Egypt and, perhaps most exciting, the UICC International Oncology Nursing Fellowship program has been launched thanks to the generosity and caring of ONS and ONCC.

During this time the Oncology Nursing Foundation was also growing. I am gratified that as of this writing the Oncology Nursing Foundation has distributed 127 academic scholarships, 60 research grants, and 36 other awards for a total of $652,500. For my part, the foundation has honored me by giving me their prestigious award, the Friend of the Foundation.

Other wonderful moments in my career include the recognition by colleagues, friends, and family at a celebration of my 10th anniversary with ONS. The way I felt seeing my daughter, Cheryl Satryan, holding her baby son and talking about me and my contributions is indescribable. Cheryl often had to wait as a child while I spent all my energy on patients. Too often I told her to be thankful she didn't have the really serious problems that my adolescent patients had. Somehow, even as a child she seemed to understand. I love and appreciate her support and good humor. Cheryl was also in attendance during another happy day when I was inducted into the American Academy of Nursing in 1993.

My fondest memories also include recollections of Bobbie Scofield, the first president of ONCC who died from cancer, and Ellyn Bushkin, second chair of the Oncology Nursing Foundation, who also died of cancer. Both were visionary, warm people who are greatly missed. I also want to mention how important is my association with Connie Henke Yarbro, Judy Johnson, Colette Carson, and with my dearest colleague and friend, Deborah Mayer.

Today the quality of oncology nursing care is so different from when my mom had cancer and this is in great part due to ONS and its influence. The ONS conferences, publications, practice and education standards, guidelines, and research mentoring all reflect ONS's desire to affect care and to help the front-line nurse. I believe this is also a reflection of my philosophy of nursing and of my vision for ONS.

30

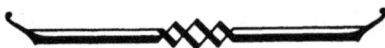

Catherine O'Brien

Growing up in the Bronx in the 1950s as the oldest of three daughters of Irish immigrant parents was in many ways like growing up in a small town. New York is really a collection of neighborhoods, more so in the outer boroughs of the Bronx, Brooklyn, Queens, and Staten Island. We described ourselves as BICs, or Bronx Irish Catholics, and our community as our parish. Although a three-room apartment was crowded for a family of five, it was a far cry from the two-room cottages my parents grew up in. Since most of our neighbors lived in equally crowded circumstances, we considered this the norm for the working class community we all strove to escape.

Grammar school days in a parochial school led to a scholarship to a small Catholic girls school. I was always an avid reader and attempted to read my way through the local public library before realizing the impossibility of this and becoming discriminating in my reading. I was one of those children who read under the covers with a flashlight to the constant admonitions of my mother that I was destroying my eyes.

I never thought of any career other than nursing from my earliest days. Of course my generation was socialized to nursing, teaching, and the telephone company as appropriate career choices. I never considered a baccalaureate program and opted for a hospital-based diploma school in a county hospital. This suburban setting seemed like "country" compared to a city hospital. There were few baccalaureate programs and they required five years of study rather than three in a hospital where we were trained rather than educated. We never heard of the nursing process or nursing theories. We were taught to obey doctors' orders and not to question them. A good ward looked neat and tidy with all patients buffed and puffed, medications and treatments given on time, and doctors' orders carried out promptly. Running smoothly meant for the doctors' benefit rather than the patients'.

I was married the month before graduation to a boy I had known since first grade. Only senior students could live at home if married, others continued to live in the dorm even when married. I worked in a local community hospital, floating—med/surg, nursery, pediatrics, recovery room. There was little specialization—a nurse was a nurse was a nurse. My husband was attending college at night and the plan was that I would go to college when he completed his education. By the time he finished law school, we had two children and I was pregnant with another.

I had continued to work at the local hospital part time. Two spontaneous abortions while working in the recovery room were probably the result of occupational exposure to ether although my correlation of this was dismissed by physicians as not possible. Later research has shown a correlation. My third child had lived only two days after a breech delivery. The most empathetic neonatal ICU staff member was the unit secretary. Nurses looked at me seemingly afraid to say anything.

Rather than my returning to work after our fourth child, my husband taught evenings at the local community college. He made more money teaching one and a half hours than I could working eight hours. My life was busy. I moved to the suburbs, took a few college courses, had another baby, took some more courses, considered majoring in history or political science, and then decided to return to work. I took a refresher course since I was afraid nursing had changed drastically during my hiatus as a mother.

The refresher course gave me confidence. This was the first I heard of the nursing process. We had used the nursing process intuitively; we just didn't know its name. This was the first time I truly saw nursing as a profession, independent and autonomous.

My return to work in a small community hospital as a med/surg float led me to focus on cardiac nursing in a telemetry unit and later to postanesthesia nursing. Without a dedicated oncology unit, oncology patients were "all over the house," frequently cared for by staff who thought cancer equaled death. Patients were seen at diagnostic workup, surgery, treatment failure, and death. As ambulatory and office care increased, inpatient nurses saw most of the failures and few of the successes.

My diagnosis of inoperable lung cancer was a learning experience both professionally and personally. I dismissed my shoulder pain as a result of lifting patients since I had injured my other shoulder previously this way. My cough I attributed to a cold (Yes, I was a smoker). I thought the weight loss was great. My denial was absolute.

My diagnosis at the institution where I worked stressed all staff members from porters to physicians. As a small institution we considered ourselves a family and the illness of one affected all. Most cried with me and told me to pray to St. Jude, the patron of hopeless cases.

Transfer to a teaching hospital revealed the complexity of a large institution. I was being entered in a clinical trial (radiation versus radiation and a radiosensitizer) which required a CAT scan of the abdomen before entry. The scan was canceled twice until an assistant director of nursing (a true patient advocate) on patient satisfaction rounds intervened. At my small institution, my wait for a CAT scan was dependent only on whether or not I had to fast.

During my workup, I was surprised at how uncomfortable maintaining my position for various scans was. Never again would I say, "It's just a picture." One radiologist recognized my difficult role of health care professional as patient. He fully explained a test as though I was a neophyte stating, "Doctors and nurses receive less information than any other patient."

I knew very little about radiation and considered it palliative rather than curative and was surprised when the physician stated he was going for cure. I researched lung cancer and treatment options through library and computer searches. Part of me still denied how sick I was as I read everything as though I had stage II disease rather than the stage III I actually had. Since radiation was given during my period of "existential plight," I remember little of the nursing care and teaching. Periodically a word or concept will trigger an "I remember that."

I was completing my bachelor's degree in health care administration and taking my last two courses when I was diagnosed. One professor came to my home and I took my final in my dining room. The other final was an oral exam in the professor's home. My research topic was the relationship of nurses' smoking practice and their knowledge of smoking-related cancers and frequency of smoking cessation teaching.

I had a squamous cell tumor of the right upper lobe with mediastinal nodes, compression of the trachea and esophagus, and extension to T3 vertebra. After completion of radiation, I returned to work in the PACU. Two weeks later, I returned to the hospital with possible spinal cord compression. Terror reigned again—death seemed easier than dependence. The feared "three Ds" of cancer are death, disability, and dependence. Again I returned to work (the diagnosis had been radiation myelopathy) only to have herpes zoster two weeks later. Since pain preceded the rash, I was sure it signaled rib metastasis; I was ecstatic to see the herpes rash.

Based on a post-treatment CAT scan, a diagnosis of residual tumor was made and surgery was suggested to remove as much tumor as possible, place radioactive implants in the unresectable tumor, and remove T3 and replace it with methylmethacrylate and rods from T2 to T4. All biopsies were negative and revealed pulmonary fibrosis. Assuming an error when the T3 biopsy was negative, T2 and T4 were also biopsied and T3 location confirmed by a cone X-ray of the vertebra. The OR must have looked like a comedy scene of people tripping over one another in the crowd—thoracic surgeon, radiation oncologist, neurosurgeon, anesthesiologist, scrub nurse, circulating nurse, and residents for all of the above services following their attending like baby ducks follow their mother. Then the chiefs of the involved services were called in to decide what to do. After biopsies of lung, pleura, mediastinal nodes, clavicle, and aforementioned vertebra, the incision was closed. An overheard report of "a thoracotomy for biopsies" was accurate and not the "open and close" I assumed. I was intubated and unable to question why implants had not been placed.

I never expected negative biopsies—I had expected a few more "good" years but not the absence of disease. It took me a while to realize it was real. I continued working in PACU and searching for knowledge about cancer. I expanded my focus from lung cancer treatment options to a knowledge base of pathophysiology, characteristics of major cancers, treatment modalities, and nursing management. I became a resource for staff and patients.

I attended a one-day seminar on oncology nursing which whetted my appetite for the study of oncology nursing. The speaker described ONS and suggested joining, which I did. I still felt "job lock" and was afraid to change jobs and fulfill a pre-existing condition requirement or be placed in an HMO without access to the physicians responsible for my survival. As I studied the various options available for studying oncology nursing, I realized a graduate degree as a clinical nurse specialist in adult medical/surgical nursing was my best choice.

Several schools refused to even speak to me on the phone since my undergraduate degree was not in nursing. I was willing to take all required undergraduate level courses if necessary. I decided to attend Pace University which had a program specific to my needs. After successful completion of an NLN placement exam and a bridge course consisting of education, management, and community health, I could matriculate.

Since I could happily be a professional student, I was exhilarated to be back in school although I was juggling family (two children in college and one in high school) and full-time work in the PACU. Staying late with an unstable patient frequently made me late for class. As I looked at my options for a more flexible schedule, a position as an inservice educator became available. I had always enjoyed teaching so I applied for and received the position.

At the same time I became a member of the nursing education committee of the local divisions of the American Cancer Society and the American Heart Association. I was overwhelmed by the expertise of members of these committees—imagine working on a committee with people who published. A chance meeting with a friend from grammar school at an ACS educational lecture led to my recruitment to the Long Island/Queens Chapter of ONS.

I continued as a resource for all staff and patients on oncology issues. Physicians, nurses, and nursing assistants consulted me for personal or patient oncology problems. Oncology patients were finally cohorted on one unit and most of the nurses attended a series of lectures on chemotherapy taught by members of the ACS nursing committee including myself. To develop my knowledge base in oncology nursing, I focused every paper or project on an oncology issue and spent three semesters with preceptors in inpatient, outpatient, and palliative care settings at a comprehensive cancer center.

As a survivor, my "experiential expertise" was an asset. I knew when patients were so terrified at the time of diagnosis that they couldn't focus on anything you were trying to explain. Cancer became their life—they ate, drank, and slept cancer. I could reassure most of them that the day would come when their waking thought would not be cancer. In fact they would even forget they had cancer at times.

With the resignation of the assistant director of nursing for education, I was promoted to that position. A disgruntled colleague stated I had received the position because I had had cancer. I found this reverse discrimination delightful. The promotion was bittersweet. Two people I would have shared my success with had died in the preceding months. My husband had died of lung cancer after a rollercoaster hospitalization of three weeks from presentation with spinal cord compression to search for the primary to death from sepsis. My close friend had been killed in an auto accident two months previously. When I was diagnosed we had assumed she would look after my four children and now I was looking after her four girls—one in high school and the others grown but still needing a mother at times.

Although my title was administrative, I continued to give direct patient care as I relieved for lunch in various units and when called for problems such as pain management and troubleshooting vascular access devices. Patient care encounters continued to be the most satisfying part of my day. I felt I had survived cancer to give back to others.

As the financial problems of the hospital increased, the education department was decimated until I was the only educator covering all shifts. After a takeover, the medical insurance of management was changed to an HMO, leaving me to pay for access to the physicians and institutions I would have chosen. I decided to apply for medical insurance with a $50 thousand deductible through the American Nurses Association. I was rejected based on my medical history although it was five years since my last treatment and I had no evidence of disease. I was devastated. Aside from my feelings of vulnerability, I felt let down by my professional organization.

Although I was involved in many oncology issues through consultation, education, clinical practice, and committee work (I had become president of the Long Island/Queens Chapter of ONS and chair of the nursing committee and member of the executive committee of the Queens Division of the American Cancer Society), I wanted to focus my career entirely on oncology. I was tired of mandatory education, troubleshooting problems, and trying to teach busy, harried nurses in an inadequate time period. Wearing many hats in a small institution, I sometimes felt my day was all meetings. After 17 years in the institution, I was very comfortable but was contemplating moving on. Everyone from the housekeeping department to department heads still consulted me for advice on cancer related issues, from risk factors and diagnosis to treatment. I was still called on to speak to newly diagnosed patients or those experiencing setbacks or recurrence. Since I had "been there" I could talk about the impact on the patient and his or her family.

All the talk about the role of the advanced practice nurse in the new health care reform proposals led me to take the exams for ANCC certification as a CS in med/surg nursing. I figured this made me more marketable. I also wanted to be more clinical and less administrative. I accepted a job as an oncology nurse clinician in a hospital-based hematology-oncology clinic. Not only does this position include direct patient care, but the open role has allowed me to act as a liaison between inpatient and outpatient settings. I couldn't think of any place I'd rather be. I love being involved with the patients one on one (not just traditional taking care of a problem and moving on). An extra perk of the job is health care insurance that allows me to choose the physician and institution.

I feel, given the prognosis at diagnosis, that I survived for a purpose and that purpose is to give back. By utilizing my personal and professional resources in oncology nursing, I am revitalized. Prior to diagnosis I was burned out, thus pursuing a degree in health care administration, looking to get away from nursing. After my illness I realized that I could make a difference in someone's life and that this is the most satisfying aspect of my career. I found new meaning in my life.

Actually I view my illness as part of the mosaic of my life. Life is a continuum of peaks of joy and depths of sadness, differing in intensity as we seek the equilibrium, only to be pulled in one direction or the other. Some are more open to the depth of emotion and some become open because of events in their life. I now always make time to "smell the flowers" and appreciate each day.

As one of the "gray gorillas" of nursing I feel we have an obligation to nurture and mentor young nurses rather than "eating our young" of which we have been accused. The support of my ONS chapter members has been a source of inspiration to me. Their expertise and caring are evident and readily shared.

In writing about my life, I was overwhelmed by the stories of nursing's leaders. But we are all leaders in our own way. We lead a profession, an institution, a department, a unit, a team, a colleague, or a patient. Every one of us makes a difference.

When my daughter decided to major in nursing I was proud she had chosen our profession, although I heard many derogatory comments about nursing from colleagues. In my discussions with my daughter, I must have conveyed the joy of nursing as well as the negative aspects. It's wonderful to have your daughter call and ask if her nursing diagnosis is appropriate.

Last year I was asked to speak at a Cancer Survivors' Day celebration before an audience of over 1,000 people. Since I fear public speaking, I hesitated. Then I thought, "If I can survive cancer, I can do anything." Cancer empowered me. I have since spoken at several cancer survivor celebrations as someone who knows cancer from both sides of the sheets. I still have a sense of awe at the road from cancer patient with a poor prognosis to someone alive and well and active in oncology nursing. When I reflect on the past few years I am reminded of a Yeats poem:

> All changed, changed utterly
> A terrible beauty is born.

31

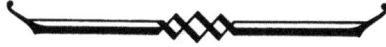

Kim Parylovich

As I reflect on my specialty choice of oncology, I realize that it was as if God gave me a sign. I had decided that infectious disease was the specialty for me until my college roommate's mother Lorette was diagnosed with lung cancer. I hadn't even considered oncology as an option for my career when all of a sudden I was face to face with it.

I took it upon myself to investigate lung cancer and found the most current magazines and books. Cancer, in general, fascinated me. I quickly learned how cancer affected a person and family. At the time, I did not understand my roommate's anger toward her mother's physician, but now I realize her anger was her way of coping and attempting to control an uncontrollable situation.

I also accompanied Lorette to her outpatient chemotherapy treatments. Throughout all of her chemotherapy and radiation treatments (she developed brain mets), Lorette was as sweet as can be. She never complained about anything the entire two years she battled oat cell lung cancer. After spending time with Lorette, I knew that oncology would be my specialty. Even though I have only been a nurse for five years, I can still absolutely say that oncology will be my specialty forever.

Lorette's death was difficult for me and I chose not to fully deal with it. I regret this. When she was admitted for terminal care, I was not allowed to take care of her because my unit manager knew she was one of my friend's mother. I did not go into her room often. During her last comatose days, I rarely visited. My friend remained angry and at that time I did not know how to deal with it so I didn't. I regret not knowing how to be there for my friend. I attended the funeral, but I never let myself truly feel the loss.

Eventually, I did allow myself to feel the loss of a patient. Meagan was her name. She was admitted into the hospital one bright sunny day in November. I was reluctant to take her as my primary patient because I didn't think I could relate well to someone my own age, or maybe it was because I could relate too well.

I decided to go for it and for the first time, I became emotionally involved with a patient. Meagan was a 23-year-old, red-haired, intelligent law student who was full of life and dreams. At first, Meagan did not require much physical care, so we would chat about our boyfriends, parents, siblings, and friends. It was almost like I had known her forever. Meagan and I would order out for pizza and watch Christmas specials together. One night she called out to the desk, "You have to send Kim in here right away." I knew why she was calling me. "The Grinch Who Stole Christmas" was on. We would talk about going out for pizza after she was discharged and made many other plans. I had found a new friend. Meagan was doing so well with her chemotherapy, I thought for sure all of our plans would materialize.

On Christmas Eve, Meagan began to have abdominal pain. I didn't think too much of it since she was supposed to be discharged right after Christmas and her blood counts looked good. She had a CT scan Christmas Day and I did not see the results because I went on vacation for a week.

Upon my return, I was shocked to learn that Meagan had relapsed and her only hope was the intense acute myelocytic leukemia (AML) regimen because her disease was very aggressive. She looked terrible—edematous and just not Meagan—but she was as happy as could be.

I met her parents at this time—wonderful people. Her mother and I talked at great length about everything—Meagan, herself, her career and how it was affected by Meagan's illness, and how the entire family was affected by Meagan's acute lymphocytic leukemia (ALL).

Meagan's physical needs became all-consuming. She had multiple IV lines (13 to be exact). She became incontinent of urine and stool, even more edematous, and her skin turned purple from the chemotherapy. She was in a tremendous amount of pain and I could not seem to give her enough Hydromorphone HCI to control it and that bothered me. To make matters worse, Meagan became confused. Her electrolytes were out of balance and even when they were normal Meagan remained confused—pleasantly confused. I remember her saying, "Since when did I get a roommate?" I answered, "Meagan, that's your mother. She is staying with you." Meagan answered, "Oh, O.K." and smiled.

Even through her confusion she would ask for me, "Get Kim in here! I need some ice!" I took care of Meagan like this day after day, week after week. I thought, "What is happening to my friend?" When I finally took a step back to really look at the situation, I realized she was dying. My first instinct was to run away from the situation, but I couldn't this time. Meagan was emotionally my friend and I could not desert her. Meagan required one-on-one care and I was in the room with her 90 percent of my shift (my poor two other patients), but she deserved my all. She helped me to realize that it's O.K. to become emotionally involved sometimes.

I bought Meagan a guardian angel pin with her November birthstone in it. She wore it at all times, though I am not sure she ever knew that it was there or that I gave it to her. Somehow I think that she did.

One day in February, I came into work and Meagan said to me, "It's O.K. for me to die at this time in my life because I am not married and I don't have any children. I have lived a fulfilling life. There are so many other sick people who have husbands and young children." Meagan had no self-pity and was always thinking about others. That day she also said that she felt content to die and told her parents who she wanted to give her belongings to. I had to walk out of the room. I knew the time had come for Meagan to die. She was ready.

Meagan's parents also realized this and hated to see her in such pain and in and out of confusion. Her parents asked that Meagan be given something stronger for pain so that she would be pain free and die peacefully. After much discussion, a versed drip was ordered. At that point, it was the end of my shift so I said good-bye to Meagan and her family, but I couldn't stop thinking about her. I called the unit several times to see how she was doing. My coworker said that Meagan and her family were reminiscing about the good times and she wasn't that confused.

At 2 A.M. the next morning, the phone rang and I knew she had died. A coworker confirmed my thought. Part of me wished I had been there when she died and part of me was glad that I wasn't there because for the first time I would have really cried; I did all night at home. The entire next day, Saturday, I wandered around feeling empty. I went up to the floor to see if any of Meagan's family were still there and they weren't, so I wandered home. I called a few coworkers for support.

The next Friday was my birthday and I was at work when I received a phone call. It was from Meagan's mother. She said, "Meagan had your birthday marked on her calendar and I know she would have wanted me to call you." I was so touched. Meagan was a true friend and I still think of her often.

Meagan kept a journal throughout her adult life. Her last entry is as follows:

"Time lost cannot be found again."

—*Benjamin Franklin (from watching "Civil Wars" on TV)*

Just a thought—this time in the hospital does not have to be and should not be viewed as lost time. I can't let it be lost time, because time is very valuable and now more than ever I have to make every second count.

I just got out of bed and turned on the light because I feel that I must express the following analogy:

> The train that is my life was on a very straight track to its destination. My illness can be viewed in one of two ways; a wreck, or a change of course. It's a change of tracks—someone flipped one of those switches at an intersection and sent me a different way. Now I have to go over a mountain instead of through the tunnel. It's a harder climb, and there are a lot more curves, but it still will reach the same destination. And I will experience a lot more along the way.

Another person who made a significant impact on my career is Mike. Mike was a 15-year-old boy from Knoxville, Tennessee. He came to my unit in Georgia for an unrelated bone marrow transplant so he was away from his family. Fortunately, his mother was able to stay with him most of the time. I was not sure that I wanted to take Mike as my primary patient either because I was not experienced or comfortable working with a teenager, but I did.

At the beginning, Mike was withdrawn. His silence bothered me because I wasn't sure what I should do about it, if anything, but I continued to reach out to him by trying to be "cool."

I can't remember how it happened, but Mike did start to open up to me. I quickly learned that Mike's goal was to live long enough to see his 16th birthday so that he could officially drive his new red truck. I knew that his goal probably wouldn't be attained, but remained optimistic. Mike had chronic myelogenous leukemia (CML) which is rare for children. He remained in chronic phase for only one month before converting to blast crisis. No chemotherapy would convert him back to the chronic phase. We were going to try a transplant and had already found a bone marrow donor for Mike. Mike did not tolerate the chemotherapy regimen well. He had very bad stomatitis and diarrhea, not to mention pain and severe nausea and vomiting. Mike never complained about any of it. He would even try to eat.

Mike liked a candy called MegaWarheads. They are hard candies. Some are very very hot and some are very very sour depending on which flavor you choose. Mike's mouth could not tolerate the candy because of the chemotherapy, but he thoroughly enjoyed watching other people (mainly nurses, doctors, and ancillary staff) try the candy. I was one of the first victims and tried the hot orange. I thought I was eating a jar of chili powder. After two seconds, I spit it out. Mike laughed and laughed. It was nice to see, although my mouth didn't recover for a while. Next, I tried the blueberry sour. That was worse than drinking a bottle of lemon juice. I couldn't finish that one either. Everyone who went into Mike's room was offered a MegaWarhead. Most people accepted and were sorry that they did. Mike wasn't sorry. As a matter of fact, the MegaWarhead time period was the happiest time for Mike. I could see pure enjoyment in his eyes.

Mike and I never became really close like Meagan and I, but we definitely had an understanding and trust. Mike trusted me to give him quality care with a twist of fun and I trusted that he would tell me when something was wrong. He shared a lot of family stories with me. He told me about one time when his mother had told him to clean the fishbowl and he had refilled the bowl with hot water so the fish wouldn't be cold. Next thing he knew the fish were floating dead on top of the water. To hear him tell the story was hilarious. I can still hear him now.

Mike couldn't tolerate much eating, but he seemed to tolerate Mayfield banana popsicles well. These banana popsicles were difficult to find in the grocery store—every once in a great while the store would carry them. I can't remember if it was the secretary or Mike's mother who called up the company and asked where the popsicles could be purchased. The Mayfield company said that they would do better than that and have a man personally deliver some banana popsicles to Mike in the hospital. The delivery man came one night with 10 boxes of banana popsicles. There was barely enough room in the unit kitchen freezer for them. Mike was thrilled. I was thrilled to see Mike thrilled.

Mike was much wiser than his age. He knew that things weren't going well for him physically even though no one told him outright that the treatment had failed. Finally, his physician told him that a transplant was out of the question. At this point, Mike had three options: he could go through another round of chemotherapy, try an experimental chemotherapy, or nothing. Mike was devastated, but told me he already knew in his heart that he would not be able to receive a transplant.

I told Mike that it was his decision to make about the chemotherapy. I informed him of the facts of each option so that he could make the best decision. Although he was never very expressive with his gratitude, I could feel it. He chose the experimental chemotherapy because it virtually had no side effects. He said he could not tolerate another round of heavy chemotherapy. I believed him.

Mike knew he was going to die. During the next couple of months as he received the experimental chemotherapy, he was also mentally preparing for his death. He expressed to me and his family what personal belongings he wanted to give away, to whom, and why. It was touching. I had never looked at children before as knowing what life is all about, but now I do. Now I always do. I never gave children enough credit in general for appreciating life. Now I do. Mike helped me have a better understanding and appreciation for children.

Unfortunately, Mike passed away long before his 16th birthday, just after I had moved across the country. Mike's mom had my address and wrote to me that he had passed away and sent me a huge bag of MegaWarheads. I cried then and still have tears when I think of him.

Dawn, 30, came to my unit for a bone marrow transplant for recurrent Hodgkin's disease. The entire process was flawless until Dawn developed hemorrhagic cystitis from the Cyclophosphamide. Her counts returned in about two weeks and she could have been discharged shortly after if she had not had hemorrhagic cystitis. She was on a high rate of IV fluids and then a continuous bladder irrigation (CBI). As soon as the CBI was discontinued, the blood and clots would return. We repeated the process several times, but each time the CBI was discontinued, the blood and clots would return. Dawn even went to surgery to remove the clots, but nothing worked. To think she could have been home weeks earlier was really frustrating and disappointing for both of us. What kept Dawn sane was my spending lots of time with her just talking about hobbies, men, friends, and good times. Finally, Dawn was discharged even though the blood never completely disappeared from her urine. She did well at home for three months. I talked to her frequently on the phone. When I moved across the country, we exchanged addresses. She said that she would call me first. So I waited and waited but she never called. Then I received a call that Dawn had relapsed and died quickly. I couldn't believe it because she had looked so good when she had left the hospital. I think back and say, "Wow, what a wonderful person I knew. I was lucky to have known her even for such a short period of time."

Carita, 28, was a newly diagnosed AML patient who was also 18 weeks pregnant. There isn't much literature about chemotherapy and pregnant women and its effects on the unborn child so her physician was unsure what to do. Carita decided to abort the baby, but no physician in the town would abort an 18-week fetus, so Carita decided to carry to term and take the necessary chemotherapy for her to live.

AML induction chemotherapy has a 10 percent mortality rate for the patient so I was worried about the fetus. Carita tolerated the chemotherapy well, but after a while did not have enough amniotic fluid to support the baby. Her obstetrician decided to induce her labor at 24 weeks. I was scared. I thought for sure the baby would be stillborn. I was totally wrong. Carita delivered a 1.5-lb baby girl who had no blood counts. The baby remained in the hospital for months, recovered her blood counts with the help of multiple transfusions, and gained weight a little at a time. No one could be certain about long-term defects, but at the time there appeared to be none. Carita was the happiest mom I've ever seen.

The challenge of oncology nursing for me is maintaining a positive attitude about chemotherapy treatment. Not that I think chemotherapy is ineffective, but it is difficult to see it fail. Also, there are situations when I question why we are giving it at all.

What helps me maintain a positive attitude about chemotherapy are the new agents that are being trialed at this time for more resistant tumors and the new biological response modifiers. It's amazing and exciting to me what is being discovered.

National Cancer Survivors' Day is a time for us to celebrate. I have attended two celebrations for survivors' day. You would never know who had cancer by looking at people. I had difficulty recognizing former patients who now had hair and a healthy glow. The joy felt from these celebrations is unexplainable.

Oncology is a specialty and I believe it takes a special nurse to work with people who have cancer. It is an emotional bond that an oncology nurse and patient feel. Rather than being a sad place to work (which is what the majority of the population thinks), an oncology unit is a happy place to work because the patients continue to live their lives to the fullest even in the hospital. What continues to amaze me is how nice and sweet the majority of the cancer patients are. They endure so much and continue to smile.

I have recently begun a new role in my career as an oncology clinical nurse specialist. Intellectually, I easily made the change from staff nurse, but I miss the interaction and emotional bonds that I had on the bone marrow transplant unit. Although I interact with patients, I am no longer a primary nurse on a unit where the patients stay at least a month.

In my current position, I have had the opportunity to teach ICU nurses about chemotherapy and general oncology. I never realized how different two kinds of nursing mindsets could be. The focus of the oncology nurse is the patient's quality of life and emotional state of mind. The ICU nurse focuses on the technical details and how to perfectly perform these tasks. I had to change my entire way of teaching to include wordy handouts and an overabundance of unnecessary technical information just to get their interest.

The people I have known and experiences I have had have affected my life in a positive way. I will never forget them, especially Meagan, Mike, and Dawn. They taught me what is important in life—family, friends, and to live your life for you. I have also learned that there are a lot of caring people in this world. I feel privileged to know an abundance of them.

32

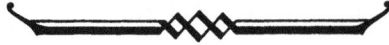

Karen Pfeifer

Like most little girls growing up in the late 1950s and early 1960s, I revelled in the idea of "playing nurse." I had the traditional "nurse's kit" and recall receiving an entire nurse's uniform for Christmas one year to extend my fantasy play. However, *unlike* most little girls growing up during this time period, being a nurse when I became an adult was *not* one of the careers I seriously considered. This factor is probably even more surprising when one knows that my mother is a registered nurse.

My mother, Daphna Bell Burns, was born and raised in a small farming community in northeast Texas. Her parents were cotton farmers, and my mother began picking cotton in the fields at the age of six. She continued to participate in the activities of the farm until, when a senior in high school, she saw an advertisement for the United States Cadet Nurse Corps. My mother's acceptance into and enrollment in this program provided her the needed funding for nursing school. She was accepted into the three-year diploma nursing program at Wilson N. Jones Hospital in Sherman, Texas, with the understanding that, should the United States still be a part of the events surrounding World War II upon her graduation, she would be obligated to enter military service in repayment of her financial debt.

I listened to the many stories my mother told of her experiences in nursing school and after graduation, not understanding until later in life that my mother was a significant part of nursing history. Even more important, little did I know how much I was being influenced by her love for nursing. I only *thought* I wanted to be an artist or astronomer when I grew up!

By the time I entered junior high school, my mother's many stories led me to at least acknowledge that I might be interested in the health care field. Again, however, nursing was not one of the options. I spent the summer between the eighth and ninth grades volunteering in the laboratory at Lowell General Hospital in Lowell, Massachusetts. I quickly decided, though, that my interests were not in that area. In my mind, I would definitely need more "human" contact in the career I selected.

I spent the remainder of my high school years unsure of what direction I would take in my life, although I continued to focus my time and energy within the sciences. Without a doubt, two singular events occurring near the end of my high school years brought me to where I am today. The first event, a fiery car explosion occurring near our home one fall evening, allowed me to witness firsthand the intense pain and suffering individuals sometimes face. As neighbors gathered together to render help and support to the two strangers burned in the explosion while we waited for emergency help to arrive, I began to grasp the essence of what it meant to my mother to be a nurse . . . and I wanted to be like her. The second event, one which was much closer to home than a random car accident, was my first experience with the potential loss of a loved one. Between my junior and senior years in high school, my father, Robert M. Burns, was diagnosed with a vocal cord malignancy. My father traveled on business frequently in those days. Upon returning home from one of his trips, he was obviously hoarse and said he had been hoarse for the majority of the trip. As always, my mother acted promptly and had my father in to see a doctor immediately. Because of her prompt response, radiation therapy and constant vigilance over many years have brought my father to the status of long-term cancer survivor, having been diagnosed 22 years ago.

Although the ending is certainly a happy one, the months of anxiety, pain, and anguish endured by my family during my father's radiation therapy forever changed us. The isolation we felt because cancer was in our midst is a feeling I will never forget. It is undoubtedly these feelings of overwhelming fear and isolation that cemented not only my desire to enter nursing, but led to my ultimate involvement in oncology. I was determined to make a difference in the lives of individuals faced with the same diagnosis, to break down the barriers for them, to ease their sense of isolation.

Needless to say, when I announced to my parents in the fall of my senior year in high school that I was going to become a nurse, my mother was quite surprised! As I look back on my decision, I recognize that, by virtue of my youth and naivete, there were other health care careers overlooked. Yet after 17 years of observing and working with experts in other health care disciplines, I can unequivocally state that my decision to enter nursing would be the same.

As my mother often did at important junctures in my life, she provided sage counsel when I was faced with the task of selecting a nursing school. It was she, not some high school guidance counselor, who advised that I seriously consider a four-year baccalaureate nursing program. By my senior year in high school, a dear friend, also named

Karen, was in her first year of a three-year diploma nursing program at a nearby Catholic hospital. I was ready to follow Karen into this program. My mother, always being knowledgeable of important trends with nursing, gently guided me in the direction of a four-year nursing program. For this reason, I applied to and was selected for admission into Harris College of Nursing at Texas Christian University in Fort Worth.

Needless to say, my mother served, and continues to serve, as my first significant role model in nursing. Although she worked in a variety of areas within nursing over the years, surgery is her area of expertise and first love. So much did my mother influence me that my first position within nursing was also in the operating room. The two clinical days of observation within surgery while a junior nursing student were not enough to satisfy my intense curiosity. And I argued then and continue to argue to this day that the operating room is not a place devoid of the nursing process. Indeed, what I consider to be one of my great professional accomplishments was my successful lobbying for a perioperative nursing elective at a baccalaureate nursing program where I would later teach after completing my graduate education.

The registered nurse in surgery is a vital link in the perioperative process for any individual exposed to this intervention. The greatest illustration for this fact is the surgical case I clearly remember where, when acting in the role of circulating nurse, I prepared a woman for a laparotomy. Upon admitting her into the operating suite and completing my nursing assessment of her, I was aware that her anxiety level seemed greater than usually seen in patients immediately prior to surgery. My perusal of her chart and gentle probing revealed nothing out of the ordinary, but I knew differently. I made a special effort to be by the woman's side during induction of her anesthesia; I sensed her isolation and fear. Imagine my shock when the surgeon later announced after the case began that the woman's husband had died on the operating table six months earlier! No wonder her anxiety level was sky high! Had this vital information been a part of my assessment data from the beginning of my interaction, my nursing care would have been more focused, pertinent, and not based on an intuitive feeling.

My experiences in the operating room led to an unexpected opportunity to work with a Fort Worth surgeon, the majority of whose practice was surgical oncology. This experience was truly the practice of perioperative nursing, as I assisted patients through the entire spectrum of activities. I saw patients during their office visits, preoperatively, intraoperatively, and postoperatively in the hospital and, again, in the office. This unique perspective allowed me to mature as a nurse and an individual. In addition, this surgeon embodied the ideals of medical practice, and I was fortunate to have had the opportunity to work with and learn from him. However, after a period of time, I was drawn to explore other options, namely graduate school. When asked by the surgeon why I wished to pursue a master's degree in nursing, I responded with the typical academic jargon of wanting to "increase my knowledge base." I will never forget the look on his face as he heard my response. He leaned forward and reminded me of the importance of saying what I mean; if I wished to return to school to "learn more," then say it. I have never forgotten this wisdom and try to apply it daily in my nursing career.

Of all the patients I cared for during my perioperative nursing experience, three patients during my final week will stay with me forever. Two of the three patients were women; the third was a young girl, only 11 years old. Of the two women, one was in her 70s, the other in her 30s. Both women were scheduled for breast biopsies. Based on the preliminary information available, it was our hunch that the older woman's tumor was malignant and the younger woman's tumor benign. Of course, the frozen sections proved us all wrong. As we closed the biopsy incision on the older woman and rejoiced in her good news, we were soon to discover that our joy would be short-lived. On the same day, the news would not be good for the younger woman and, as we moved immediately from the biopsy into the radical mastectomy (keep in mind that this was the late 1970s), I reflected on the injustice that someone so young should have her health stripped away. Later that final week, we would perform a bilateral radical neck dissection on the 11-year-old girl for thyroid cancer. That was the longest surgical case I ever scrubbed for, in so many ways. I felt physically ill as the case progressed. One lymph node after another came back positive and, with each positive node, the extensiveness of the surgery increased. At the time, I was not yet a parent; I hope I never have to learn where a parent finds the strength and courage to help a child cope with chronic disease and trauma. I do not know what the long-term outcomes were for the young woman or little girl, but I carry them with me always in my mind and heart. I hope that, for the brief time spent with them and their loved ones, I broke down some of the barriers for them and eased their pain and isolation.

Throughout my nursing career, I have occasionally been responsible for the supervision of others, be they nursing students, registered nurses, licensed vocational nurses, secretaries, nursing assistants, or others. The individual who most impacted my style of supervision and management was an instructor in my basic nursing program. My knees literally knocked when she arrived on the unit, as I knew my knowledge of the patient and nursing care delivered and documented would be closely scrutinized. Yet despite my fears, I enjoyed the challenges she set for me. Needless to say, because of her high, but realistic, expectations, I learned a great deal from her about nursing. And she always had a smile for me, the other students, the patients and families we were responsible for, and the staff on the clinical areas. I would hope that staff whom I have been responsible for would agree with my statement that I have set high, but reasonable, expectations for them to meet and done so with a smile. As a matter of fact, I still have a copy of a newspaper article given to me 10 years ago by a dear friend and colleague, Shirley E. Otto. In this newspaper article, the author penned his views that the more effective supervisor was the one who managed with a smile. On the newspaper article, Shirley wrote, "A validation of your style." This was one of the highest compliments a colleague could have paid me. Obviously, it means a great deal, as I have kept the article all these years and prominently displayed it in the offices where I have worked. It is important to remember to pat each other on the back once in a while. Something that probably took no more than 10 minutes of Shirley's time has stayed with me for 10 years.

I hope that staff for whom I have been responsible would also agree with the following statements: I am always willing to do myself what I ask of them, and I am always willing to leave the paperwork behind and provide assistance when needed. As a nurse manager, it is important for staff to see that you are willing to help when they are drowning, whether that help is administering chemotherapy, answering emergency bathroom lights, or teaching a class. I believe this makes you approachable as a nurse manager and opens up avenues of communication between yourself and your staff that might otherwise remain closed. For the nurse manager with direct responsibility for a clinical area, I believe this also makes you more approachable by the individuals for whom your staff is caring. As the nurse manager of an oncology department for a regional medical center in Wichita, Kansas, I recall many patients feeling comfortable enough to simply wheel their IVACs into my office and just sit and talk. This was certainly the highest compliment a patient could pay me as a nurse manager, and the many conversations I had with these individuals will be pleasant memories of my career in nursing that will last my lifetime.

One particular patient with whom I had many talks in my office will always be very special. I will call her "Bear," as that is the nickname she had been given by her children. She had been diagnosed several years earlier with breast cancer. However, she had not allowed this life-altering experience to affect her usual love for life. Bear was full of life, joy, and will to live. You always knew when she arrived on the unit, because you could hear her all the way down the hall, laughing and visiting with the staff who had become her dear friends over the years of treatment and relapse. Bear eventually lost her life in her battle against cancer, and it was difficult to watch that happen to someone to whom I had become very close. But I was healed when I attended Bear's funeral and participated in this formal good-bye to her. I will never forget the image of the tiny stuffed bear her children had placed on her shoulder. This is a comforting image to me, and it is one I would not have if I had not gone to Bear's funeral. It is not earthshaking news to state that oncology nurses form intense, close relationships with the individuals in their care. Although there is great debate about the value of a nurse attending the funeral of someone for whom s/he has cared, it is an effective way for me to close one chapter so that I have the continued strength so important in oncology to tackle the next chapter.

If I have learned anything else in oncology, it is *not* to predict the end for someone living with cancer. Many individuals have proven my prediction wrong. I recall one patient who, like Bear, had been diagnosed with breast cancer years earlier. Near the end of her life she suffered a massive intracranial bleed that, from examination of her test results, she should not have survived at all, let alone for an additional seven weeks. And throughout this seven-week period she remained lucid and an active participant in her care and pain control. I am continuously amazed by the endurance of the human body and spirit since my entry into oncology.

Speaking of endurance, I am also continuously amazed at the endurance of the oncology nurse, as s/he tends to both professional and personal lives. It is also not earth-shaking news to announce that it is difficult to juggle both a career and personal life. For many of us, that means job, spouse, and children. I am no different, as I have a husband, Ken, and son, Adam. The time I found the juggling act to be the most challenging was the period when I commuted 120 miles daily to work. This long commute, combined with the usual rigors of a demanding position in nursing, was stressful but also provided many humorous moments. The need to leave for work early in the morning to avoid traffic meant that my son was still fast asleep when I left home. Thank goodness for cellular phones, as I served as his wake-up call each morning. One particular morning, as I drove 65 MPH down the interstate and began to encounter the Dallas rush-hour traffic, my son, who was then seven years old and in religious education classes every Wednesday, announced to me over the car phone that he was supposed to have the Ten Commandments memorized for his religion class later that day. Keeping in mind that we would have had one week to prepare for this event had Adam informed me a little earlier, I knew we were in trouble when he asked, "Mommy, what *are* the Ten Commandments?" Now, I regard myself as a spiritual person, but I have to admit that it had been a while since I had named each of the Ten Commandments. So, picture me dodging rush-hour traffic trying to remember them, one by one. When I finally came to "Thou shalt not commit adultery," Adam shot back with, "Mommy, what's *adultery?*" To which I could only reply in exasperation, "Ask your father!"

These humorous moments in our personal and professional lives serve to keep us motivated, renewing us to go on and deal with the stresses of assisting persons with cancer. It is also important to have someone to mentor you throughout your career in nursing, not just when you first graduate from your basic nursing program. I have mentioned two mentors who have shared of themselves so that I might become a better nurse. The first is, of course, my mother. The second is Shirley E. Otto of Wichita, Kansas.

I first met Shirley when she interviewed for the oncology clinical nurse specialist position at the same regional medical center in Wichita where I was then serving as the nurse manager of oncology. I was immediately impressed by her expertise in oncology nursing and recognized her value to our institution and department. Fortunately, Shirley accepted the offer of employment made by the institution, and she and I quickly became colleagues and close friends. Although my employment at the regional medical center ended years ago when my family and I moved to Texas, Shirley and I have maintained not only a close friendship but a professional relationship. This professional relationship is based on mutual projects that have allowed us to continue to collaborate in nursing. One example is a pre-Congress session we gave in 1991 in San Antonio. Perhaps an even more dramatic example is in the area of writing.

Although Shirley has mentored me in many ways over the years, nowhere has her mentorship and belief in me been more steadfast than in writing for publication. Shirley is the editor of *Oncology Nursing,* and I am proud to say that I am one of the contributing authors to both the first and second editions of this text. When Shirley first called several years ago and offered me the challenge of authoring two chapters in her next text, I was flattered that she would even ask me. After all, I had no writing experience and certainly am not one of the recognized experts in the field of oncology nursing. But Shirley's belief in my writing ability and knowledge of oncology opened a door for me that might otherwise have never been opened. At that time in my life I was not actively seeking to become published. After all, who would be interested in reading what I wrote? At the time, I was a clinical nurse specialist in a small community hospital in Texas. Without Shirley's offer and continued encouragement throughout the entire editorial process, I would have continued to think I had nothing of significance to write. And because of Shirley I have been bitten by the writing bug, so to speak. It is my goal to have my first journal article published in a refereed nursing journal within the next year. Ideally, that journal will be the *Oncology Nursing Forum.* We all need our Shirley Ottos—people who believe in us and have faith in our abilities, people who push us beyond what we think we are capable of doing.

Shirley's dedication to and support of the nurse directly involved in the care of persons with cancer have had a profound impact on my practice. It has become increasingly apparent to me over the years that the majority of cancer care is not delivered by those of us who think of ourselves as experts in the field of oncology. Indeed, in my experience, the care is most often given by the nurse who is an expert medical/surgical nurse but not necessarily an oncology expert. Nowhere did this become more apparent to me than in my position as a clinical nurse specialist in a small community hospital in northeast Texas.

This position provided my first taste of a small institution and, for the first time, *I* was the nurse in an outlying area. Prior to this, I had been the "expert" based in the large regional medical center, providing guidance and direction to nurses in outlying areas who, for example, were searching for information about a particular device a patient had brought into the office. Now the shoe was on the other foot. Although I certainly had the knowledge and skills to assist the nurses in the care of persons with cancer admitted to our institution, I was often just as frustrated because of a lack of resources.

Initially, I was surprised at the types of oncological situations the nursing staff faced on a daily basis. Many of the patients admitted to our institution received care from a Dallas-based oncologist. However, upon returning home and encountering a variety of problems, these individuals ended up in our emergency department and on our medical floor.

I used these situations as an opportunity to promote growth within the nursing staff, to help them "learn more" about oncology nursing, thereby increasing their confidence when caring for persons with cancer. I am proud of the fact that I was able to institute a chemotherapy course and institutional chemotherapy certification program, avoiding the need for the nursing staff to travel great distances for the same information and service.

I used the same situations as an opportunity to enhance physician knowledge of oncology, particularly pain management. While facilitating an American Cancer Society Dialogue program within our institution, I met a young couple; both husband and wife were in their 40s. The husband had been diagnosed with leiomyosarcoma earlier and had exhausted all treatment options at M. D. Anderson in Houston. They had been married for a short period of time, and this was a second marriage for both spouses. They came to Dialogue seeking comfort in their long struggle that had come to an unhappy conclusion. Both knew that the husband would not live long, and they were feeling very alone. As always, I grew quite close to them over the weeks and was drawn into parts of their lives.

One morning, about seven weeks after our initial meeting, I received a call from the wife. She was on the medical unit of our institution, and she frantically explained that her husband had just been admitted. She said he "looked bad" and had been bleeding all weekend. Fearing the worst, I immediately went to the medical floor and spoke with the wife in the hallway. She said he appeared to be in great pain. I remembered him having a vascular access device (VAD), as he took great joy in demonstrating how to cleanse and care for it during one of the Dialogue sessions. As I entered the husband's room, I was shocked to see a member of our nursing staff administering an intramuscular injection. The husband was semicomatose, and he responded by nearly coming off the bed. A quick questioning of the nurse revealed that she had administered a commonly-used combination of medications that I knew would be ineffective in controlling the husband's pain. A quick assessment told me that his VAD had obviously been discontinued at some point in the past seven weeks.

I was then faced with the dilemma of how to approach the husband's family practice physician with my recommendations for more effective pain control. I have never had any significant problems with physicians; I have treated them as I wish to be treated, and that philosophy has generally been effective. Yet I always have a knot in my stomach when making such calls. However, upon contacting the physician and providing him with a complete assessment of the husband's status, including pain status, along with recommendations and rationale for a more effective pain management regimen in the absence of a VAD, I was delighted to hear that he was more than willing to institute my recommendations. I have generally found that complete and accurate information, accompanied by recommendations based on that information, is welcomed by physicians. Of course, such a working relationship does not happen overnight, particularly for a nurse in an advanced practice role. There is a certain amount of testing, so to speak, between both physician and nurse. But the rewards of that testing can be gratifying to both parties. I recall the family practice physician who contacted me at home one Saturday morning seeking information about the care and maintenance of a Groshong catheter. The fact that I was able to provide him with the needed information at an important time elevated our working relationship to a truly collegial one. Our relationship became based on mutual respect for what we each have to offer in caring for persons with cancer.

What truly is, and most likely will remain, the most significant event in my career as an oncology nurse concerns a young wife and mother, Cheryl. In 1984 she was a patient on the oncology unit of the regional medical center in Wichita where I was the nurse manager. Cheryl was diagnosed four years earlier with Hodgkin's lymphoma. At the time of her diagnosis, she was pregnant with her daughter. Our department's medical director had been Cheryl's physician from the beginning, and he had taken great pains to ensure the safety of Cheryl's unborn baby as she underwent guarded radiation therapy after her initial diagnosis. Indeed, their physician–patient relationship was a special one.

Many of the staff had cared for Cheryl throughout the entire four years and, despite the fact that I had known her for only one year, I quickly became close to her. I never really knew why I felt such a kinship with Cheryl because, after all, all of our patients were special people. Perhaps it had to do with our close proximity in age.

In March of 1984 we celebrated Cheryl's 31st birthday on the unit, all the time knowing that her condition was deteriorating rapidly. She had begun to seize frequently and spent several days in our intensive care unit. Cheryl's husband and daughter lived a great distance from the medical center and could only visit her on weekends. I guess that because her birthday fell on a weekday, we were determined to make it as special as possible.

Shortly after her birthday, staff became concerned that Cheryl's life was coming to a rapid close. Upon returning to work one morning, the night staff nurse approached me, obviously concerned about Cheryl, explaining that she was becoming weaker every hour. Immediately after hearing this report, both the staff nurse assigned to care for Cheryl on the day shift and I assessed her. We both agreed it would be wise to contact Cheryl's husband, especially in light of the fact that we both knew it would take several hours for him to arrive. I also requested our unit secretary to notify the oncology chaplain and our medical director.

As I returned to her room and saw how weak Cheryl was, I wished there was more I could do to ease her difficult breathing. But all that she complained of was being thirsty, and she asked for some iced tea to drink. As I left to find some tea for her, our oncology chaplain arrived on the unit and entered Cheryl's room. Within moments, he appeared at the nurse's station and told me Cheryl was having a seizure. When I ran into her room, Cheryl was sitting upright in her bed. As I came to her side, she began to lay gradually back onto her pillow, repeating twice, "I'm going . . . I'm g-o-i-n-g . . ." At that point, Cheryl lost consciousness and, within about 15 minutes, she had taken her last breath.

During those last 15 minutes of her life as I stood by her bedside, I found myself saying to Cheryl, "I am with you . . . you are not alone." Of course, I now realize I was transferring *my* feelings to her, because I could not think of a worse death than dying apart from loved ones. I prayed for Cheryl with the oncology chaplain and Catholic chaplain who joined us during those final 15 minutes. I have never refused to pray with a patient or family member who requested it and, although Cheryl had not asked me to pray at this time, I knew it was the right thing to do.

After all indications told me that indeed Cheryl's life was over, I had to turn to the practical matters of hospital policy and seek out a physician to declare her dead. Our oncology resident was tied up in surgery and would be occupied for a long time. Our medical director, who had been Cheryl's physician, arrived on the unit immediately following her death. I informed him of her death and, explaining why, asked if he would pronounce her dead. I knew how close they had been and how difficult it was for him to lose her, and it was obvious from the look on his face that he did not want to be the one to complete this act. But in my heart of hearts I knew that Cheryl would not want anyone else to close this chapter of her life. And I felt that, in the long run, it would be healing for our medical director to know that he had come full circle with this patient after so many triumphs and tragedies. It was gratifying to hear him acknowledge this fact in a postconference held a week after Cheryl's death.

As it always is when there is a death on the unit, it was an extremely busy shift. The staff nurse assigned to care for Cheryl had a heavy load of chemotherapy to administer, so I offered to prepare Cheryl's body. It would be several hours before Cheryl's husband arrived to see her; I would not allow her to be transferred to a local mortuary until after he arrived and took whatever actions were needed to assure this reunion. Unbelievably, two patients within my department coded on the same shift that day. Both of these codes were successful; of course, the joy felt for these patients helped to take away some of the sting caused by Cheryl's passing.

I have never witnessed a death like Cheryl's since my entry into oncology nursing, and I doubt I ever will again. Most individuals who have died in my care have been comatose for the majority of time at the end, or the death was so physiologically dramatic that the individual so affected never knew what happened. To this day, when I reflect on Cheryl's death, I still get shivers. I witnessed a person who, in the last seconds of her life, was acutely aware that life was leaving her at that moment. It was as if I could sense her soul leaving her body.

Because of Cheryl I am a better nurse, and whenever I think of death now, I am not afraid. Thank you, Cheryl. And, thank you, Mom and Dad. Had it not been for your love of nursing, Mom, and the courage you showed in your struggle against cancer, Dad, I would have never had the privilege of knowing the Cheryls of this world.

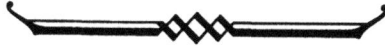

33

Joan A. Piemme

I have often thought about how I got started in oncology nursing. When did my interest begin? What sparked it? I keep remembering a specific patient I knew as a nursing student. Of course I didn't realize at the time that these experiences I had could forecast my subsequent interests, but the fact that over the years my mind always goes back to her when I think about my origins in cancer nursing, is, in my mind, telling.

The year was 1958 and I was a junior nursing student assigned to this "feisty old lady" with metastatic breast cancer. I got the feeling that no one else wanted this frail-appearing, but very outspoken retired school teacher. So I took a deep breath and went into her room. The first thing I heard after entering was a low whistling sound and I wondered, fortunately to myself, who in the world had left the window open on this blustery November day. (Yes, hospital windows opened in those days!) Well, upon checking, the window was tightly closed and it wasn't until later in the morning that I discovered the source of the whistling sound. When I changed the dressing on this lady's chest, I saw a hole in her chest. She informed me that her lung was "stuck" to her chest which kept her lung "inflated" and it had been like this since the radiation after her mastectomy. This disclosure began a series of conversations that took place during several hospital admissions over the next year and a half. She told me in no uncertain terms about her will to live and the plans she and her bachelor brother had made which she intended to complete before she died. I became very fond of this feisty, independent woman who, with her indomitable spirit, taught me an enormous amount about coping, the will to live, quality of life, internal locus of control, taking charge, and being an active participant in health care decisions long before those attributes were described or advocated in the literature. Bear in mind, this was also occurring in the era when it was "unprofessional" to get close to a patient—I was "Miss Altree" and had been taught not to reveal even my first name!

During the latter part of my senior year, my "teacher" was readmitted yet another time. This time she told me she was ready to die. Nothing had really changed in her physical condition, but she said she was tired of fighting and was ready to go. Her brother, her sidekick throughout life, agreed with her, and I knew it would be soon. She was in control. After we talked and had in essence said our good-byes, I left hoping that she would die before I returned to work. She fulfilled that wish. Today, I know that I would be able to be with her when she died, but 35 years ago, I wasn't quite ready. So you see, in my mind this delightful, feisty lady has had a lasting influence. I have thought of her often over the years and am thankful that in many ways she was so ahead of her time and that even in retirement, she continued to teach some very important lessons.

The next episode that shaped my career and chosen specialty was teaching undergraduate students at the University of Pittsburgh. While I had been in graduate school a few years before, I had focused on the cancer patient in my advanced medical/surgical nursing courses. This focus carried over to my subsequent clinical teaching with the generic students who soon labeled me as the one who *always* assigned cancer patients. I was struck with how often I needed to figuratively or literally put a firm but gentle hand on their backs to help them take that initial step into what they perceived to be an uncomfortable but interesting situation. My clinical focus was almost exclusively working with people with cancer.

While on the undergraduate faculty, I learned that Dean Marguerite Schaefer wanted to change the structure and curriculum of the graduate nursing program from an advanced medical/surgical program to one that offered role and clinical specialization in cancer, cardiovascular, or neurological nursing. I desperately wanted to be a part of this evolution. Now "desperately" sounds like a fairly strong, perhaps exaggerated word, but believe me, I was a woman with a mission and Peg Schaefer did not make snap decisions. I told Peg of my interest and ability at every possible opportunity. The most memorable was in the ladies' room in Scaife Hall when from my vantage point in an adjacent stall, I noticed the blue leather shoes that I had seen on Dean Schaefer's feet earlier in the day. I spoke right up and said, "Peg, is that you? I'd really like to talk with you more about the graduate program and my proposal to offer the clinical courses in cancer nursing." Dean Schaefer replied, "If you're this persistent about having the faculty position, we should talk." She suggested we meet in her office a bit later in the day, and soon after that I got the position.

In the fall of 1968, ten years after my first memorable cancer nursing experience, of the 24 students who entered the master's program, eight enrolled in the oncology area of specialization. Thus, the first graduate program in oncology nursing in the United States was started. And it is for the founding of this program that I was inducted as a Fellow in the

American Academy of Nursing. This honor is most memorable and significant and one for which I am deeply grateful. I am delighted to say that over the years I've been able to maintain some contact with three of the graduates of that first program—namely, Marilee Donovan, Sandy Pierce, and Ruth Mrozek. A high point for me was the dedication that was given to Nellie Abbott and to me in Donovan and Pierce's first edition of *Cancer Care Nursing*. To this day Marilee and I often reminisce and enjoy the memories of both the exhilaration and frustration of that new venture in nursing education and practice. I do have two regrets about that experience: first, I was only able to see one class through to graduation as my husband had accepted a position in Washington, D.C., which necessitated a move sooner than I had planned; and second, I did not have the foresight to realize how important it would have been to write about this program in the nursing literature.

Once I adjusted to the necessity of moving, I was eager to explore opportunities in oncology nursing in the metropolitan Washington area. Where else to start but the NIH? And so I successfully completed the first hurdle of the infamous SF171 application form and scheduled an interview. Well, this was in the days when you could not request a specific nursing service or unit; the Clinical Center placed you in the area of greatest need. "But," I implored, "how often do you have someone who requests to work with cancer patients?" "Not very often," came the reply. "And how often do you have someone apply who has academic and clinical experience with people with cancer?" I continued. "Even less often," I was told. Despite my saying that I might kill someone on the cardiac unit because I could only recognize fibrillation and standstill on the monitor, the policy was certainly not going to be altered for me!

Well, it's an ill wind that blows no man good and I found a wonderful opportunity at the Georgetown University School of Nursing. I have often said that for nurses with a master's degree and clinical expertise in 1970, the world was our oyster. Again I was teaching undergraduate students and using the medical/surgical nursing setting to select people with cancer for students' experience. Along with these responsibilities, I had the unique opportunity of working in a small task group with Dorothea Orem in a major curriculum revision which resulted in the Self-Care Theory becoming the theoretical framework of the curriculum.

During this time for me there were barely enough hours in the day professionally—the curriculum implementation was challenging and demanding, I was chairing the Maryland Division, ACS Committee on Nursing Education, and was active in the D.C. Nurses Association. In addition, personally, I was making sure that I had daily energy and uninterrupted time each day to spend with my "three-ring circus," Geoffrey, Jennifer, and Karen. At this time, I became acquainted with the projects that Louise Lunceford was directing at the National Cancer

Institute for continuing education in cancer nursing. I responded to a request for proposal in 1974 to develop an oncology nursing program at Georgetown University which was subsequently funded for a three-year period. In addition to meeting the continuing education requirements of the RFP, I was able to incorporate some specific components that were important to me in that I believed by including undergraduate elective courses in cancer nursing, students would not only gain a greater depth of knowledge and experience but might also make a conscious choice to pursue oncology nursing upon graduation. Thus I was able to provide the first senior level clinical elective "Nursing Clients with Cancer" that GUNS offered. And indeed, some of these students did pursue oncology nursing. Ricky Preston for example was as high-spirited and creative in this program as she is today! Buffy Garabedian practiced in pediatric oncology nursing at NIH and is now an invaluable resource as a reference librarian in the Clinical Center library.

The faculty I recruited for this program gave me only a one-year commitment with an option for extension. This was reasonable as we were not certain how we would all work together. It is a tribute to all involved that we share the same philosophy and vision, worked productively together throughout the three-year period and exceeded the specifications of the program. This was one of my most enjoyable professional experiences— working with a small group of committed colleagues, reaching a large number of nurses in the metropolitan Washington area, and contributing to the enhancement of the quality of care for people with cancer as well as raising awareness of cancer prevention measures.

At this same time one of the faculty members, Donna Herndon, and I initiated a service for women concerned about breast cancer which we called NURSUPPORT. This program was designed to assist women to take a more active role in decision making about their health. The service offered was primarily by phone to provide factual information and psychological support to help women cope with their concerns and fears. Upon request, either Donna or I would accompany a client to the physician's office or visit her in the acute care setting. It was during one of the hospital visits that I had an experience forever etched in my memory. After having a mastectomy, a patient was asking me about reconstructive surgery. In answer to her questions, I described the current state of the art. When I left her hospital room her surgeon approached me, told me that he had heard all that I had said, and furthermore stated, "Reconstruction is not necessary to appease female vanity because I got it all and that's all that matters." I clarified that I was not advocating reconstruction but merely answering this individual's query. I thought that was the end of it, but lo and behold, I was summoned before the hospital review board to answer charges by this surgeon that I was practicing medicine and interfering with the doctor-patient relationship. Thank goodness, I had some advance notice from the dean, whom I had told of the encounter, and I was "saved" by two recent articles on breast reconstruction appearing in *Woman's Day* and *Redbook*. I was able to demonstrate that the information was in the public domain and within my realm of practice to discuss when asked. It was a memorable experience but not one that I would like to repeat!

It will come as no surprise to readers that this was a period of great awakening for cancer/oncology nursing. We wondered, What is the best term to use? Does it make a difference? Is there enough momentum to have a specialty organization? Although I was not one of the movers and shakers, I did attend and participate in the formative discussions of the Oncology Nursing Society and am very proud to be one of the 200 charter members.

Twenty years ago—it hardly seems possible. The Oncology Nursing Society has been a significant part of my professional life, both in terms of the contributions that I believe I have made to ONS, and the benefits, experiences, and fulfillments that I have had as a member since its inception. In some ways our first official meeting in Toronto seems like yesterday, yet it is incredible to realize that actually in a relatively short span of time ONS has grown from 200 to 25,000+ members. We are such a sophisticated, smooth-running operation today, incredibly vision-ary, efficient, and diversified. Yet there is a part of me that misses the old business meetings with the unpredictable situations, arguments pro and con, and never knowing from what corner an unexpected issue may arise. We are so civilized now!

My participation in ONS has taken many forms over the past twenty years. Each endeavor has been different and each one has also resulted in forming relationships, many of which have flourished over many years. My initial participation was as a member of the education committee. Next, I was invited by Susan Baird to be on the program committee for the annual meeting which was held in Washington, D.C., in 1978. Can you imagine, Su Hubbard responsible for registration, I for local arrangements, Linda Rickle for commercial exhibits, and so on! Each of us knew virtually every centimeter of the operation—we had to! At the conclusion of the meeting, the elections were announced (Yes, in the past, the suspense was held up until the last moment). I learned that I had won the election for vice president, having been director-at-large the year before. There we were, all of the new and continuing officers properly on the stage of the Sheraton Hotel's ballroom when I received a handwritten note that seemed to require immediate attention. It read, "Joan—2 toilets have overflowed. Can VPs take care of that sort of thing if they are also local arrangements people? Should we clarify that kind of thing in the bylaws? Can Pearl do that now that she is treasurer? Should that be in the bylaws or should it come under 'Bullshit'?" I looked up to see a group of my colleagues doubled over in quiet laughter just waiting to see how I could maintain my composure. This, I think, was my first official duty as VP!

I expect I could go into detail about a variety of experiences with ONS, both official and unofficial, but I'll omit some stories so that a few of the "Don't you remembers" can be saved for the 20th anniversary discussions and beyond. One event, however, I must include for posterity. In 1980–1981 I was chair of the Congress committee with the Congress meeting in Baltimore at the new convention center in May of 1981. Four days before the Congress was to convene, the keynote speaker canceled! I cannot find the words to capture my state of mind. I will be forever grateful to Jean Johnson, who on such brief notice gave an eloquent keynote address. The Congress attendees gave her a standing ovation for her message and her rescue. She will certainly always be my vision of an angel of mercy!

A highlight of my career is the Oncology Nursing Society Educator of the Year Award which I received in 1989. It is truly a wonderful feeling to be nominated and affirmed by a group of nursing colleagues for whom I have enormous respect. An excerpt from that nomination packet continues to express my beliefs, so I would like to share that quote: "In any curriculum in which Joan has had an influence, four threads will be evident: A) The focus is people not the disease (Disease and treatment information is important but as a means to an end not as an end in itself); B) The key role of the nurse is to assist the patient/family to help themselves; C) Nursing interventions make a difference; D) Skill development is critical." I am both humbled and elated that oncology nursing leaders such as Susan Baird, Jeanne Rogers, Roberta Strohl, Marilee Donovan, Barbara Farley and Judy Spross affirmed my contributions to oncology nursing education and practice.

I have also experienced defeat during my participation in ONS. Is it really good for the soul? Who knows, but that attitude cushions the impact! I've had my share of abstract rejections and publication queries turned down. Only once did I embark on a venture where I knew the chance of success was a real long shot. In 1984–1985 Judi Johnson was running unopposed for a second term as president. I was greatly distressed that in an organization as large as ONS had become, no one seemed willing to respond to the nominating committee's request for an opposing candidate. How can we have an unopposed candidate? I asked. Well, raise the question, you'll get the answer. At the urging of some of my supporters, I threw my hat in the ring. (I still have the hat Jill Mangan gave me to commemorate that decision.) Now, please know, this was not a token gesture. Once in the running, I wanted to win the presidency and thank all those who were so enormously helpful.

The defeat did not necessitate my withdrawing from active participation in the formal organization, however. Karen Heusinkveld had asked me to be a member of the ONCC test development committee, pending the outcome of the election. So while congratulating Judi on her reelection, I entered on a five-year tenure helping to develop a certification examination that would identify the requisite knowledge, attitudes, and skills of oncology nurses, and upon successful completion of the process, foster the recognition so richly deserved.

My most enduring commitment within the organization has been with the government relations committee. This too has been an evolutionary process, starting out as the resolutions and legislative committee in 1985—a real grassroots type of effort to learn about the legislative process and how to garner effective visibility and influence for issues of importance to those with and at risk for cancer and for oncology nursing. Our expertise and sophistication has certainly grown over the years. There are a multitude of stories that could be told about this committee's efforts, but those too will be allocated to the earlier designated "Don't you remember" series—save one! In 1990 ONS held its Congress in Washington, D.C. The government relations committee held a pre-Congress workshop on the legislative process which was culminated by scheduled visits on "The Hill." The chair, Mary McCabe, who has been my professional colleague and valued friend since our days together at Georgetown, asked me to accompany a particular group which had three members known to speak up from, shall we say, "shaky" information. Mary said, "I know you can handle this and I'll buy you a scotch tonight for your efforts." I assumed my assigned responsibility and ran interference that would challenge Joe Namath. On returning, Mary asked, "How was it?" I replied, "You know that drink? You owe me a bottle!" We still chuckle over this one.

Returning to that aspect of oncology nursing that is my livelihood, from Georgetown I migrated to George Mason University for five years. During this time, Susan Baird came to NIH as chief of the cancer nursing service. In 1983 I learned that there was a new position opening as nursing educator. (Over the thirteen-year interim since my initial encounter with NIH, it was now possible to interview for a specific nursing position.) Much to my surprise, part of the interviewing process for this position included teaching a class! A topic would be chosen by the search committee from the three suggestions I submitted. Sue's philosophy was that if hiring an educator, one had to determine if that person could teach. It makes good sense, but it was a new interview experience for me! I was delighted to be able to join Sue's leadership team. I certainly admit to bias, but I believe that under her creative and visionary leadership, together with Judy Spross, Marguerite Donoghue, and Martha Gibbons, we were able to initiate some innovative programs for patients on biomedical research protocols and for the professional development of the nursing staff. It was truly an exciting and fulfilling period in my oncology nursing career.

As I think about it, one of the qualities that has facilitated my career development is that I have been open to exploring opportunities as they present themselves. That sounds a whole lot better than saying that I can't articulate my five-year goals! This is pertinent to my developing an interest in people with HIV disease. Even though the majority of patients on AIDS research protocols were being studied by NIAID researchers, NCI has a designated patient population as well. In preparation for the opening of NCI's dedicated AIDS unit, I asked to be the educator (there were now four nursing educators rather than one) for that unit. Thus began what has become an ongoing commitment to working with people with HIV disease and getting out the message for prevention. While at NIH I had the opportunity to have a 3/5 appointment as a policy analyst for nursing (a staff position) on the National Commission on AIDS. I will always be grateful to Marguerite Donoghue for suggesting my name and to Jean Jenkins, current chief of cancer nursing, for supporting this endeavor. The scope and magnitude of the epidemic became even more apparent from this vantage point. The inquiries from a variety of professional and nonprofessional groups and individuals, hearings, briefings, site visits, and the preparation of reports all indicated that HIV disease was a multidimensional problem that would not lend itself to a quick fix. The impressions from this experience will remain vivid, I'm sure.

For example, my curiosity was coupled with cold fear when I visited an open-air drug market with street outreach workers in Puerto Rico. Jason (my coworker) and I had been told to dress in casual clothes—no suit and tie or skirt and heels—so that we wouldn't stand out as possible law enforcers or other unwelcome strangers. We were also told that we would ride in the outreach van because it was known in the community. After getting into the van with one broken seat in the back and an engine that was reported to be on its last leg, I doubted that it would run long enough to get us in and out. However, after driving through six blocks of slum housing with groups of young men on every corner staring at the van as we drove by, we stopped and parked next to a shell of a building. We went up two flights of stairs into a room whose roof had long since been lost to fire. There were two men who had just finished "shooting" and a rather large woman who seemed to be running the operation. I noticed the bandages on the woman's legs and asked about these (my questions and comments were translated into Spanish by the outreach worker). The woman showed me her leg ulcers and seemed quite pleased that I said they looked free of infection and that she was obviously taking good care of them. When I asked the translator to thank this woman for allowing us to come, the woman (without benefit of translation) said, "You may come back anytime." I suddenly realized that this woman understood everything Jason and I had said during our visit and that unbeknownst to us, she was scrutinizing our credibility and concern from the moment we arrived. I was so struck by a real glimpse of a life that I had only read about. I also realized how important it was to our safety that we remain silent about our candid observations until after we had left the area. Little did I realize that this experience would be valuable a few years hence.

Another aspect of this experience on the commission staff that continues to be important is knowing that there is an array of people, from renowned scientists and clinicians to unsung heros and heroines who are committed to harnessing this epidemic, and although the statistics may appear to contradict this, I believe the efforts are making a remarkable difference. Shortly after my tenure on the commission staff was completed, I realized I wanted to concentrate my efforts working in this area of health care. Because of the multiple needs of the cancer nursing service, it was not possible to pursue this interest in my current position. As luck would have it, the VA Medical Center in Martinsburg, West Virginia, was looking for an HIV coordinator, as this patient population was experiencing a decided increase in number. The decision to leave NIH was not an easy one to make, but the challenge of working with a very different patient population, along with the opportunity to design the parameters of this new position, were very attractive. If I thought this was what I wanted to do, I had to be willing to take the risk!

Now I must say at this point that many nurses have asked me how I could "leave" oncology nursing. I don't feel as though I have left. Aside from the fact that the specialty sees this type of nursing practice within its purview, I have found that the knowledge and skill pertinent to the care of people with cancer is equally applicable to those with HIV disease. Many of the psychosocial aspects are identical as people deal with such issues as effective coping, quality of life decisions, ethical ramifications, legal issues, and economic concerns. And so I believe that I am able to use all of my experience in oncology nursing as I address this epidemic.

One of the rewarding aspects of my most recent position as HIV coordinator is that I have been able to design the scope of my practice. My primary responsibility is akin to a nursing case manager for now approximately 75 veterans—a large number for a relatively rural setting. The patient population at the VA is very different than the patient population at NIH. NIH patients having biomedical research studies generally are knowledgeable about their disease and aggressively seek the latest in medical treatment and information. The veterans that I see often have multiple diagnoses, including post-traumatic stress disorder and polysubstance use. Many are or have been homeless and/or incarcerated and have frequented drug markets similar to that which I described earlier. Sometimes I feel as though I can almost hear my mother saying, "Young lady, do you know what you are doing?"

As outrageous as it may seem at first, the diagnosis of HIV disease has been a catalyst for some of these men to find meaning and purpose in their lives. As I carry a message of prevention into the elementary, middle, and high schools in the eastern panhandle in a program entitled "Let's Talk About It," some of these veterans who accompany me are my very best teachers—they really reach the children. In addition to my responsibilities at the VA, the opportunities that I've had for teaching in the schools and in helping to establish a local community-based organization have been enormously rewarding. There is such a need, and truly, for the most part, people are receptive and eager to learn. There is much yet to do.

Finally, I would like to acknowledge my family who has been very supportive of my nursing career. Nearly 30 years ago when I decided to continue to work after having my first child, Geoffrey, I experienced a lot of criticism. That's hard to believe today, but 30 years ago, once a woman had children, she was expected to be a homemaker. My mother and father provided unfailing encouragement, surprising since they themselves had been quite "traditional" in their roles. My father was British and my mother a first-generation German-American, so it is easy to deduce that I was raised in a family where discipline was the watchword. That value was imbued, however, with both love and nurturing. My former husband was supportive in that he felt that we could both pursue professional careers. My daughters, Jennifer and Karen, followed quickly on the heels of Geoff with just three and a half years separating their births, thus my pet name of "my three-ring circus." After a series of babysitters/childcare folks, I was very fortunate to hire Jennie Hall who had taken care of a colleague's son prior to their relocation. Jennie came highly recommended, and indeed she was with us for 12 years. Having a consistent, responsible, and loving person for childcare really enabled me to enjoy both a professional and family life that did not require an enormous amount of juggling. My children are both proud of my achievements and appreciate that at home I always made sure I had the energy and uninterrupted time to devote to them and to their activities. They have now all flown the nest and are pursuing their careers in Washington, D.C., Boston, and San Jose. I am as proud of them as they are of me.

Reviewing my career has been a wonderful experience for me. Like most of us, I doubt that I would have taken the time and effort for reflection had I not had a reason. It has been a timely affirmation for me of the significance of my practice, and I appreciate the opportunity.

34

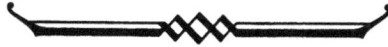

Nita Kay Schulz

I was a new grad from a community hospital-based diploma program. The year was 1972 and one of my first assignments was team leading on a medical/surgical floor in a large "downtown" Los Angeles hospital. The hospital itself was a monument in antiquity. The four-bed wards were an obstacle course of safety hazards: divided hand-rails that fell off; gas wall heaters that you burned yourself on if you weren't careful; windows that would not close; and dumbwaiters sending food trays that never came. Long before oncology units evolved, I cared for one of my first cancer patients.

I knew little of the pathogenesis or treatment of cancer when I cared for a patient with head and neck cancer in a ward bed next to the window. Her fragile, emaciated limbs were in restraints. She did not speak. I assumed her to be mentally incompetent. As I went about performing personal care tasks, I became aware of her eyes watching me. As I moved on to her oral care, I was moved to tears to discover that it had been completely neglected. As I began cleaning her mouth, teeth, and tongue, I apologized to her for the lack of attention and told her what I would do to make her more comfortable. I felt sure she understood.

Her doctor came in after her care was complete. A radio I had left at her bedside played softly. He was well pleased with the work I had done for his patient. Little did I know that within the year I would be working for that surgeon, administering chemotherapy, assisting in minor surgeries, and providing comfort and support in an office practice. So began my oncology nursing career.

When I accepted the office nursing position, I knew only that I was to give chemotherapy for a group of four surgeons for whom "the novelty of administering chemotherapy had worn off." Feeling a little over-whelmed and a little underprepared, I asked if they were sure I had the necessary skills. My dear Dr. Sakulsky answered, "Well you're a nurse aren't you?" As I was unable to dispute this logic, I began a journey with this group that would last 20 years. Taking only a small cut from my hospital salary, I went to work in ambulatory care for $835 per month.

The first five years went very quickly. I was assisted by an X-ray technician who, when she wasn't taking pictures, helped me attend the four doctors using six examination rooms. We assisted in breast biopsies. We snipped off skin lesions right and left, learning the difference between a nevus, a basal cell skin cancer, and a melanoma. We did sigmoidoscopies with rigid scopes on tables you could not adjust. I learned to debride a skin graft and aspirate a breast cyst or a seroma. We did pelvic exams, thoracenteses, corporate physicals, and the like. The practice also provided radiation therapy utilizing a cobalt 60 and ortho voltage machines and those patients too passed through our exam rooms. I ordered drugs and supplies, stocked rooms, sterilized and made surgical packs, refilled prescriptions, drew and submitted lab samples, and filed reports. And I also gave chemotherapy.

I remember my one and only training session in chemotherapy administration. The senior partner stood behind me and guided my hand as we entered a patient's vein with a needle attached to a syringe full of 5-Fluorouracil. Butterfly needles, chemogloves, vertical flow hoods, and OSHA guidelines were the ghosts of oncology nursing yet to come. For the time, we would prepare small piles of syringes prefilled with cyclophosphamide, methotrexate, and the like, and hope that the needle would stay in the vein while disconnecting the syringe from the needle and reconnecting the next syringe for multidrug chemotherapy. The day I gave the "red medicine" that came from the National Cancer Institute, I was particularly nervous and stayed with the patient throughout the infusion. At least by that time I had a butterfly needle.

I don't remember the names of many of the patients from those early years. A 40-something woman named Carol Ann with breast cancer metastasized to bone exemplified the scope of the challenge to my nursing care. But I do remember vividly the net effect of five years of caring for patients like Carol Ann. Lying in bed, waiting for sleep to come, I would begin to sigh. As the sighing got heavier and the breathing more rapid, the palpitations began. My legs and arms were tingling and I was sure I would faint. When the medical exam, blood tests, and X-rays were complete, the results were reassuring but troubling: gastritis and anxiety attacks. At this point in my oncology nursing career, I was certain that my knowledge and skills were pitifully inadequate to care for the complex needs of my patients and their families.

I was indeed burned out. I wanted to quit. I felt alone. My husband had suggested early on that at social events I give my profession as that of a "ballerina" so as not to bring the conversation to a grinding halt. Unfortunately, I bear little resemblance to a ballerina.

My redemption came in the form of the Macomber Oncology

Nursing Course at USC. My redeemers were a group of nurses much like myself and our nurse instructors, Julena and Joanne. As we sat like little sponges soaking in the body of knowledge barely covered by our nursing schools, the healing that comes from sharing began to take place. I had a taste of what I needed to go on. I had information, I had resources, and I had colleagues. When our physician practice moved to a building adjacent to our admitting hospital, another nursing hand was waiting. It was Pam's.

She was the clinical nurse specialist on the newly formed oncology unit. Her friendship and support combined with a burgeoning cancer program in providing me with many opportunities for growth as an oncology nurse. A CHOP grant (Community Hospital Oncology Program) from NCI would lead to a later CCOP grant (Community Clinical Oncology Program) and a new role for me as protocol nurse for research trials. An award from the American Cancer Society, California Division, launched our cancer rehabilitation team which still exists 12 years later. Participation on this team was the answer to a prayer from the early days when I felt I must have all the answers and provide all the services. The circle of communication created by including hospital staff, office staff, and home health services set a standard of patient care that I continue to strive for in ambulatory care practice today.

As the oncology program grew at our community hospital, the size and composition of our office practice also changed. The radiation therapy department gained a physician trained in radiation oncology. Our first hematologist/oncologist also joined the practice. The nursing staff grew. I stopped thinking about changing jobs. The diversity of the patient population and the cornucopia of services provided within our practice made every day challenging and a learning experience.

I loved the puzzle of trying to fit a patient to a research study even though one could spend all day on the task and find the patient ineligible in the end. There was so much satisfaction in being in the minor surgery room when the frozen section came back with a biopsy proven benign. But if the lesion was proved positive, to be able to tell that patient you would be by her side from post-op to chemotherapy to radiation therapy to celebrating the first haircut when it grew in again was a gift for an oncology nurse. There are so many gifts in oncology nursing. I try to be gracious when accepting thanks and praise from patients and their families and others outside of the profession. However, I usually find myself compelled to share with them that there are far greater rewards in the caring than any amount of pain or sacrifice made in the course of treating the patient. I am convinced that if life could be sustained without money, nurses would rather pay to practice oncology than do anything else.

I am sure that is the way Pam felt, and because of her efforts I met 24,000 more nurses like her. It was she who convinced my employer to allow me to attend the Fifth Annual Congress of the Oncology Nursing Society in San Diego. At that time, I joined the organization knowing little of what it was all about. At congress, I was fairly overwhelmed. I had never heard so many acronyms. I thought these nurses were speaking a secret language. The research presentations left me mystified. Just what were they trying to say with those statistical slides? Everyone seemed to have a degree and they seemed to think it should be mandated that I have one too. I was not sure I really belonged in this group.

However, there was something else. There was the adrenalin rush when we stood together at the opening and closing ceremonies; the inspiration of the keynote speaker; the fun and relaxation of enjoying the time off and meeting new people. Some of those nurses shared their experiences, their successes and failures. They shared their aspirations, both personal and professional. The experience of Congress planted a seed of professional growth that would be nurtured by my colleagues and by personal determination. The fertilizer soon followed in the form of an oncology nursing interest group that within a year would become the greater Los Angeles Chapter of the Oncology Nursing Society. Pam had an active part by volunteering as program chair. Blessings to all current and former program chairs. Naturally, I had to assist her. It was gracious of her to appoint me chair when she resigned after successfully running for president. That year the chapter wanted to rotate meeting sites so I had to set up meetings all over Los Angeles County.

Pam and I spent the night together in a hotel in Pasadena the night before the symposium my committee had planned. We were so nervous I don't think we slept. What a joy the next day was! The parking lot was full before half of the participants arrived so the majority had to park throughout the surrounding neighborhood. The first speaker was my own physician coworker who was on crutches following knee surgery. My deodorant immediately failed me as I ran around the parking entrance trying to catch him and park his car so he could get to the podium. When he did get there he had to shout because the microphones didn't work. The speakers before lunch had to raise their voices as well, for the thin collapsible room divider did little to drown out the clanging of the silverware as the busboys set the tables. By the time the last speaker arrived without her handouts for an interactive presentation, I was oblivious, having indulged in two glasses of wine with lunch. When I was asked if I wanted to run for vice-president the next year I thought, there is a job for me.

Another source of inspiration for me was a feisty little Ecuadorian, a rehabilitated ICU nurse named Patty. She came to work with me in the early 1980s and not long after, having been a hospital school of nursing grad herself, came to show me a brochure for a consortium B.S.N. program. Bolstered by the support of my employers, my colleagues, and my family, I took the plunge with Patty. For 18 months we did nothing but study. Every five to eight weeks was a new course with written assignments, reading assignments, oral presentations, group projects, and special projects. Every holiday and every vacation was spent in the library or writing. Thursday nights I would drive home after 10 P.M. with my brain either in a state of mental ecstasy or terror at the prospect of being unable to complete the assignments. My patient experiences at work brought an important focus for the material I was learning and served as subjects for endless reports.

It was an extremely emotional time as well. The patients in my reports were not numbered research subjects. Their stories were very real to me and my studies drew me even closer to them. I was especially involved with Mary Jo, a 34-year-old divorced pediatric nurse with ovarian cancer. She was loving and giving and very brave. She continued to work and she lived life to the fullest. In the last weeks of her life, her friends and I rotated shifts at her home. Mary Jo and I slept together on a sofa bed in the living room and I can still see her sitting on the edge of the bed looking as though her spirit would ascend any moment. How ironic that before her death I would come to tell her that her doctor, my mentor and friend, had died before her of a glioblastoma at the age of 49.

That same doctor who had proclaimed that if I was a nurse I could give chemotherapy, was gone. He had seized while driving to work in February and just after Father's Day he was dead, leaving a wife and two children. He had showed me the difference between a nevus and a skin cancer. He let me suture and showed me a fluid wave. We palpated lumps and bumps and made rounds together. He yelled at me and made me cry. I called him a chauvinistic pig and made fun of his height. He wrote a beautiful recommendation for me for my B.S.N. program. He sometimes threw instruments and got angry without cause. I called him an SOB into a live microphone while whispering to my nursing colleague during a quarterly staff meeting at the hospital. I sometimes dream that I see him again and tell him how much I have missed him and about all the advances that have been made in oncology since he left.

If the death of these individuals were not enough, I became pregnant a year into my B.S.N. program. The pregnancy was unplanned. My husband's wishes had forced me to give up the dream of motherhood. My nurse friends once again became my counsel. My resolve to be a mother was short-lived as I miscarried in the tenth week. But my goal was now set. My husband was helpless. He said, "When I looked at you coming out of surgery after the miscarriage I knew we would have a child." When I graduated with my class the following summer, I was five months pregnant. When my daughter was born in December of 1987, nothing I had learned so far in life had prepared me for the experience. I think I am a much better nurse than I am a mother. She knows I love her though because I hug and kiss her every day.

She was three months old when I went back to work. Dr. Kennedy let me use his office for my electric breast pump. I can't say I blazed any major oncology nursing trails the first couple of years of her life but I did at least mentor the hospital staff nurses by providing a practical experience for their chemotherapy certification course and a chance to verify their skills. Eventually I returned to ONS Congress and my local chapter meetings. The size of our office staff was now 17 and there were 14 doctors and 7 offices. We received grants for drug company studies and I attended investigator group meetings. After completing my own research project for my B.S.N. program I wasn't quite so lost anymore with statistics. I found eligible patients for nursing studies for my colleagues Linda and Margie at UCLA. I helped the hospital put on oncology nursing symposia. I served as a consultant for pharmaceutical companies. I lectured for ACS and for hospice volunteers. I never considered myself exceptional. I felt lucky to be surrounded by some very dedicated medical and nursing professionals who provided me with a wealth of opportunity and encouragement.

My belief in the exceptional qualities of oncology nurses was further validated in 1991, the year I was honored with the American Cancer Society Lane Adams Award. Accompanied by Dr. Robert McKenna, my nominator and a booster throughout my career, I listened as the character and contributions of 19 other awardees were described. I especially remember the hospice nurse from Hawaii who gave her home number to all her patients and their doctors and drove to every shack and mansion on the island in her four-wheel-drive vehicle. I also remember the nurse from Seattle who helped pioneer central line placement and had excelled in the bone marrow transplantation unit since its inception. She had been a nurse for 50 years. Hearing the stories of these oncology nurses, I knew my own story was not unique. As I write now, I believe it is only an example of how so many of us "fell" into oncology nursing and stayed because we loved it. We loved it because the patients gave us back more than we could ever give them and because our colleagues gave us the kind of recognition and encouragement that no one else could.

I received that kind of encouragement last year when I served as president of my local Oncology Nursing Society chapter. I expected to start my year as president full of confidence and with the support of my employer and staff. Instead, I was in a state of emotional upheaval as I watched the medical group I had worked with for all these years suffer a deep and painful split. I left the comfort and familiarity of my professional "home" and threw my hat into the ring with a small band of dreamers to launch the practice of a single oncologist.

Throughout my transition period, my ONS board was the greatest. Our two- to three-hour meetings on Saturday mornings were full of laughter, enthusiasm, and sharing. An ad hoc committee planned our ten-year anniversary. They gave 110 percent of themselves to the project. Sharon, the immediate past president, was a great mentor of leadership skills. At the same time, I was able to use my experience to mentor one of the program chairs and other first-time board members. What a pleasure to receive calls from nurses new to the organization and to extend a welcoming hand. I am thankful to the oncology nurses who helped me along the way.

So how are things going and what will the future bring? What pearls of wisdom do I have to share with future oncology nurses? Well today I am happy to say I work with a group of people who make going to work a pleasure. You don't have to make your coworkers your friends and confidants. Courtesy, respect, and team spirit go a long way in providing job satisfaction. You don't have to work in a state-of-the-art cancer center to provide good patient care. In our new office we provide hugs, jokes, comedy videos, *Eric Clapton Unplugged*, fish tanks, juice, popcorn, lots of phone access, and the best medical and nursing care we know how to give.

How do you avoid burnout? Once every month or so you hang out with nurses like yourself who respect what you do. You laugh at yourself whenever possible, meaning you don't take yourself too seriously. You make sure you have a life outside of your work. There is only one Mother Teresa. As for motherhood, ask Betty Ferrell. She tells the best stories about motherhood and nursing I ever heard. How do you keep your heart from breaking when the patient you come to care about so deeply is dying? You give them all the physical and emotional support you have to give. Then when you go home and you watch the news or some silly TV movie, you let the tears fall. And you renew your hope and faith by rejoicing in things around you that you love.

As for the future, I plan to be in nursing until I retire. By that time I expect there will be major attention to wheelchair access at congress due to the advanced age of so many of us. I hope to go back to school again. Mostly, I would like to teach. In the meantime, the most important role in oncology nursing for me is that of patient advocate. While the winds of reform are blowing, I will be on the phone with the case manager, utilization reviewers, or anyone else who might threaten to compromise the standards of care we have all fought so hard to achieve.

35

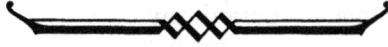

Judith A. Spross

Where does this story begin? About eight years ago, I went to a reunion of the eighth grade class of the parochial school I attended. There I was reacquainted with two women who had been the girls I played with back then; I had moved away after eighth grade graduation and after a few years we had lost touch with each other. They were surprised to learn that I was a nurse; both remembered that I had often talked of being a television newscaster—a memory totally obliterated in my own consciousness! How did I move from that childhood dream to the very different reality that is mine in nursing? There were no nurse relatives (or other health care providers). My mother worked part time as a waitress—work she loved and continues to do. My aunt was a businesswoman—a result of being abandoned by her husband and needing to support her child. I think she liked her work but it was an unplanned life path. In high school, the idea of becoming a nurse formed. In my mind, the only alternatives I had were being a teacher or a nun. No one ever suggested to me that I might put my skills to other uses—I had done well in biology, math, and English. I think the idea of being a newscaster was socialized out of me. For some reason, I was wise enough to test my hypothesis that I would enjoy nursing and be good at it. There was the Future Nurses Club; I joined and through that activity volunteered at Fitzgerald Mercy Hospital. That led to a position as a nurses' aide as soon as I was old enough to work. Since the beginning of my sophomore year in high school, I have been involved in nursing.

As a nurses' aide, I was fortunate to work with some very fine nurses and nursing students from Fitz's diploma school of nursing and Gwynedd Mercy's A.D. program. As I got to know the Fitz students, they encouraged me in my work and in planning for my future. Several encouraged me to get my B.S.N. "upfront." They let me know that the profession was headed in that direction; they foresaw themselves having to "go back" and wished that they had had similar guidance when they were making plans. Between my home, volunteer, and school responsibilities, I was somehow sheltered from the issues that drove many students during my high school and college years (1966–1974)–the Vietnam war, the women's movement. Part of my postcollege informal education meant getting caught up on these things—my intimates tease me that I must have slept through the 1960s.

As a nurses' aide, I worked every other weekend and worked hard. It was still the era of team nursing. We got report; the RNs gave me my assignments. For a long time, I kept many of those pieces of paper. I'm not sure why. Mr. K., an amputee, "a partial bath; VS qid; I & O; bed to wheelchair; S(ugar) & A(cetone) q 4h;" Mrs. C., a woman with gnarled digits, wizened and whining in pain from her arthritis; Mr. G., a man who was five years postlobectomy for lung cancer, still smoking! As I recall those times, I remember the nurses I worked with as being happy. Betty Lazarro was a role model of encouragement; to any evidence of a patient's progress, she'd say, "That's the ticket!" Sr. Marie Peter was young, vibrant, happy. I can still see her standing with the med cart in front of her, in a room with eight (I think) beds, bantering with the men, kind and firm. Barbara Strohl became an evening supervisor over the time I knew her. She was smart, a good teacher, supportive of staff, and helpful. She and another evening supervisor left me with a firm idea of what it meant to administer, a committed and involved supervision. I remember Peggy Prokapis dashing to a room and initiating CPR, when as a new nurses' aide, I told her this patient wasn't responding. Peggy Di Enno was the RN with whom I worked nights one summer, the two of us caring for 40 patients. I was an LPN then, having sat for the LPN boards between my junior and senior years of college. When I told her how difficult I found it to sleep during the day, she said, "Go home and have a beer and a sandwich."

One challenge that summer was a man who had Guillain Barré syndrome. He was paralyzed from the waist down, and was about 50 years old with white hair. It was a very busy night. He put the light on; he needed the bedpan to move his bowels. When I went to get the bedpan, he was shocked. I was "too young;" couldn't I get someone else? I knew I couldn't ask Peggy and I knew that I could easily be in this situation again and somehow I had to make it O.K. I don't remember exactly what I said but it was along the lines of, "I know this is difficult for you; you're used to doing this on your own; it's embarrassing," acknowledging how difficult it was and assuring him that his dignity was important to me, somehow trying to communicate that my youth belied my maturity and competence. He seemed O.K. then. The funny thing is I can still recall very graphically the bedpan I removed—details I will spare the reader! I helped him resettle for the night and I know I cared for him many more nights after that and that he felt comfortable with me. I often think of this, especially when someone associates nursing with tasks, such as toileting, that are regarded as menial. It took everything I had learned in school and "on the job" to respond to this man in a way that preserved his dignity.

At the age of 42 I think about the parts of my career that were planned and those that were unplanned. Decisions "made" in the early years were often caught up in relationships with significant others. I wasn't planning for a career in nursing; I was merely preparing for a useful occupation for the few years between college and the script of marriage and children that the society and culture of which I was a part offered me. Nursing was always something I could "go back to." It's not that the script is a bad one; what surprises me is that *that* Judy Spross never questioned it, never thought there might be alternatives, was so *unthinking* about it. When I was on the precipice, at the age of 20, of living out that unquestioned script—a decision surely destined to end in pain and misery—something happened. I went to a conference at the University of Pennsylvania. Among the panelists were Ingeborg Mauksch, Hans Mauksch, and Claire Fagin. I am not certain of the subject; I am fairly sure that Ingeborg Mauksch talked about nurse practitioners. It seems to me that some of the content had to do with change. I think seeing the two nurse leaders, hearing their vision, and appreciating their scholarship offered me a glimpse of another alternative. It was vague, very vague, but I think it is what gave me the courage to break off the engagement. As I move back and forth in my mind across the landscape of my career, I see that other conferences were turning points also.

In my experiences at Fitz, I always liked caring for cancer patients. I was challenged. I felt that even in my role as a nurses' aide I could offer comfort—care that was vital but did not depend on the knowledge and technical skills and responsibilities of an RN. In my junior or senior year in college, I had a wonderful med/surg instructor, Jean Maurer. I especially remember caring for Mr. T., a man in his late 40s or early 50s who was married and had a teenage daughter. He had a brain tumor and was dying. I received a lot of support from Jean—something intangible. Although I don't remember the details of a particular conversation in which we talked about what I was doing, I remember thinking that how well this patient was cared for depended a lot on me, the nursing care I planned and provided. The doctors had nothing to offer. It was a good time to be in nursing; I had been exposed to Kübler-Ross's work. I didn't feel helpless. I worked with that family and I believe I made a difference. This was the beginning of my "specialization."

I tried to be a good student. Clinically, I was very good—it was reflected in those grades. I lived at home—a "dayhop," as commuting students were known. I had received some financial aid; otherwise my school expenses depended on what I could earn. At one time I was holding three part-time jobs as well as going to school full time; my nonclinical grades reflect this workaholism! I would go home and study on some days and then leave the house at 9 P.M. to work at a pancake house until 2 or 3 A.M.; sometimes I worked this shift on my weekends off from Fitz. I also worked at a department store near Villanova that I could go to directly from school. I worked in books and stationery. I enjoyed all of these jobs and liked meeting so many different people. Eventually, I just worked at the department store during school breaks and gave up the waitress job. I was having fun, too; family events, dances, football and basketball games. I marvel at this person who needed so little sleep! I can count on one hand the number of times I've stayed up until midnight in the last 16 years!

Another event that occurred in my work experience at this time that was influential was an experience with a patient, Jimmy, who was an age peer and also a substance abuser. Probably because of the closeness in age, we connected—not in anything but a professional way. No doubt I had an inflated idea of being able to rescue him from his habit. One of the RNs warned me about getting too "involved with patients" based on whatever she was observing in this situation. I think this incident was the beginning of my developing a questioning and critical mind.

The curriculum at Villanova was based on Peplau and Travelbee. I knew about the idea of "professional distance." I was never sure exactly what it meant. I translated it as maintaining a boundary such that my needs and the patients' needs did not become confused or blurred and that the relationship was therapeutic, but not cold or distant. As I grew in oncology nursing and learned about the joys and sorrows of caring for people with chronic illness, I knew that professional distance meant nothing to me; it defied feelings of warmth, love, caring, grief, and loss. So what I kept before me, in the midst of the many feelings I experienced in so many situations, was, "Is the focus here on the patient's needs?" Martocchio's Mara Mogenson Flaherty article on authenticity, closeness, self-representation, and belonging captured so beautifully my own conclusions about what oncology nursing is all about. To me it is a classic; one I return to often. As an educator, rather than put a student or young graduate in the position of being reprimanded for "getting too close," I would talk about the one-sided intimacy that seemed to characterize nursing. I'd explain that the feelings they might experience with patients would feel like feelings evoked in their closest relationships; what was different was the absence of mutual and similar expectations and responsibilities. The feelings are powerful; it is folly to ignore them; being aware of them and tending to them is important. Often, expressing them to patients (feelings such as sorrow, joy) would be therapeutic for the patient; at other times it would be a burden on patients and families. I would tell my students that part of clinical judgment was learning this kind of distinction and identifying personal and professional supports for taking care of themselves so they could continue to care. I get concerned about theorists who try to use friendship as a paradigm for the nursing relationship. In my opinion, it is a terribly misguided and misleading analogy. Travelbee remains the most eloquent writer about the nature and power of the nurse–patient relationship.

I graduated and stayed on as a GN, then RN at Fitz (now Mercy Catholic Medical Center–Fitzgerald division). I considered Sloan-Kettering and went up for an interview. I don't know why I didn't go to Sloan-Kettering. It wasn't time to leave Philadelphia yet. It was a good decision to stay in a place that was familiar. The biggest challenge was supervising the nursing assistants who had been my peers and were older than me—Bea, Cass, Gene, and Kate. I still had the immediate and tangible support of family and friends.

Within months of graduation, I became the evening charge nurse and began orienting other new grads. I got involved in the primary nursing committee and helped develop the first primary nursing job description for our agency. I still have the letter I received from the director of nursing, Mary Ann Morgan, regarding my involvement in that project. I was proud of my work. I loved the autonomy of the evening shift, the unfettered collaboration with the house staff, and the opportunity to *really* get to know the families of patients. I liked not being caught up in all of the scheduled tests that make mornings so busy and chaotic.

Some of those evenings were powerful. I remember Vince who came in through the emergency room with what I can only call "raging diarrhea." He was married and middle-aged. The diagnostic workup was unrevealing. What might have been a four- to seven-day hospitalization turned into weeks. One night he had a fever of 104 degrees. His wife was angry; she raged at me. I didn't get flustered; I knew uncertainty and the failure of the diarrhea to abate were wearing and frustrating. By now he had lost several pounds. I listened to her as well as doing all of the appropriate diagnostic and comfort measures for Vince. In retrospect, I think the fever must have represented an omen to her; her rage masked her dread which, as events proved, was well founded. Her rage was continual and it was accompanied by Vince's own helplessness to help her, I think. I stuck with both of them, challenged by trying to comfort in the face of the unknown. Vince died a few weeks later. I don't remember whether the diagnosis was known just before he died or from the postmortem. It was a gastrointestinal lymphoma. Some time after he died, his wife returned to my unit to talk to me. She gave me a present with a lovely note. The gift was a sterling silver ankh on a chain, an Egyptian symbol of hope. I wore it for many years—until I lost it. I've lost things over the years but I don't think I've missed anything quite as much. I think it is why I still weep at the end of the ONS video, "Those Were Hard Days" when Virginia Barckley holds up the "gold" button given to her by a young patient.

I wasn't fully aware of it at the time—I learned to appreciate it more when I was in graduate school—but one of the pioneers of leukemia treatment, Isaac Djerassi, M.D., was working at Fitz and its sister hospital, Misericordia. When he began to try methotrexate in adults, my unit got many of the patients. Suddenly I was seeing things I hadn't seen. I don't think I learned much about the leukemias in school because they were less common than solid tumors, and, in adults, not particularly treatable. I began to see how much I didn't know. Joe was a young man with AML who loved his motorcycle. He was on high-dose methotrexate. Among his responses was a horrendous stomatitis (treated with gentian violet) and a cutaneous reaction like a severe sunburn. He developed several infections. This was my first encounter with amphotericin B. I didn't think he'd leave the hospital alive. All he wanted to do was get on his bike again. As it turned out, he achieved a remission. He left and came back to see us with bike tales related in his leather jacket, *healthy*. The remission was short-lived. It must have been a matter of months, at most a year. I took care of him while he was dying and he died before I left Fitz, 15 months after I graduated from college. Vince and Joe are probably why I chose to specialize in oncology when I went to grad school but that was only part of my so-called "decision" to return to school.

It wasn't all work during those 15 months post-Villanova. I played on Fitz's bowling league, arranging to have that night off every week. I accepted a dare from my college friends to try a computer dating service. The service mostly missed the mark as far as I was concerned but I met one man whose influence, unknown to him perhaps, was central. As I got to know him, I learned what it meant to "plan a career." His goal was to be the youngest person to get a Ph.D. in his field. We had a lot of fun; he was a graduate student. I got to know something about his life and he, mine. Among his fellow doctoral students were several women, none of whom I got to know well but, as a group of women, they again represented some alternative I had not considered. These observations were not at all conscious at the time but as I've reflected on my life I've come to understand how I came to make choices and live this life which was not the script offered me. At 22, however, I was still rather unquestioning, at least as far as the social script I "was supposed to follow." This man seemed a likely candidate to play the opposite role but as time went on it became clear to me he had no particular script. When I talked about going back to school for a master's degree, he was supportive and unthreatened, even though I was considering going away. I can't say that my reasons for going back to school were well thought out; a seed had been planted in my professional issues course at Villanova and nurtured by my exposure to Ingeborg Mauksch. My friend made advanced education seem exciting.

My best friend and roommate was getting married so I would need to do something about the apartment we shared—give up the lease or find a roommate. When the time came to make a decision (I had been accepted at Catholic U and the University of Pennsylvania, in addition to MCV as I recall), I chose MCV, not for any specific reason though I have made some deductions about the likely convoluted subconscious reasons. The fact that there was funding and a stipend thanks to the federal nurse traineeships was probably a factor. Suffice it to say, it was time to try my wings. It was a fortuitous decision.

The first year was hard personally; I underestimated the impact that the loss of my personal supports would make. I traveled home many weekends from Richmond to Philadelphia. I joked that the new car I'd bought (a Ford Pinto) had become a dependent. It broke down a lot; eventually, I went to work part time to support it. My rent for a townhouse off Horsepen Road was $150; I was amazed—newly sanded hardwood floors, two bedrooms, and two floors. A deal compared to the nearly $300 I had paid in Lansdowne for a cookie-cutter apartment.

I loved school. Pathophysiology was challenging, as the sciences had been at Villanova. I particularly remember the young professor with a British accent teaching about acid base balance and describing how one set of ions "mop up" the other. Though MCV didn't have an oncology program per se, I was fortunate to be there. They were among the first to have federal monies to establish a comprehensive cancer rehabilitation program which was under the direction of Dr. Susan Mellette. Barbara Satterwhite and Ann Pryor, ONS members, taught me how to give chemotherapy, a new role for nurses. I remember the first doses of vincristine I gave, afraid I'd extravasate. I was fortunate to have such calm, competent mentors. Marilyn Dunavant taught me all about stomas. Dr. Lawrence Brown was one of the surgeons; he went on to be a leader with ACS national. Virginia Wessels and Tina Bear taught me about interdisciplinary teamwork, outcomes, quality assurance, and continuity of care in cancer rehab. Rehabilitation was the underlying philosophy of my cancer education. As I see how the history of oncology and oncology nursing has unfolded, my choice of schools was auspicious, the beginning of durable, sustaining connections that I cherish today, and a practical philosophy regarding cancer care.

My sister students were a great group. About seven of us hung around together, three of us with an interest in oncology. Pat, Ann, and I heard about an oncology nursing conference that was going to be held in Toronto in the spring of 1976. We began to make plans to drive up. One of our friends, Sue, had family in western Pennsylvania and she arranged for us to stay there on our way up, to break up the trip. About three days before our departure, Ann found out that I did not know how to drive a car with a stick shift. There ensued a crash course in driving a standard in an empty parking lot. Sorry to say, it wasn't until 1982 that I mastered this fine art. Poor Ann survived my encounter with the mailbox at Sue's family home in Pennsylvania and a Chinese fire drill on a teeny hill in the middle of rush hour traffic in Philly on the return trip. My driving was not the only source of laughs. Ann, a contact lens wearer for years, was not in the habit of carrying her glasses or a spare pair of lenses with her. So in Toronto, when she lost a lens in the ancient plumbing of the Old Vic Hotel, she was devastated. The fact that I was totally green at driving a standard probably increased her motivation to solve this minor disaster, since she couldn't drive one-lensed. She consulted with the concierge, who assured us that on a Saturday, no plumber could be found. To his credit, he suggested the local hardware store. We went to the store and purchased a long piece of tubing—narrow enough for the drain and wide enough for a lens. The three of us taking turns at siphoning the contents of the drainpipe was quite a sight! The lens was retrieved and we did not come down with any disease!

What was more important about Toronto were the lectures we heard and the discussions regarding an organization for oncology nursing. Katherine Nelson talked about the merits of using the term *cancer nursing* as opposed to *oncology nursing* in naming such an organization. I was new at this. I hadn't known about the earlier national ACS nursing meeting. I am sure people who came to be influential in my career were at that meeting but it wasn't time to meet them yet. The Three Musketeers returned to Richmond re-energized. Certainly my commitment to oncology nursing was solidified. I still had another year to go in grad school.

Around the same time, I learned that both of the doctorally prepared med/surg faculty members were leaving and who the faculty would be for my second year was up in the air. I had been in graduate school long enough to be so elitist as to think that only doctorally prepared faculty should be teaching in my program. I kept my ear to the ground during the summer to see who was hired, prepared to leave Virginia and transfer to another program. When I heard that a person with *only* a master's degree had been hired, I was chagrined. Before making a final decision to leave, I thought I should at least meet her before making another big change in my life. Sometime in August, we met for lunch. When I tell you that the person I met was Ann Hamric, you can guess that I stayed. I had no clue that we would write a book together but I did realize that I could learn a lot from her. I did and I have and I still do! Another thing that happened that summer was that the IV nurse where I worked was going on vacation. Because of the initiative I had demonstrated in starting IVs, which she had taught me how to do, I was asked to cover for her during her vacation—doing all IV starts including children and post-op patients. It was satisfying because it meant I had mastered a skill so important to my future in oncology.

While in grad school, I took ice skating lessons to relax—one foot glide, two foot glide, front swizzle, and back swizzle. I had been a self-taught skater, able to stay up, glide forward, and stop. I enjoyed learning a different set of skills. How much of this was influenced by the potluck gatherings Ann, Pat, other students, and I had while watching Dorothy Hamill skate her way to an Olympic championship in 1976, I don't know!

In the summer of 1977 I had to decide—do I stay in Richmond to work as an oncology clinical specialist or do I go to rural New Hampshire for a similar position? I chose New Hampshire—there was little difference in money and I had a good feeling for both of my prospective supervisors. I don't know exactly what led me to New Hampshire. I was uprooting myself again to a place where I knew no one. Perhaps I was buoyed at having successfully weathered the difficulties of my first transition and the conclusion that it was the first year that was the hardest. The fact that Dartmouth Hitchcock Medical Center was an academic medical center had some appeal. I knew something about moving that I couldn't have known before Richmond. Living in a rural area seemed like a personal adventure I couldn't resist; besides I hated hot, humid summers.

The five years I spent in New Hampshire were particularly heady, full of personal and professional opportunities and risks. The director of nursing, Marilyn Prouty, and the associate director and my immediate boss, Sarah Jo Brown, were strong and assertive women, incredibly supportive. These mentors continued to model and support some self-discovery that had begun under Ann Hamric's guidance. I took risks. I took stands. I navigated conflict instead of ignoring or suppressing it. The two head nurses with whom I worked, Lorraine Baker and Marilyn Bedell, I think would agree that we built a strong unit, a strong staff, and pretty effective nurse–physician collaboration.

I don't think we ever counted how many staff went back to school—the ward clerk who went for an A.D., the diploma grads who pursued B.S.N.s, and the college grads who went on for master's degrees. Many have sustained their commitment to oncology nursing and have been involved in ONS at the local and national levels.

I learned about research and received both practical and further academic preparation in ethics. The clinical specialist group was strong. My officemate, then friend and colleague Shirley Girouard, Ph.D., R.N., was the med/sug CNS. Sarah Jo made sure I met with Susan Baird early on. That relationship flourished into a wonderful mentorship and friendship. She helped me through my first publication—the one on superior vena cava syndrome. It is notable that I didn't have enough confidence to think I could write the article by myself so I collaborated with an oncology fellow. The physicians were great; they cared a lot about patients. They got used to having me around, asking questions. I could write a book about all of the patients and the extraordinary experiences I had. As Ann Hamric had taught me, I kept logs of my practice—which I still have. These data later were the basis for the Schering lectureship.

In addition to being mentored by Sue Baird, in so many ways—publishing, research, lecturing, ACS activities, editing (I remember helping her paste up issues of the journal in her New London kitchen, shortly after she assumed the editorship of the *Oncology Nursing Forum*)—there were other important events. I got involved in ONS—the journal (including those productive, wonderful board meetings at Moose Mountain) and the nominating committee (I was not elected the first time I was on the ballot but was the second time). I volunteered for ACS, participating in the teaching "travel teams" that brought cancer nursing CE to the far reaches of rural New Hampshire. These travel teams were an innovation that can be credited to Sue Baird and Pat Champagne.

I mentioned that we had a strong CNS group. One event that occurred was our deciding that we needed a conference for CNSs in our region. As we began planning, I wanted them to meet Ann Hamric, to be exposed to her vision of specialty practice. One of the issues we were struggling with was evaluation and Ann had spent a lot of time on this in my program and had at least one publication on the topic at the time. That first conference was held at the Lake Morey Inn in Vermont. It was exciting. There may have been 30 or 40 attendees. The content was so compelling that Ann was interested in seeing whether we could publish it as a monograph. There is more to the story but our search for a publisher for the monograph led us to Carol Wolfe at Grune & Stratton. Carol saw its potential as a book and encouraged us to find some other contributors so that we could have a book-length publication. It was a challenging project; Carol mentored her two novices along. The text became one of G & S's top-ten sellers.

Another turning point, which occurred early in my CNS position at Dartmouth, was attending a workshop given by Margo McCaffery. Her teaching joined Ann Hamric's—the two of them provided me with the most empowering experiences of my life. Pain was a common problem in my clinical practice. Thanks to my clinical experiences with Mario Kuperminc, M.D., and Joanne Kyle, R.N., N.P., at MCV I felt reasonably competent to help patients. Of course, much of it was based on using methadone and dosing round the clock. McCaffery's workshop gave me so much more. Her teachings immediately translated into practice. I got the psych CNS, Anne-Marie Barron, to help me practice relaxation skills. My first clinical use of the technique was apocryphal—in using it to ease the anxiety of one hungry, irritable, and elderly gentleman on call for a gastrostomy, I inadvertently "relaxed" the three other men in the ward. The evening staff were eager to have me use my newfound skill over the intercom nightly! Margo's teaching gave me so much more courage and skill to deal with the conflicts that often arose around pain management. If my voice in this project is nothing more than a testimonial to the influence she has had on our profession and our involvement in pain management, my reflections will have been worth the time to capture them in writing. My own passion for the issue can be directly traced to that long-ago workshop and her willingness to be available to those who attended.

I applied for the NCI foreign nurse fellowship. I didn't get it the first time. Sue and Sarah Jo both encouraged me to reapply. One of the lessons of this period in my life was in not feeling defeated if I was not successful the first time I tried something. My second application to NCI was accepted. I could go to London, Amsterdam, or Brussels. I wanted to go to Brussels and use the four years of French I had studied in high school. In September 1980 I went to Brussels to work at Institut Jules Bordet, taking a leave of absence from my CNS job. I was young in research and my career. What came out of this investment was a small study on preventing and treating stomatitis and an abstract presentation at ONS on applying Orem's self-care model to bone marrow transplant patients. I gave several talks on a variety of oncology and advanced practice topics in Belgium, Holland, and England—several in French. I implemented a CNS role working with staff and caring for patients at Bordet.

I returned to Dartmouth in April 1981. Over the next year there were some key nursing leadership changes. The combination of these administrative changes and my recent, novel overseas experience interacted to make me restless, feeling ready for a change but without a clear direction. I'm sure I discussed my restlessness with my mentors. One aspect of reality shock in this first CNS job was the realization that I had learned little about education (except for patient ed) in grad school. What I acquired about the technical and cognitive aspects of CE and student education was strictly on-the-job and hit-or-miss. A post-master's program in oncology nursing education had been funded at two universities. I began to investigate and apply.

I mentioned that New Hampshire was an enriching time for me personally. That was my athletic era. I played volleyball and learned how to cross-country ski in the middle of the 1978 blizzard. The latter had been an invitation from the first head nurse I worked with, Lorraine.

I had a feeling that there was more riding on this than the overt social aspects. Lorraine was an excellent skier. I did not allow the snow "squall" to deter me. I still had my (rear wheel drive) Pinto and drove the ten hilly miles from Hanover to Woodstock. We skied; she was a good teacher. I had to ignore my terror on the narrow tracks that went by what looked to me like bottomless ravines. I cringed when I saw the black signs that meant "most difficult" trails. I did not have the courage to insist on the easiest; there seemed to be more at stake than whether I just skied. I found myself wishing for windshield wipers for my spectacles! We skied; we had a delicious lunch at her home; I drove home. The storm that ended up paralyzing Boston and much of New England did not paralyze me. I attribute the considerable success Lorraine and I had during her tenure as head nurse to whatever we accomplished on that ski tour. I made forays into downhill skiing but never took to it the way I did to cross-country skiing.

I continued to skate; I ran; planted my first garden ever and enjoyed its bounty; learned to play racquetball; and began taking voice lessons. When Shirley Girouard, a former Rainbow choir girl, respectfully asked me to refrain from singing "Happy Birthday," I decided to do something about it! After a year or so of lessons, I was in the chorus of a Gilbert and Sullivan play. I also participated in a life-changing reading group that focused on women's literature. In our early years as CNSs, Shirley and I started the Upper Valley party circuit to help us adjust to the absence of urban distractions. This group has gone on for quite a while; through it I met my spouse, Joe Barry (summer 1981). It's funny; I had abandoned the script society had given me. I loved my work and couldn't imagine a relationship that could support what I hoped to do. Joe was as interested in reinventing the scripts for marriage we'd been given as I was. We married in March 1982 and have been reinventing ever since! We left New Hampshire in August 1982 so I could enroll in the post-master's program in oncology nursing education in Birmingham, Alabama—a nine-month stint. I left the door open to return to Dartmouth (not necessarily in a CNS position if my position were filled) by taking another leave of absence.

The experience in Alabama filled in some of the gaps I noted above. With the exception of Joe, who accompanied me, I felt as though I had taken a leave of absence from everything else in my life—committee work and volunteer work. I started a book group similar to the one I left. I did some CNS consulting and worked part time as a hospice nurse. I made a wonderful friend as well as some terrific colleagues in oncology nursing. In December 1982 Susan Baird let me know that she would be moving to Bethesda to assume the chief of cancer nursing position at NCI. She didn't know what positions would be available but hoped that I would consider applying for an oncology CNS position. I was intrigued;

I had done a brief practicum in the outpatient setting at NCI while I was at MCV—with Bonny Johnson and Susan Hubbard as guides.

I applied for an NCI clinical specialist job—a unit-based position for a new unit that would open in a few months. During the nomadic months between my being hired and the unit opening I got involved in the new population we were seeing—those with AIDS. I learned a lot about the disease, its treatment, diversity, and tolerance, lessons that have served me well in my professional and personal life. The unit for which I was hired never opened so Susan "detailed" me to the surgical oncology unit.

I don't think Rachel Brown, the head nurse, was sure she wanted me or what to do with me if she did! Surgical oncology was low on my list of desirable areas to work in or develop, and it was certainly the area of oncology that I was least competent in. It had been ages since I dealt with stomas in a consistent, "expert" way; the power sprays of my grad school days were rusty. I had observed Shirley's efforts to work on surgical units at Dartmouth; I didn't feel up to those kinds of challenges. On the other hand, I had just moved and couldn't move again; I wanted to work with Susan and the team she had put in place; and simply put, I needed a job! I quickly decided that the solution was not to try to become an overnight surgical oncology nursing whiz kid—the staff was highly skilled and talented, not to mention perceptive. So I focused on figuring out how my medical oncology background could fit in.

As it turned out, pain was a major issue; the surgical oncology branch was developing clinical trials on biologicals; and there was more and more post-op chemotherapy. The emphasis on surgery was decreasing but not absent. I learned what I needed to from the staff about caring for the surgical patients so I could care for them at least as competently as the proficient surgical nurses. I reviewed the tube and drain class Shirley had incorporated into her orientations at Dartmouth. I remembered her basic approach to surgical nursing: "Surgical nursing is easy, Judy—you just need to know what part was operated on, what it was supposed to do before surgery, how the surgery alters normal functions, what can go wrong, and what is considered normal post-surgical function." I was particularly challenged by the patients with pancreatic cancer who had complicated surgery and intraoperative radiation therapy. My inability to find much in the way of nursing literature is what led to the article in *Seminars in Oncology Nursing* which I wrote with two of the staff. Working on this unit was very satisfying for me. Rachel and I worked well together and witnessed a lot of growth in the staff. When Susan left NIH though, I knew I would not be far behind her. I yearned to go back to New England. I left in July 1985 to go to, of all places, MGH in Boston, a career switch to graduate educator.

The time I spent at NIH also is associated with some key career events and transitions. I was in the middle of a clinical center CNS meeting, when I got beeped and answered a page from Judi Johnson. She told me that I was the board's choice to be the first recipient of ONS's Schering award for excellence in clinical practice. I was stunned. On what basis was I chosen? I wondered. I went back to the meeting dazed but thrilled; my colleagues congratulated me warmly. Some readers will remember the lecture I delivered on pain. I never worked so hard on a lecture in my life. The topic emerged from a review of the many clinical logs I had kept in my seven years as a CNS, my memories of my most challenging clinical experiences, Amy Valentine's use of the Dickinson poem at a St. Anselm conference, and conversations with colleagues. Why was it such a problem, when, as McCaffery had shown me six years before, so much knowledge was available to treat pain? There had been an article in *Image* that had used literature and legend to explore a topic; my title was an expansion and adaptation of that article's title. I am a voracious reader (or was until I began doctoral studies!), so my leisure reading for the next few months was every nonclinical account of pain and suffering I could find. I probably cited half of what I found—I couldn't use everything.

This began what has become a sort of professional hobby. I keep a file now of writings on the subject of pain and people who know me send whatever they come across. In 1990 I updated my Schering lecture in an article in *Dimensions in Oncology Nursing*. My original Schering lecture is often cited in the literature. I received some warm, wonderful, and moving letters from people who heard it. I hesitate to say that it was a turning point, not just for me, but for our specialty but it's an impression I get from what kind people say and the events that followed.

It wasn't just the preparation that was demanding; I also practiced and practiced my delivery for I wanted the words and emotions of the patients and families who had suffered with cancer pain, often need-lessly, to be heard as their words, not my translation. So I had to get into those moments/centuries of suffering with them—to find *their* voices and *their* anguish. At the same time, I had to sustain myself so I would get through the speech. I was so frustrated during the speech, the slide projector that had worked when I checked it just prior to my speech failed and I couldn't advance the slides myself! I had to develop a signaling mechanism so that the performance aspects of my presentation would not be jolted by, "Next slide please."

The event was overshadowed by the presence of a nurse whom I had met on an international tour I had led. Shortly after that trip her long marriage had broken up and she was devastated; this was her first ONS Congress. Though I didn't know her well, I was familiar to her--her pain was tangible and hardly bearable. The Congress seemed ludicrously irrelevant but here she was. I made sure she met good people who would help her feel secure, engage her, and show her around if she had the energy to do so.

I wanted to arouse the kind of passion for addressing the pervasive problem of poor pain management as Margo McCaffery had done for me. I wanted to do it at a gut level as well as a cognitive level. What I remember most about the lecture was that there were many people in tears. There are other things I remember; Susan Baird, mentor extraordinaire, gifted me with a trip to the hairdresser. Marie Bakitas and Marilyn Bedell stayed with me when the lecture was over; kind attention that I sorely needed. The lecture, regardless of how many times I had practiced it, had the same power, even on that day, to make me feel incredibly sad. Joe sent me flowers ("Knock their socks off"); my NIH and Alabama colleagues presented me with flowers afterwards. The day had the emotional roller coaster quality normally associated with weddings.

Part of the post-Schering experience for me was a letdown phenomenon. It was as though I had established a standard for myself and subsequent lectures were not meeting it. This lasted about two years; my passion for the topic made me continue to try to get the message out. From the perspective of wisdom that eight years has given me, I can see that the Schering lecture was a special one requiring a special approach. Now and then I have to call on the particular skills I developed for that day and can reasonably hold myself to that standard.

Around the time of the Schering lecture, planning for the second edition of the CNS book began. It came out in 1989. The content for the third edition is being planned.

The move to graduate education at the MGH Institute of Health Professions was a great one. It was a wonderful opportunity to get to know Debbie Mayer, hired at the same time. Prior to this we had just known each other from prior conventions, a loose connection based on the fact that we both came from the Philadelphia area. Based on a colleague's suggestion, it was Debbie I selected to co-lead the 1984 tour to the Far East with me. Again I had a wonderful director, Elizabeth Grady, who supported me, and like other supervisors, gave me enough rope to do what I was capable of doing.

I am most proud of the three-credit graduate course on pain that I started with a physical therapy colleague, Terry Michel. She and I also collaborated on a funded symposium to teach faculty and clinical preceptors about pain assessment and management.

This position at MGH was also the source of a wonderful personal and collegial relationship with Sheila Norton, a nurse–midwife. We could write several books, among them *Adventures in Teaching*, which would be about innovation in methods of teaching and curriculum development. Another would be about the similar issues we face in each of our specialties. What we did write about was role development of clinicians who become faculty members and incorporating concepts of women's health and psychological development into our methods of preparing nurses who are mostly women. With Sheila's help, I have also begun to bring the message about cancer and chronic pain management to advanced practice nurses in primary care. She and her eight-year-old daughter are family now. Joe and I live downstairs from them.

I am most proud of the ONS position paper on cancer pain. I feel fortunate to count as colleagues the leaders of the Wisconsin Pain Initiative, another group (Charlie Cleeland, June Dahl, Dave Joranson, Sandy Ward, Sophie Colleau) whose influence on my professional life has been profound. I am grateful for whatever forces brought us together at that first international conference on cancer pain in Rye, New York. I was proud to be asked to deliver the keynote address at their fifth anniversary celebration, a presentation which deserved and got the special "Schering lecture treatment."

I am finding it difficult to capture 20 years of experience, of patients, colleagues, mentors, friends, and family who have made my career in oncology nursing so enriching and rewarding. In fact I am a bit impatient, for I realize how much more I need to do. Debbie McGuire, Debbie Mayer, Betty Ferrell, Margo McCaffery, Regina Schmitt, Carol Curtiss, Pearl Moore, Trish Greene, Margaret Barton-Burke, Nancy Hester, Joan Piemme, and other colleagues in and outside of nursing have done much to shape the part of me that pursues the issue of cancer pain relief.

Because of oncology nursing, I have a deep appreciation for the fleetingness of life. I have witnessed too many who have said, "I wish I had . . ." and, "If only." I try to appreciate every day as a gift and my friends and family as precious. My career has instilled in me an understanding of the life of the spirit in ways that were wanting in the religious education of my youth. I have tried to give up the workaholism of my early career; mostly I am successful. If at times it seems I am not, it is a purposeful, conscious reflection of what one set of choices means for the roads not taken. Alleviation of cancer pain and advanced practice issues (in that order at the moment) are the polestars that guide my professional choices. And nurturing my relationships and caring for my own health are my personal priorities.

It is interesting to be at a point where I have goals but no script. My career began with many unexpected twists and turns. By the time I had been in New Hampshire a year or two, there was more deliberation and planning. I still try to keep a flexible and open attitude about the paths that lie ahead. People ask me what I'll do when I finish my doctorate. I don't know but I can see the seed of future opportunities being planted. I have liked just about everything I have done in oncology nursing so I can't imagine that the right kind of work won't present itself.

I have many stories to tell: holding an original letter of Florence Nightingale's and listening to her voice on tape while at the University of Alabama; seeing her hospital, St. Thomas' in England, for the first time, making so real the wisdom of her writings; the first and second OCNS conferences; Ann's diagnosis of breast cancer while we were in the middle of the second edition of the CNS book during which I became one of her many "teachers;" and finally, becoming an educator like Ann Hamric (unlike her I was not a born teacher but she is the standard I aspired to). It took a couple of years and several mistakes to synthesize intelligence, caring, humor, and flexibility—taking what was good about how I had been taught and abandoning old unworkable rules (another script perhaps?)—into a meaningful, coherent role that felt as comfortable as my CNS roles had felt. I can believe I was a born nurse, even a born CNS—but a born teacher I was not! I wondered whether education was where I belonged and was grateful for the opportunity of a joint appointment. I collaborated with physicians to establish MGH's cancer pain center. It's no coincidence that my teaching improved while in this role, though other factors played a part as well. Some of my classroom students were precepted by me in the pain clinic. I remember theology and philosophy courses at Villanova. As I grew in nursing, in oncology nursing, where life and death and the big and little moments in between are full of meaning, poignancy, and nearly every emotion one can think of, those courses assumed a new relevance. I began to speak of nursing as "applied philosophy" and tried to convey this to my students. Writing this, I realize I am full of moments, stories that are all a part of who I am and also a part of what oncology nursing is and can become.

Oncology nursing and nurses continue to inspire me. I am grateful for the gifts of friendship and professional support and opportunities that those named above and so many others have given me. The generosity within our specialty (both among individuals and within our specialty organizations) is a source of wonder to many in other specialties. When I was going to graduate school, my father said, "Why? If you're going to spend that kind of money and time why not go to medical school?", a question I know many others have been asked. I tried to explain but did not feel terribly successful. If my mother wondered, she never asked, content to have me follow my heart. There is no doubt in my mind that my father has been able to answer his own question for a while now. Oncology is where the "rubber meets the road," so to speak. Oncology nursing is about rhythms, music, *life*: Who could ask for more?

36

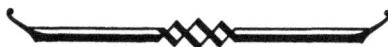

Shirley Stagner

I always wanted to be a nurse. Part of the desire must have stemmed from my admiration for my mother who is now retired after a nursing career spanning 28 years. She was actually a specialist nurse, spending 21 years of her career caring for the mentally ill.

During the 1950s and 1960s when I was making this life-shaping decision, accepted career options for women were fairly limited—nurse, secretary, teacher, or housewife. Anything else was pushing the envelope. I just liked taking care of people, being helpful. And, though perhaps not at the forefront of my decision, there was the fact that my mother always had money. She did not have to ask my father for money; she had her own money.

Whatever the conscious or unconscious reasons for the choice, it was a perfect choice.

Recently, through some intensive seminar work, I was forced to put my personal mission for my time on the planet into words. For some in the seminar it was very difficult. For me it was easy. My mission, my purpose in life, is to serve others through my love, my faith, my courage, my wisdom, and my passion. What other career choice would have offered me the myriad opportunities to fulfill this purpose? I am grateful. Through all the uncertainty and turmoil that is a part of life, I have never really had to grapple with the great question, Why am I here? I have known.

Serendipity has played a big part in the direction of my career. I chose to get a baccalaureate degree in nursing not because I thought one type of nursing education was better than another, but because I wanted a college degree. People in my circle went to college. My family expected it and I was not into disappointing my family, especially my father.

Even though this great plan was interrupted after one year of college by marriage and the birth of my daughter, Sema, I never let it go. When my husband finished his degree and informed me that he wanted to stay where we were so that he could go on for a master's, I balked. I had already been accepted to the University of Tennessee in Memphis and I was not waiting any longer. I didn't.

However, I have always been thankful for the precious 18 months I had with my beautiful daughter. I did not have a job and only went to school part time. Essentially, I was always there. Whatever she wanted or needed, I was there to take care of it. After the move to Memphis in 1967, that special time came to an abrupt halt. I was ALL school and in life up to my elbows.

Even while getting my degree, my vision for myself in nursing was stretching the boundaries. I can remember writing a paper about how I saw my role after graduation. The paper described something much like the current clinical specialist role in mental health nursing. I remember writing that I would "sell" a hospital on this role. In those days, I thought all things were possible.

Somewhere in the process of doing clinicals, I learned that my love was pediatrics. I loved the children: holding them, calming their fears, playing with them—making an unpleasant situation a little better.

Oncology just sort of happened to me. I had done a rotation at St. Jude Children's Research Hospital, and I knew I wanted to work there. It had children, and it was the only hospital I had seen that matched the idealistic picture I had developed of health care during my years at UT. There were multidisciplinary conferences and nurses who were really involved. I knew I would have good role models. I only planned to work there for a year or so until I felt secure in my skills and well grounded as a professional nurse. Then I was going to go out and reform health care, at least one little piece of it—our local city hospital.

When I returned from my job interview at St. Jude, my husband who had supported us for three years was very interested in how much money I would make. I had forgotten to ask! (In 1970 it was $7,600 per year.)

I got the job. In a short time I was hooked—hooked on St. Jude and hooked on oncology. My odyssey really began.

Advances in therapy for childhood acute lymphocytic leukemia (ALL) were beginning to take hold. When I began working at St. Jude in 1970, no one talked about curing ALL or much of anything else in childhood cancer. In the early 1970s, Dr. Donald Pinkel, the medical director of St. Jude and the idea man behind the successful St. Jude ALL protocols, published the first article that reported an 18 percent cure rate for childhood ALL. Cure! What would everyone say? Would anyone believe us? We were all abuzz.

I thought it very gutsy for Dr. Pinkel to make that unequivocal statement. There was data to back it up, but to use the "C" word. . . . I knew he believed it. The fact that he believed ALL to be curable is a major reason why it is curable. And I believed it. I was living it every day, providing care according to clinical protocols, recording and inter-preting data. Children with leukemia were living longer and doing better than anyone would have expected even five years before. They were growing up.

But in the early 1970s it was a new way to think.

Early on, I was feeling my way along as a staff nurse. Pulling daunomycin into a syringe, dislodging the plunger and spilling hun-dreds of dollars worth of the drug on my shoes. Giving chemo into an antecubital with the patient wearing the tourniquet. Some days were scary.

Other days were terrifying. Finding a patient dead. My first. Listening, feeling, watching. Not wanting to say she was dead. What if she wasn't? Could an 11-year-old child possibly be dead? She was.

Jane Berg and Robbie Simpson were my trainers, my mentors. I still love them both. Jane seemed to always have the answers to my questions and she was always patient. Jane is now in Alaska. Her first husband died of cancer and she left oncology. We correspond at Christmas.

Robbie and I often worked 3–11 together. Two RNs and 25 critically ill children. (St. Jude only had 25 beds at the time.) What a team. Our operation was seamless. With the help of our trusty house officers, we could handle whatever happened. Robbie was just about the best nurse I have ever seen.

During the time Robbie and I worked together in 1970–1971, I would describe myself as a weekend hippie—too goal-oriented to drop out and too full of life and rebellion not to be part of the times. Robbie was a lovely, southern, Christian young woman with no aspirations to hippie-dom. But she liked the clothes. My sweetest memory of her is our shopping trip to the Highland Strip, our local hippie and pseudo-hippie haven, for the latest in flower-child fashion. We had a ball; she looked a little uncomfortable but adorable in her new outfit.

Six months later she was dead from hepatitis at the age of 23. She probably got it at St. Jude but we never really knew. As I sat by her bed on the night before her death and watched over the writhing, orangey woman who was my friend and colleague, I had my first really close encounter with helplessness and grief. It still brings tears to my eyes and yet my image of her is surrounded by a beautiful golden light.

After working as a staff nurse for about a year, a big opportunity opened up for me. A physician colleague, Dr. Jim Sumners, happened to be sharing an office with the then head of hematology, Dr. Joe Simone. Jim learned that the leukemia service planned to add a nurse practitioner. He thought I was perfect for the position. I don't remember if I said it out loud (I hope not), but I thought, "If they want me, they will ask me."

Fortunately, I recovered my senses and went after the position. I spoke first with Andi Wood, the very first nurse practitioner in pediatric oncology. Thankfully for me, she also thought I was an excellent candidate. She went to bat for me with Dr. Simone and within a short time I had the job.

In November 1971 I began a six-month intensive on-the-job training program at St. Jude to become a nurse practitioner focused totally in pediatric oncology. At that time there were very limited opportunities to obtain nurse practitioner training and whatever was available was focused in primary care. Actually, there were very few nurse practitioners and none in pediatric oncology except at St. Jude where I became the fourth in history.

Nurse practitioners happened at St. Jude because of Dr. Pinkel. He was familiar with the original training program in Colorado. Dr. Pinkel believed there was a place in the care of children with cancer for nurses in an expanded role. Having few clinical trainees on board probably also had some influence on this decision.

In my undergraduate years I had been an outstanding student academically and otherwise. I think the faculty viewed me as a nurse with a promising future. When I moved to the nurse practitioner role, there was a definite shift in the attitude of many of my admirers. I had gone over to the other side. I had abandoned nursing to play doctor. There was much debate in the general nursing community about whether the nurse practitioner role was really a nursing role.

I was too excited, too busy, and having too much fun to pay much attention to the negative babble. Sometimes a person just has to take the risk and *do* something. I was learning, learning, learning. I was participating in the care of children and families in a way that was extremely meaningful and rewarding for me.

I never forgot I was a nurse. I was not "playing doctor;" I was contributing to the creation of something valuable to patients and nursing. All this was not entirely clear to me at the time. I just knew that I was in a role that I could shape—a role where the walls were not as high as they had been in staff nursing. I could directly influence and in many instances independently make decisions which promoted high quality, loving care for the children.

Now nurse practitioners have attained a level of acceptance which is rapidly expanding. Nurse practitioners are respected and many nurses aspire to this level and type of practice. Graduate programs all over the country are providing educational programs that lead to the role of nurse practitioner.

It took two years of seeing patients every day, reading nothing but journals and texts, attending meetings, and asking thousands of questions of my physician and nurse practitioner colleagues before I felt truly competent. Nursing programs in the 1960s taught almost no physical assessment. It was pulse, respirations, temperature, and blood pressure.

The rare nurse owned a stethoscope. I had to learn all about physical assessment, as well as acquire much more knowledge of childhood cancer: treatment; protocols; procedures such as lumbar puncture and bone marrow aspiration; and childhood development and adaptation to illness. It was exhilarating, frustrating, and often overwhelming. And it was wonderful.

I will never forget the first patient who loved ME the most. Not the other doctors or nurses, but *me*. He was five years old with ALL, very smart and very cute. He and I had many adult conversations about leukemia, therapy, and life; and we played silly games. We hugged a lot. I was into hugging before it was fashionable. Some of the things I did or ordered done caused him pain and made him cry. Somehow he understood and loved me anyway. And I would make a balloon for him from a sterile glove and draw a funny face on it. He knew it was a love offering, and we kept on fighting together. Since he loved me, his parents did, too. We were a team in a real sense with me as player–coach.

That wonderful little boy taught me a lot. He died at age seven of varicella. My primary emotion at the time was anger, mostly directed at a particular physician. Before leaving the hospital for the evening, I had directly requested that this physician call me if Glen died during the night. I thought it would be a great comfort to his family if I was there. When I made rounds the next morning, Glen's room was empty and cleaned up. I had not received a phone call and Glen's parents were gone. I immediately went to the physician and asked why he had not called me. He said that he had not wanted to wake me up. I said, "Who the (bleep) do you think you are to make that kind of a decision for me?" I used language that was not even part of my vocabulary at the time. I expected to be taken seriously as a professional accountable for and to my patients. Later, that physician and I became loving friends.

I took very little time to grieve over this terrible loss. There were too many other children and parents who wanted and needed my guidance and care. Really, I did not know how to grieve. I had many opportunities to learn.

I don't remember being frightened that there were so many people who depended on me for so much. I can remember feeling burdened at times, but not frightened. Where did all that self-confidence come from? It must have been from not knowing any better.

And I was not alone. There were others to follow—nurse practitioners Andi Wood, Clara Mason, and Ellen Shanks, and Drs. John Aur, Manuel Versoza, and Rudy Jackson. There was support—people who wanted me to succeed. Stretching the limits was expected and encouraged.

In 1972 Robbie Simpson reappeared in my life. She was much loved, much admired, and much missed. Why not establish a fellowship in her honor that would offer nurses an educational experience in pediatric oncology? The Robbie Simpson Fellowship in Childhood Cancer Nursing was established. Announcements and requests for applications were placed in several oncology journals. It was a competitive fellowship that paid a $2,000 stipend for a three-month period. One fellowship was awarded in the spring and one in the fall. Think about it. How many nursing fellowships existed in 1972?

The nurse practitioners assumed primary responsibility for the fellowship. We developed the curriculum, participated in and eventually took over the selection process, and did much of the actual teaching.

The fellowship had an auspicious beginning with Trish Greene, now the national vice-president for patient services for the American Cancer Society, as the first Robbie Simpson fellow. Trish helped to set a tone that the nurses selected for this fellowship were special individuals who could hold their own in a sophisticated, complex clinical research environment. It gave me a very warm feeling when I once heard Trish acknowledge me as a mentor. That has worked both ways.

During my tenure at St. Jude, many outstanding people were awarded the fellowship. Pat Klopovich from Kansas, Mary Lauer from Wisconsin, Lucy Barksdale from Vanderbilt University in Nashville, Betsy Manchester from California, Ralph Vogel from Washington state, and Eileen Hourigan from Canada are just a few. Many of the fellows established practices as pediatric nurse practitioners in oncology, sometimes against great odds. When there was opposition, usually it came from nursing. But the fellows prevailed.

For me, the fellowship offered an opportunity for special teaching and mentoring. One of the nurse practitioners had primary responsibility for each fellow. Although over the course of three months a fellow would spend time with many people doing a variety of things, the principal relationship was with this nurse practitioner. There was ample opportunity to model this exciting new role. Several of the nurses who came were skeptical about the nurse practitioner role. Resistance varied with individuals and with regions of the country. Some nurses wanted only to learn about childhood cancer and not learn nurse practitioner skills. Others who began as skeptics saw that through the nurse practitioner role they could utilize their nursing skills more fully than before. The most timid became the most confident and the most determined. It was fun. After a while I learned to say, "I am going to the bathroom now." Our visitors stuck so close that they would end up there with us.

The Robbie Simpson Fellowship was a catalyst for many outstanding careers and long-standing friendships. For me, it was a singular opportunity to share hard-won knowledge and a certain wisdom about caring for children with cancer and their families, about the value of clinical research, about relating to physician and nurse colleagues, and about a new role for nurses that held much promise.

St. Jude always had a lot of visitors. Physicians, nurses, researchers of all ilks came for a day, a week, a month, a year. Virtually everyone spent time with a nurse practitioner. We were good teachers, knew the protocols inside and out, loved to talk about our patients and about St. Jude; and we were unique. The nurse practitioners were beginning to get a little attention around the country and sometimes people came just to spend time with us.

One of the most important visitors in terms of the ongoing development and proliferation of the role of the nurse practitioner in pediatric oncology was Jean Fergason of Children's Hospital in Philadelphia. After visiting St. Jude in 1972, Jean returned to Philadelphia and took the necessary steps to establish a three-month continuing education program to train pediatric oncology nurse practitioners. This program operated under the auspices of Philadelphia Children's Hospital from 1976 until 1980 when it was incorporated into the master's program of a local university. Jean is directly responsible for the development of 94 people as pediatric oncology nurse practitioners. When I called Jean to clarify for myself exactly how all this got started, without hesitation she said, "You and Andi and Clara were absolutely the inspiration for my program. I loved the role. I could see that it really benefited the children." Thank goodness for Jean, her vision, and her courage.

When you consider the Robbie Simpson Fellowship, Jean Fergason's program at Philadelphia Children's, and the numerous nurse and physician visitors who were introduced to the role of the nurse practitioner in pediatric oncology through the St. Jude nurse practitioners, it seems safe to conclude that those early days at St. Jude were the start of something big in pediatric oncology and in nursing. Andi, Clara, Ellen, and I not only pioneered a role and contributed to the successful utilization of this role in pediatric oncology programs nationwide and internationally, but we may have been among the first nurse practitioners to manage patients with chronic illnesses. Not a bad beginning for a career. I was in the right place at the right time.

In the early 1970s, though pediatric oncology was a recognized specialty, nurses working in this area were scattered around the country at various institutions. Some nurses were privileged to visit other institutions; but in general, nurse-to-nurse communication was minimal. There were no oncology nursing journals. The *American Journal of Nursing* would have the occasional heartrending story about "my little patient who died" and that was it.

There were no oncology nursing organizations. The national organization that attracted a smattering of pediatric oncology nurses was the Association for the Care of Children in Hospitals (ACCH). In 1973 Trish

Greene from Grady Hospital in Atlanta, Andi Wood and Ellen Shanks from St. Jude, and June McCalla from the National Cancer Institute had lunch together at an ACCH meeting in Atlanta. To have oncology nurses from different institutions together to share information and offer support to each other was unusual. This was the impetus for Trish to begin writing letters in an effort to determine the level of interest in creating a national organization for pediatric oncology nurses. Such an organization could do much to promote communication and overcome the professional isolation experienced by most pediatric oncology nurses.

A similar movement was taking place in the adult oncology nursing arena.

The first organizational meeting for what was to become the Association of Pediatric Oncology Nurses (APON) was held in May 1974 in Chicago during the national ACCH meeting. The concept was enthusiastically supported by the 40 nurses in attendance. I was elected chair of the nominations committee and directed to prepare a slate of officers for a fall meeting in Atlanta.

It was exciting to meet so many oncology nurses for the first time, to renew friendships with some of our former St. Jude visitors, to swap stories, to be with people who really understood. After the meeting, we began what became the traditional move to the hotel lounge. Everyone had a favorite child, a sad story, a moment of inspiration to share. At some point in later years I became a dropout; I had too many stories of my own.

The fall meeting was held in November 1974 in Atlanta, chaired by our newly elected president, Trish Greene. For most of the morning we were coherent but toward the lunch hour we began to deteriorate into jabbering, interrupting, arguing. After lunch, the die was cast. I do not know if I had already been elected parliamentarian or not, but based on experience gained through attending one national Sigma Theta Tau meeting, I declared myself the person to bring order to the beginnings of chaos. I stood and announced the rules of procedure to be followed for the remainder of the meeting. I did not stop there. I actually enforced the rules! That began my four years as parliamentarian.

I got another assignment, too. I was to oversee the development of bylaws and the incorporation of the organization. APON was incorporated in the state of Tennessee in 1976. Developing the bylaws started my 13-year stint as chair of the bylaws committee. I also served APON as vice-president and in 1979–1980 as president. I am still a member and feel sort of motherly—or perhaps grandmotherly—about the group. I am very proud.

Looking back I feel the deepest affection for all those nurses who were part of the beginnings of APON. Such loving dedication, such willingness to serve, to put self in harm's way in order to care for and comfort others.

Many of us were in harm's way. We gave all we had; too young and full of enthusiasm to hold anything back. "Taking care of yourself" had not become the catchphrase. There was virtually no emphasis in nursing education or in institutions on developing coping skills and support for caregivers. Whatever support we got was from each other and family and/or friends who could bear to hear about children with cancer.

An amazing piece of my history is that I survived those intense early years without a relationship with God. Organized religion had ceased to have any meaning for me. It was fashionable at the time to question the very existence of God. A popular expression of disillusionment was, "God is dead." I do not remember so much questioning God's existence as just not thinking about God at all—for years.

I can remember getting to work one morning, heading for the clinic, and stopping dead in the hallway with the blinding realization that I was ablaze with anger. It just was not fair: little children suffering and dying; families torn and broken apart. Who was there to blame? It must be God. That was one of the few thoughts I had of God.

Eventually the depth of my suffering about the loss of so many children led to a faith more profound than I could have imagined in my early life. I have thought over and over again, "How did I survive all those years without faith?" I may have turned away from God, but God never turned away from me.

With much difficulty, I left St. Jude in 1980. I received the most powerful acknowledgment of my contribution to children with cancer almost five years after I left. I requested a letter of recommendation from Dr. Paul Bowman, one of my most respected colleagues at St. Jude. I had worked beside him for three years and never really knew how he viewed me as a professional. His letter has warmed my heart for years. He said, "I had the opportunity to work very closely with Ms. Stagner in the management of children and adolescents with acute lymphocytic leukemia. During a time in which the emphasis was primarily on survival, Ms. Stagner was one of the first individuals to consider the importance of the quality of that survival and the child's adjustment to school and society in general. We were beginning to recognize at that time the presence of ill effects on learning and intellectual function in children receiving aggressive treatment, and it was largely through Ms. Stagner's initiative and leadership that prospective studies of psychological functioning were undertaken in this patient population. In addition, as a result of her efforts, increasing attention was paid to the individual child's function in school with conferences held with teachers and other educators to help them deal better with the problem of the child with learning handicaps as a result of radiation therapy and chemotherapy."

In the 1980s things began to shift for me professionally. I decided I had to go to graduate school. There were too many rumblings about educational requirements for nurse practitioners. Not being one who likes her options limited, I took the plunge. I was fortunate enough to get an American Cancer Society scholarship which added to my self-confidence as well as my pocketbook. I had a daughter in college. Although I worked full time, things would have been really uncomfortable without the scholarship.

In 1985 I graduated with an M.S.N. in maternal–child nursing with a focus in oncology. I had worked with my department chair to assure that every class and every clinical had a primary oncology focus.

Following graduate school I embarked on a 13-month job search. It was very enlightening. Though I interviewed all over the country for positions in pediatric oncology (Oakland, Denver, Phoenix, New Orleans, Milwaukee, Tampa, Iowa City—the list goes on) everything seemed pretty much the same. Just as I was adjusting my thinking and preparing to take a job that was not *the* job, I found a mass in my breast.

Talk about serendipity, or perhaps divine intervention. The mass was a cyst and I was reunited after more than a decade with a medical oncologist, Dr. Kirby Smith, and a radiologist, Dr. Lou Parvey, who had been at St. Jude during my years there.

After a couple of months of negotiation, I became the director of quality of life services at The Memphis Cancer Center, an outpatient treatment center for adults with cancer. It was *the* job. There was enough freedom and support to allow me to use all my life learning, both professional and personal, to develop creative means to better the lot of those with cancer. A new position to shape. As Kirby puts it, I am "the only one in captivity." We created the job title to fit our vision of the position.

In this position, I have developed programs, activities, and systems to address the nonmedical needs of people with cancer. We have been steadily building an array of support services that is unequaled in any hospital, clinic, or other facility in our area. There are support groups; an annual event in honor of National Cancer Survivors' Day; a Thanksgiving dinner for our patients and their families; and a full-time staff member whose background as a minister, cancer survivor, and bone marrow transplant recipient uniquely qualifies him as a counselor and friend to our patients and families. We have a foundation that is working to establish a free-standing support center for people with cancer in our area. I have produced a 30-minute educational and inspirational film. Between 3,000 and 4,000 copies have been distributed nationwide. Our nurses and physicians are strongly focused in education and support and are given the resources to do good work in these areas.

Many in the local health care community were skeptical and kept looking for our hidden agenda. After seven years, the picture is changing. Other physicians even refer their patients to our support services.

Dr. Smith and I and all the staff at the cancer center want to improve the quality of life for people with cancer through whatever means available. Again I am blessed. I am on another odyssey.

Whatever you can do, or dream you can, begin it. Boldness has genius, power and magic in it.

—*Goethe*

37

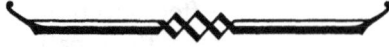

Debra Thaler-DeMers

I was a sophomore in high school when I decided I did not want to be a nurse. I had always been fascinated by medicine and wasn't fazed by blood and gore. During my high school days, I spent nearly 2,000 hours volunteering in the local hospital, observing medical personnel, and assisting wherever I could. During this time, I observed that the nurses followed the orders of the physicians, that they were not always appreciated by those same physicians for their efforts, and that patients tended to venerate their doctors. I decided that, given the choice, being venerated sounded like the better deal to me. By the time I graduated from high school, I was president of the future physicians club and had been accepted into a six-year B.S.–M.D. program that would involve nonstop studying and clinical experiences for the next ten years or more of my life.

My complete disenchantment with medicine began with my interview with the dean of the medical program. After asking the usual academic questions and praising my grades and test scores, he asked me what form of birth control I planned to use while I was studying for my medical degree. I was so taken aback by this question, I couldn't think of anything to say. He must have noted my surprise, because he continued to explain that the school would have a lot of time, effort, and money invested in my medical career and so they wanted to ensure that I completed the program. Up to this point, my goal had been acceptance to medical school. Now I was only a step away from that goal, and the dean was assuring me that I was just the type of student they were seeking. It was at this very moment that I realized I did not want to become a part of the venerated fraternity of medicine.

A natural disaster delayed the start of the academic year and provided me with the opportunity to explore other career options. I enrolled at the University of California, Berkeley. My father was very disappointed; he had been looking forward to distributing business cards engraved with the words "My Daughter, the Doctor" to everyone he knew. It took some adjustment for him to let me journey 3,000 miles across the country to attend a school he knew little about except for the student unrest that took place there during the 1960s.

Berkeley was a wonderful place for me. For the first time, I had the freedom to study whatever I wanted. Chemistry and mathematics had been my favorite high school subjects and I pursued both of these with new excitement. Many of the students in my chemistry class were pre-med students and the competition was fierce. I found that the focus was not on learning as much as possible, but on getting the highest grade possible, no matter what that entailed. The observation of one pre-med student in near hysterics after having been caught cheating on a laboratory experiment helped to finalize my decision to avoid medicine as a career. I pursued a degree in theoretical mathematics, graduating in 1976.

Aside from academia, there are not a lot of jobs available for theoretical mathematicians, so after a summer of camping and exploring the United States, I took a job in an international law firm. I found a use for my math skills while helping my boss on a case and soon found myself working for the senior partner as his secretary, researcher, and administrative assistant. David was a brilliant attorney, but was legally blind and extremely disorganized. I have always loved doing library research so a job where I could spend time in the law library doing research was ideal for me. After a year of learning to write briefs and legal memoranda, I decided to pursue a career as an attorney. I had visions of becoming a partner in a large and prestigious law firm some day. In fact, I began to plan out my life for the next ten years or so.

I had recently married and purchased a small home in the San Fernando Valley of California. Two young lawyers associated with a large firm approached me about helping them start their own practice. It was hard work as I was their only employee, but they allowed me the flexibility to attend law school at night. I felt I was working toward a bright future and the few years of hard work and long hours would pay off in the end. I had no way of knowing that my dreams would never materialize.

By March of 1980, I had moved on to a large law firm in Century City, working in the tax and estate planning department, an area where my math and organizational skills could be put to use. My boss was a partner in the firm—highly skilled and highly disorganized. As April 15 approached each year, our work days became longer and I liked to come into the office as early as possible to work while the phones were silent and few people were in the office. On a typical day, my alarm would startle me into semiconsciousness at 4:30 A.M. and I would slip out of bed, trying not to disturb my husband, and stumble toward the bathroom in the early morning darkness. As I reached for my toothbrush, I'd flip on the light and peer out from under my half-raised eyelids.

Monday, March 17, 1980 began as any other day until I glanced at my reflection in the bathroom mirror. I was startled into full consciousness by the image of a young woman who appeared to have a golfball lodged in her neck. It looked as if she had attempted to swallow the golfball and it had gotten stuck at the base of her neck. My mind flashed back to a conversation I'd had with my cousin Steven many years ago and my heart began to race. I was instantly afraid.

Steven was my older cousin whom I had idolized as a child. I liked to play with his pet hamster and waited anxiously for him to get home from school because I knew he would buy me a soda at the corner candy store. Steven was eight years older than me and was the first person in our family to move from New Jersey to California. During my freshman year at the University of California, he died after a long battle with Hodgkin's disease. I hadn't known he was sick until I moved to California. Cancer was not a subject that was openly discussed in our family. Once I was in California and observed the many medications Steven carried with him wherever he went, he sat down with me and told me all about his illness. Initially, he hadn't felt sick, he'd just woken up one morning and found a lump in his neck. He didn't remember it being there when he went to bed, but it was definitely present when he woke up. This was the conversation that was replaying in my mind as I stared at the reflection in the bathroom mirror.

"Oh, my God," I thought. "I have cancer." This was immediately followed by the idea that this was a ridiculous concept. I couldn't possibly have cancer—this was all just a bad dream. I decided if I went back to sleep for another 30 minutes and started the day all over again, I'd discover that I'd just imagined the whole episode. I put my toothbrush back in its holder, turned off the light, and slipped under the covers. I dozed off for about 20 minutes and then rushed into the bathroom, still hoping to avoid rush-hour traffic on the way to the office. I flipped on the light switch, grabbed my toothbrush, and tried to avoid looking in the mirror. But the reflection in the mirror was like a magnet, pulling at my consciousness until I could no longer avoid it. The golfball was still lodged in my neck. I told myself emphatically that I was being hysterical, exaggerating a small irregularity in my neckline. There was nothing wrong with me. I was just tired from so many long days at work. All I needed was a little more sleep. So I headed back to bed. By now the sun was coming up so I pulled the covers all the way over my head and huddled down into the bed. Just another half hour of sleep and I would be fine.

In 30 minutes I cautiously headed for the bathroom once again. I no longer had any interest in brushing my teeth—I just wanted to look in the mirror and see the "old me" staring back. My heart was pounding; I wanted to look but at the same time I was afraid to glance up from the sink to the mirror. My reflection once again had that pesky round outcropping at the base of my neck. I forced myself to remain calm. "It's probably just some kind of localized infection," I told myself. "I'll just call in sick today and get lots of rest; everything will be back to normal tomorrow." I called the office, told my husband I was taking a sick day, and went back to sleep. Any time I woke up during that day, I would go into the bathroom and check my reflection in the mirror. Whenever I saw the lump in my neck, I would conclude that I needed more sleep and head back for my nice warm covers.

Tuesday morning I got up early and went through most of my usual routine except that I carefully avoided my reflection. I arrived at the office early, made myself a cup of hot tea and started sorting through Monday's pile of mail and memos. As people arrived in the office and stopped by my door to say hello, I would casually inquire as to whether they noticed anything different about me. The first three people I talked to asked about my clothes or my earrings. Dorothy, one of the older secretaries in the office, stopped by to see if I was feeling better. We chatted for a few minutes and then I casually asked if she noticed anything different. "Let's see," she said. "I've seen the dress before, your hair is the same, the earrings aren't new—no, nothing except for that lump there in your neck." I was stunned—Dorothy had seen it! It was really there! Dorothy was saying something, but I was lost in my own thoughts. I managed to bring the conversation to a close somehow and then sat at my desk and tried to think about what I should do next. I was afraid that I had Hodgkin's disease, just like Steven. I didn't want to verbalize my fears—I just wanted it to go away. At the same time, I knew that I had to find out for sure whether the lump was significant.

When I visited my internist, I tried to be casual about the lump. "It's probably just some kind of infection draining to that spot," I told him. He agreed that it could be an infection and asked his partner, a specialist in infectious diseases, to take a look. They both poked at it, examined me, and then decided to try a course of antibiotics to see if it would go away.

Ten days later, the lump was still there. I was sent over to the hospital to get a chest X-ray. I stood in the hallway in my hospital gown waiting for the film to drop out of the developer. The technician slid the X-ray onto the view box and flipped on the light. My first thought on seeing my chest X-ray that day was, "I'm going to die!" In what I hoped was a calm and casual-sounding voice, I pointed to a large, dark circle in the middle of the film and asked the technician, "What is that thing right there?" She quickly grabbed the film from the view box and headed down the hall, calling to me with her back turned, "You'll have to call your doctor for the results—probably tomorrow." I ran after her but before I could catch up she had disappeared into an office marked "Radiologist Reading Room." I knocked. The technician poked only her head and shoulders out from behind the door. "I'd like to talk to the radiologist," I informed her. "He can't talk to you," she said. "You'll have to contact your doctor for the results. He should have them in the morning." She then disappeared behind the door.

The next few weeks were filled with long hours at work interrupted by X-rays, scans, blood tests, and finally a biopsy of that lump. I wanted to be awake for the biopsy and I wanted to see the lump after they removed it. I arranged to have the procedure done in a surgeon's office with a local anesthetic. I went back to work the next day and waited for the pathology report—and waited and waited! I called the surgeon and my internist almost daily. The pathologist was having difficulty with the slides and they didn't want to tell me anything until they were certain of the results. My parents had flown out from New Jersey to be with me for the biopsy and its results. They were scheduled to leave and I hadn't yet received the results. If I was going to require more extensive surgery, my mother was planning to stay in California to help take care of me. If the biopsy was benign, she would fly back to New Jersey with my father. I called the internist again on Friday afternoon. He suggested I come in for a conference on Monday. I told him I needed the results immediately so that my parents could finalize their travel plans. "It's malignant, but we're not sure yet what we're dealing with. We can talk about it in more detail on Monday." I thanked him and hung up. I felt as if he had reached through the telephone and physically slapped me across the face. My total experience with cancer to that point had been Steven's illness and death. I was 25 years old and felt certain I was going to die before I got much older.

Monday's conference with the internist was followed by a conference with a hematologist and five days in the hospital for more tests. Then I was referred to a surgical oncologist and surgery was scheduled for the end of May. I was told that my laporatomy was an "elective" procedure and four weeks was the first available time for scheduling the surgery. During the time I was waiting for my date in the operating room, my aunt, Steven's mother, suggested I fly to New York to see an oncologist at Memorial Sloan-Kettering Cancer Center for a second opinion.

It was during this time that I learned for the first time that Steven was not the only member of my family to have had Hodgkin's disease. My cousin Frank had been diagnosed with Hodgkin's disease while in medical school. Few people in the family knew about it and he had been in remission for several years. Frank called me and asked what I had been told so far. He shared his experience with me and told me what I could expect in the way of treatment. He answered my questions and got me the most current information on Hodgkin's disease. The mere fact that he had Hodgkin's disease and was still alive and healthy years after the diagnosis was the best news I'd had in weeks. Frank was my life preserver—a symbol for me that I could survive this illness.

For the first time, I began to think I could live a few more years. Still, fear was a constant companion during this time. Each day that I waited for the surgery, I felt as if the mass in my chest was growing. I could not understand why my surgery was urgent only to me. My oncologist assured me that I had a slow-growing cancer and a few weeks would not make a difference in treating me.

I had never been seriously ill before nor had I ever had major surgery. I entered the hospital on a Thursday with surgery scheduled for Friday morning. I fully expected to be home, resuming my normal activities by Monday at the latest. I was not prepared to wake up with tubes, drains, and IV bottles appended to my body. I felt as if I'd been split down the middle and trussed up like a Thanksgiving turkey.

Once all the pathology slides were analyzed, the medical oncologist met with my husband and me to discuss the treatment plan. I was still in the hospital and the oncologist wanted to start radiation therapy right away. My husband, who is trained as a physicist, asked about the dose of radiation to be used. He then asked about the harmful effects of so much radiation and whether there were any alternatives to this treatment plan. The oncologist became annoyed, looked at both of us and stated, "She does this or she dies. Those are the alternatives." He then got up and left the room. He returned several hours later to ask me if my husband was really a scientist. Thirteen years later, a study would be published in the *Journal of the National Cancer Institute* documenting the increased incidence of breast cancer among women who had received high-dose mediastinal radiation as treatment for Hodgkin's disease. My husband's question, so easily dismissed by the oncologist, has come back to haunt me. But it has also taught me a valuable lesson. *All* questions are valid and should be answered with care and consideration. I encourage patients and family members to ask any question they are thinking. I feel the term *stupid question* is an oxymoron. A question is an opportunity to provide new information or to clarify information previously received.

During the next six months I was in and out of the hospital for various complications from treatment. My oncologist maintained the philosophy that informing patients of all the possible side effects of treatment would cause them to worry themselves into having all of these side effects. Consequently, I was not prepared for many of the physical symptoms I was having and did not always attribute them to the treatment I was receiving. For example, I called the office one day because I had what I thought were scores of insect bites on my legs that itched like crazy and kept forming pus-filled scabs that would rupture and then just fill up again. I'd been scratching for a couple of days and now my skin was looking raw and was fairly painful. I also had a terrible headache which nothing seemed to relieve, but I failed to mention this on the telephone as I didn't think it was relevant. By the time I got to the oncologist's office and waited over an hour to see him, my head hurt so badly I could barely hold it up. My "insect bites" turned out to be shingles and I learned from reading my medical records several months later that the headache was herpes zoster encephalitis.

Of all my stays in the hospital, one incident stands out in my mind. It was close to midnight and the night shift nurse was making her rounds. The lights were off and she had a flashlight in her hand. When she saw that I was still awake, she asked me how I was doing. Just as I started to answer her, I heard the sound of someone sobbing. I listened again—the sound was coming from me! All of the emotions that I had kept tightly controlled for months came pouring out of me. I couldn't stop crying. I couldn't even form the words to tell her what I was feeling. I'd never seen this nurse before but I will never forget what she did. She sat down, wrapped her arms around me, and just held me while I cried it all out of my system. When I was finished, I actually felt much better. I felt lighter, as if a weight had been lifted from me. I realized that, after months of having my life disrupted by surgery, medical appointments, treatments, nausea, fevers, and infections, I was *sick of being sick!*

After completing my radiation therapy treatment, I began attending a local support group for people with serious illness. The group was called "Make Today Count" and it met at a local hospital. It was run by the patients with a social worker in attendance but the basic philosophy was that the patients were there to help each other deal with their illness. At 25, I was the youngest person in attendance by about 20 years. The person closest to me in age was a Hodgkin's patient in his early 40s who always brought a new joke to the meeting. Allan also talked a lot about his oncologist, whom he referred to as "Gary." Allan was always telling me Gary's opinion about Hodgkin's disease and its treatment.

I was very frustrated with my own oncologist, mostly over our lack of communication. I felt that he withheld information and that I was in the position of not even knowing the questions I needed to ask to understand what was happening to my body. In addition, I was very angry about some information that I felt should have been discussed before my treatment started. Instead, it had become a festering emotional wound that surfaced during a follow-up visit with the radiation oncologist. I mentioned the fact that I had not had a menstrual period since the month prior to my surgery and asked if my periods would resume now that the radiation therapy was completed. The radiologist seemed surprised that I did not know I could be infertile as a result of my treatment. He asked me if my oncologist had discussed this with me and then suggested I talk to my oncologist again.

My first reaction was shock, quickly followed by anger. I went to the medical library and read everything I could find about fertility and cancer. There wasn't much information available. When I confronted my oncologist about his failure to discuss with me the possibility that I would not be able to have any children after my treatment, his response was to flip through the pages of my chart. He found what he was searching for and pointed out to me that infertility was listed as one of the possible side effects on the consent form I had signed before starting my treatment. I looked at the form; there it was in fine print along with all the other side effects. I hadn't bothered to read the form at the time I had signed it. After hearing the words "she does it or she dies," I had simply signed all the consents. On that day, I probably would have jumped off a bridge if the oncologist had told me it would enhance my chances for a cure. Now I found myself facing the possibility that I would never have children. I felt betrayed. At 25 years of age, an important decision in my life had been made without the opportunity to discuss available options. My impression of my oncologist's attitude was that he felt the issue of fertility was insignificant in light of the fact that by following the recommended protocol, I could be cured. I agree that cure is the desired goal, but it does not negate the importance of discussing fertility with a young patient. Preserving fertility and achieving a cure are not mutually exclusive goals.

This incident severed the relationship I had with my oncologist. I felt betrayed by him and I was tired of having to extract information from him. I called the office and canceled my next appointment. I never made another appointment and I have always wondered why no one called me to find out why I had stopped coming in to the office. At the next "Make Today Count" meeting, I asked Allan how I could get an appointment to see his oncologist.

Dr. Gary Dosik was everything Allan had described and more. He was open, honest, and communicative. During my first visit he explained to me that we had to work together as a team. Since I was the only person residing in my body, he would rely on me for certain information only I could provide. I could rely on him to interpret this information and we could then work together to plan a course of action for my treatment. Gary taught me many things over the next few years, but two things that he did for me changed the course of my life. The first was to ask me if I was interested in participating in a study to see if it would be beneficial for cancer patients to participate in an assertiveness training course. At the time, I was a shy, introverted person who would go to the library and research the answer to my questions rather than come out and ask the question. I agreed to participate in the class, feeling

I had nothing to lose and that if Gary was suggesting it, he must think it has some merit. That class would give me the skills I needed several years later to challenge a major medical center in order to obtain needed treatment for my younger sister. My own training has given me the tools to teach other cancer patients to assert themselves and make their needs known. Today I provide workshops for cancer patients that include ample opportunity to practice assertiveness in the medical setting. I also advocate for cancer patients both as an oncology nurse and as a member of the board of directors of the National Coalition for Cancer Survivorship and as the chair of its national speakers' bureau. I travel throughout the United States educating health care professionals on the issues that face cancer survivors, including the issue of fertility after treatment.

This brings me to the second major contribution Gary has made to my life. He was perceptive enough to realize how important the issue of infertility was to me and to refer me to his good friend, Dr. Charles Gassner, who happened to specialize in infertility. Three years after my diagnosis, I gave birth to a healthy baby, Joshua; two years later, my daughter Gabrielle was born.

During the time that I was pregnant with Joshua, I received a telephone call from my younger sister Terri. She had recently graduated from college and was working as a temporary employee for a large corporation in New Jersey. This was to support her passion in life—international folk dancing. Terri had just returned from a folk dance performance in Iowa and was feeling a bit run down. The reason she was calling was that she had noticed a lump in her neck just below her ear and was wondering if it could be an ear infection. I was the family medical expert and since she had no medical benefits through her employer, Terri was asking me for advice. The word "lump" stuck in my mind; I asked her to describe the location, size, shape, and feel of it. "Skip the internist," I told her, "Get in to see an oncologist right away." I then called my cousin Frank, described the situation to him, and asked him to refer Terri to an oncologist.

Terri saw both a medical oncologist and a surgeon who performed a lymph node biopsy which revealed Hodgkin's disease. Since she had no medical insurance, her staging was done on an outpatient basis. Both her oncologist and the surgeon were aware that she had no insurance and both assured her that they would deal with the financial matters later and that she should not worry about them. However, before her diagnostic testing was completed, the cost of multiple CT scans, X-rays, tomograms, and blood work had depleted her savings. She was unable to work consistently and had run out of money. I was in New Jersey by this time and assisted her in applying for Medicaid. She was informed by her oncologist that if she could no longer pay for her appointments, he could no longer care for her as he did not accept Medicaid patients.

We transferred her care to another facility. After her first appointment, it was determined that she needed to be hospitalized for pneumonia. Admission to the hospital was scheduled for Sunday afternoon. When we arrived at the admitting department, we were informed that Terri could not be admitted because she did not have any medical insurance. We informed the hospital that her Medicaid application had been processed and we were only waiting for the card to arrive. They continued to deny her a bed. My father offered to put up his house as collateral for the bill. The hospital refused to accept this offer. I became assertive and informed the hospital that I had no intention of allowing my 22-year-old sister to die because she did not have medical insurance. I knew that the hospital received federal funds and therefore had to admit indigent patients. The hospital continued to refuse. I called my brother, a newspaper publisher. He made some phone calls and I then informed the hospital that if my sister did not have a bed by 8 A.M. Monday morning, my brother, the newspaper publisher, together with his contacts at two major New York area newspapers, and my cousin, the city editor at a third New York area newspaper, would ensure that a story concerning the matter would be prominently printed in all three newspapers.

Early Monday morning, I received a phone call from an official of the hospital inquiring about the difficulties we had encountered on Sunday afternoon. This official assured us that there would be no problem admitting Terri to the hospital that afternoon. We had no further difficulties with medical insurance matters until Terri required a bone marrow transplant three years later.

Terri had developed an aversion to medical procedures early in her life. As a child, she would faint when told she needed to have a blood test. I knew that chemotherapy was not going to be accomplished without some outside help. I contacted the social services department at the hospital and they put us in touch with a very talented social worker, Matthew Loscalzo. He helped desensitize Terri to the medical procedures to the point that she was able to inject her own bleomycin. Together, Terri and Matthew made a film to teach other social workers about the technique used to help Terri master her fear of needles and injections.

Through three years of radiation, chemotherapy, and finally a bone marrow transplant, I helped Terri with her treatment as much as possible. I used my own experiences as a patient to help her. I had no formal medical training at this time. It was during her bone marrow transplant that Terri told me, "You're pretty good at this nursing stuff. You ought to get paid for it." Some time after her death from graft versus host disease in 1986, I started to think about what she had said. I had felt comfortable taking care of Terri, glad that I was able to do something to help her. I had shared my own experiences as much as possible, so that she would know what to expect and to help her avoid as many of the pitfalls along the way as possible. She had told me that this helped her—it took away some of the anxiety and fear.

In 1989 I decided to obtain a second university degree—this one in nursing. I had come full circle—back to the profession I had decided against as a sophomore in high school. My perspective was vastly different now. I was coming to nursing as a cancer survivor. I was older and wiser, more assertive and outspoken. In the years since my diagnosis I had become active in organizing local cancer support groups based on the "Make Today Count" model and in having the more than 300 local MTC chapters communicate with each other through an inhouse newsletter for chapter leaders. I had given workshops on assertiveness training techniques for cancer patients, passing on the knowledge and skills that had helped to change my life so dramatically. I had drawn attention to myself and my experiences at one of the early meetings of the National Coalition for Cancer Survivorship and had then become involved, first as a member of the board of advisors and then as a member of the board of directors and chair of their national speakers' bureau. I had shared the story of Terri's illness on national television in order to make people aware of the issues we had faced and to draw attention to the need for everyone to have a durable power of attorney for medical care. I had compiled a three-page list of questions for newly diagnosed cancer patients to take with them to the doctor's, so that they would at least have enough information to know *what* they should be asking. I had spoken to health care professionals, community groups, public and private school students, cancer survivors, and newspaper reporters about the issues people have to deal with when faced with a diagnosis of cancer.

Now I felt ready to take the next step. I wanted to be there at the bedside for cancer patients. Part of my motivation for becoming a nurse was to gain access to as many patients as possible, in order to bring them the information and the support they would need to deal with their illness. I knew I could master the technical skills based on my experience with Terri during her bone marrow transplant. I'd had to learn about Hickman catheters, ventilators, TPN, infection precautions, blood counts, and many other things. I had coped with my unresolved feelings and questions following my own treatment by spending days in the medical library at UCLA reading everything I could find about Hodgkin's disease and its treatment.

I had to complete some prerequisite classes before I could apply to nursing school. Anatomy, physiology, microbiology, public speaking. Normally this would take three semestrers because anatomy was a prerequisite for physiology but I petitioned to take them at the same time and saved some time that way. I was nervous about returning to school after so many years away from academics. I wondered whether I could compete with 18-year-old students fresh from high school. My anxiety was relieved as I entered the parking lot on the first day of classes. I had to laugh as I looked at the date on my daily parking permit—August 34, 1989.

When it came time to apply to the nursing program, I learned that there were far more applications than there were spaces in the program and that, even though I had a 4.0 grade point average, I might have to wait several semesters before I could be accepted to the program. I was also advised by a fellow student not to disclose that I had cancer as I would probably be rejected in favor of a healthy applicant. This made me very angry but I decided to do whatever was necessary until I was accepted into the nursing program. Then I planned to take on the issue of discrimination based on a medical history of cancer.

For my application physical, I went to the student health service and saw a physician who did not know me. I didn't exactly lie, but I didn't reveal anything that wasn't asked either. The physician asked if there was any reason I could not perform the requirements of the nursing program. I said there wasn't and she signed the health form.

Managing the daily routine of being a wife, mother of two young children, and a nursing student was definitely challenging. My children were included in my study time. We made up songs about the bones of the body and how cookies made their way through the body. My study group sometimes met in my home and we had a CPR certification class in the living room. My daughter was able to resuscitate Annie, the CPR mannequin, at the age of five. Her vocabulary was also a little more technical than most kindergarten students.

Initially I was cautious about disclosing that I was a cancer survivor. Members of my study group knew, but they were sworn to secrecy. Most of the students and faculty knew that my sister had died following a bone marrow transplant for Hodgkin's disease. The week before final exams in my first semester of nursing school, my daughter came down with chicken pox and I noticed that I had also been scratching. On closer examination, I saw the row of vesicles that indicated I had shingles—for the first time in years! My nursing theory exam was in two days! Classmates had volunteered to take turns watching my daughter so that I could take all of my exams, but now I was faced with a dilemma. I met with my instructor and told him that I had come down with shingles and that my daughter had chicken pox. He allowed me to take the exam the following week. A positive side effect of this incident was that my classmates were able to see what shingles vesicles look like and to learn about a disease they might not have otherwise encountered in the clinical setting.

The issue of revealing my identity as a cancer survivor came to a head as I was about to begin my pediatrics clinical rotation. Obtaining the clinical placement you wanted was always a challenge, matched only by the attempt to schedule the rest of your life around the times set for your clinical experience. I was excited about having obtained a pediatric clinical at the county hospital where I felt I would be exposed to a broad range of experiences. The clinical instructor was a pediatric oncology nurse and I hoped I would get the opportunity to care for children with cancer. Two days before the semester began, the class was informed that everyone had to present proof of rubella immunization in order to participate in the pediatric rotation. I had not been immunized for rubella prior to having Hodgkin's disease and the vaccine is not recommended for use in patients with a history of Hodgkin's disease. I called my oncologist and asked if there was any way I could safely take the rubella vaccine. He told me the manufacturer of the vaccine specifically advised against it. I explained my problem to him and he gave me a letter that stated I could not have the rubella vaccine and that I was not posing any significant risk to the patients by not having the vaccine. I was aware of the risks to my own health and felt that I could take adequate precautions to protect myself from contracting rubella.

With this letter in hand, I met with the associate dean of the nursing program who coordinated clinical placements. For the first time, the administration of the nursing school was aware that I was a cancer survivor. The associate dean listened as I presented the problem to her, shared with her the letter from my oncologist and another document I had brought to the meeting. It was a copy of a California law which prohibits discrimination based on a medical disability, which includes a history of cancer. As long as I was physically able to perform the duties of a nursing student in the clinical setting and did not pose a risk to the patients, I felt I had every right to maintain my place in the clinical placement. I held my breath as I waited anxiously for her reaction. She agreed wholeheartedly with my position. She would contact the county hospital and if they had any further problem with my being part of the clinical placement, she would inform them of the California law and the fact that the nursing school would be willing to file suit to ensure my participation in the clinical experience.

I had finally revealed my identity as a cancer survivor to the faculty of the nursing school. I hoped that I would not be treated any differently than any other student in the class. I was at the top of my class academically and was fairly assertive as a student representative at faculty meetings. When discussions became disorganized, I generally asserted myself to summarize what people were vocalizing and plan a course of action. One result of my illness is that time is a precious commodity for me and if I feel it is being wasted, I will take action.

In my clinical experiences, I sought out patients with cancer. For my public health rotation, my experience was with the Visiting Nurses Association hospice team; for my last semester, I chose the pediatric oncology and bone marrow transplant unit at Children's Hospital.

As a nursing student, I rarely told patients that I had cancer. One exception was an eighteen-year-old patient with osteosarcoma. When Penny had been presented with the fact that her left leg would have to be amputated above the knee, she had asked the medical team to find another alternative. As a result she had received a cadaver bone graft and chemotherapy for her disease. I spent as much time talking with Penny as I could. She wanted me to meet her mother and I stayed at the hospital after clinical one night so the three of us could share fast food and talk. In many ways, Penny reminded me of myself after Gary became my oncologist. She was able to make her needs known and was not afraid to challenge the medical staff to find ways to make her treatment compatible with the way she wanted to live the rest of her life. I admired her for this and told her so. I learned a great deal from Penny and I have shared what she taught me with other young cancer patients.

Learning from my patients has been a key part of my experience as an oncology nurse. I know that my experience as both a cancer patient and the sister of a cancer patient can be a benefit to the patients and families I care for. I also know that I am just one cancer patient and that every person's experience is unique. I am careful to tell patients that I am a cancer survivor only if I feel it will be of benefit to *them*. I want to help my patients meet their needs. If caring for them brings up unresolved issues related to my own illness or to my sister's illness, I must be careful to work through those issues on my own time and not at my patients' expense. I must also keep in mind that I cannot resolve my patients' issues for them. Each person must work through his or her own issues. I can be a resource for them, but they must walk their own path.

This is particularly difficult for family members who are having a hard time letting go when their loved one is dying. A patient's wife once asked me to help her escape from the situation of dealing with her husband's impending death. "The only way out," I told her, "is to put one foot in front of the other and walk through it. It won't be easy, but it is the only escape. Some days you will take one step forward and two steps backward. Don't worry about it. Just keep going. If you need help along the way, don't be afraid to ask for it. One day, maybe when you are not even paying attention to the journey, you will find that you have come to the other side."

Her husband, Jerry, had been very interested in my work with the National Coalition for Cancer Survivorship. He was a five-year survivor of lung cancer who had a recurrence with bone metastases. He told me his goal was to finish treatment and come back in five years to give me a big hug. In his mind, a survivor was someone who had achieved five years of cancer-free survival. In fact, NCCS defines survivorship from the moment of diagnosis, and for the balance of the individual's life. Patients undergoing treatment are in the acute survival period. At the end of treatment, survivors enter the extended survival period and when cancer is no longer the major focus of the person's life they have entered the permanent survival period. Cancer survivorship is a process rather than an outcome. It is the experience of living with, through, and beyond cancer. After I explained all of this to Jerry, I told him I wanted my hug right then and there; I didn't want to wait five years for it.

When I started working as an oncology nurse, I did not tell anyone that I was a cancer survivor. I was not sure how the patients and my coworkers would react and I wanted to be sure that I was covered by the hospital's health insurance policy before I became too vocal about my medical history. I work the night shift and at 5 A.M. I make rounds to draw blood from central lines for morning lab work. One morning I was drawing blood from Barry's central line, chatting casually with him as I did so. Barry was a long-term survivor of colon cancer who had developed a second primary cancer as a result of his initial treatment. He was in his early 40s and had been hospitalized for many weeks for complications related to his pancreatic cancer. As I inserted the second syringe into his line, Barry reached up and flipped over my Medic Alert® bracelet. There was nothing I could do as he started to read it. "What is Hodgkin's disease?" he asked me. I told him. He wanted to know more—how long ago did I have it, how was I treated, was I a nurse when I was diagnosed? He had a long list of questions. I answered each question openly and without reservation. About 20 minutes after this conversation took place, I was standing outside his room at the med cart, drawing up his morning insulin. I overheard him talking excitedly to his wife on the telephone. "You have to come in early and meet this nurse," he was telling her, "She had cancer ten years ago and then went to nursing school. When can you get here?"

When I came back to work that night, there was a note at the nurses' station for the charge nurse. It was from Barry's wife and it was a request that I be assigned to take care of Barry every night that I worked.

Barry and I became good friends. I learned a great deal from him and I believe he learned from my experiences too. By taking the initiative in reading my Medic Alert bracelet, he showed me that my patients could benefit from knowing that I was a cancer survivor. When Barry died, I extended my understanding of cancer survivorship. As I continue my work in oncology nursing, Barry continues to survive because of the influence his life has on my practice of nursing.

Jack was an older patient who was being admitted for his first chemotherapy treatment. He had mixed feelings about it, having been told by friends and relatives of the horrible side effects of treatment. "I don't know why I'm even bothering with this chemotherapy," he told me. "No one ever survives cancer anyhow." Without thinking, I blurted out, "I beg to differ with you. If no one ever survives cancer, then you're talking to a dead person." Instantly I began to wonder if I'd said something wrong. Jack turned his head and stared at me with eyes opened wide. "*You* have cancer?" he asked.

"Ten years ago," I told him.

This opened up an opportunity for Jack to ask me the questions he'd been holding back. I told him, as I tell all my patients, that he could ask me about anything. I would not be embarrassed and if I felt I didn't want to answer something I'd tell him and I'd tell him why. There is no such thing as a stupid question. Any question that a person has deserves an answer.

Many times, when patients ask me questions in the middle of the night, I wonder aloud why they haven't asked their oncologist about the things that they are worried about. My patients tell me that they don't want to take up the doctor's time; that he is in and out of the room so quickly in the morning that they don't have a chance to ask; or that they don't think of the questions while the doctor is in the room. I encourage patients and family members to write down their questions so they have them handy when the doctor arrives. I also teach them that they are employing their oncologist. Since they are paying for his services, they have a right to expect that their concerns will be addressed. This does not mean that they can monopolize the doctor's time. If they have a lot of concerns or questions, I suggest they tell the doctor this and ask if there is a time they could meet to talk.

One of the reasons that I work the night shift is because I remember what that night shift nurse did for me 13 years ago. When family is not visiting and things quiet down in the hospital, patients have time to be alone with their thoughts. This can be a painful time for them, physically and emotionally. Despite what others may think, the night shift is not an "off shift." Patients are awake and in need of nurses who have the skill to handle a crisis with minimal resources. Pain can be more intense at night because there are fewer distractions from the painful sensations. People can become more aware of their body's sensations in the stillness of the night. People can also be more agitated and frustrated by the amount of noise and their inability to enjoy an eight-hour block of uninterrupted sleep. Hospitals are not the best places in the world to rest.

The slower pace of the night gives patients the opportunity to process their thoughts and emotions. You might be surprised at how much patient education goes on between 11 P.M. and 7 A.M. Much of this is re-education and clarification of information previously received. I have learned that the message a physician, nurse, or social worker intends to convey to a person is not always the message received by that person. It is rare that health care professionals take the time to verify that the patient or family member has heard the information conveyed accurately. We forget that the words, phrases, and abbreviations that we use every day are equivalent to a foreign language to the average person. If we stop to think about how difficult it is to understand something said in a language that is not our primary language, particularly if the tone is soft or the pace of the communication is fast, we will have some understanding of what it is like for the average person to try to understand a conversation spoken in "medicalese."

Something that I learned from the night nurse in the ICU where my sister was a patient has stayed with me through the years. My sister had developed respiratory difficulties and was transferred to ICU and placed on a non-rebreather mask. I had been up with her for 48 straight hours and was slumped in a chair beside the bed with my eyes closed. Terri started pounding on the bed and yelling, "I want my sister right here, right now." I heard the nurse tell her that I was asleep in a chair beside the bed. Terri continued to pound the bed and repeat over and over, "right here, right now." I got up and went to the side of the bed. I tried to comfort her but she kept pounding the bed and repeating, "right here, right now." The nurse turned to me. "She wants you to get in the bed with her," she told me. I didn't think family members could do that—climb in bed with a patient in the ICU with all its monitors and equipment. The nurse started moving things to make a spot for me in the bed and I climbed in. Terri instantly calmed down. She started to talk to me. I didn't understand what she was doing at the time, but many weeks later I figured it out. She knew she was dying and she was saying good-bye to me. She wasn't saying it directly, but it was so important to her that she convey this message to me that she had been willing to use up her limited amount of oxygen to ensure that I got in the bed with her and heard what she had to say. I will always be grateful to that ICU nurse for her insight into what was happening. A few hours later Terri lapsed into a coma and never spoke again.

I learned two important lessons from this experience. There is rarely a reason for not allowing family members to sit on a patient's bed or to get in bed with a patient. I can think of several times when a patient has been near death and I have encouraged a spouse or significant other to lie in bed with them and hold or touch them. I have seen a positive effect on the patient and on the family member when this is permitted. If a person is not able to die at home in their own bed, they should be allowed to die in the manner that is most comfortable for them. Even when patients are not near death, sharing their bed with a loved one can bring positive results. I have set up private moments for patients and their spouses to enjoy each other's company without fear of interruption. Intimacy can be achieved on the oncology unit without disturbing the normal staff routine if the staff engages in a little ingenuity and planning.

Early on in my nursing career, it was reported to my immediate supervisor that I had been seen in bed with a patient. The patient in question had been in the midst of a panic attack; no family members were present. I gave the patient a sedative and then held him in my arms and talked to him until the medication took effect. When I explained the situation to my supervisor, she gave me her full support. I don't know what the patient reported to his physician, but I saw his progress note for the day which indicated the patient had received "Ativan and TLC" for his panic attack.

I love being an oncology nurse. Nurses from other departments ask me if I find it depressing. They tell me that they could never be an oncology nurse and hope they don't have to float to our unit. Yes, sometimes the work is sad; at times it is stress-filled; but I do not find it depressing. I can think of no other profession where I can meet such a wide variety of people and interact with them in such an intimate manner. My patients come from many different ethnic backgrounds; their careers range from circus performer to nuclear physicist. In the hospital setting, they must exchange their familiar clothing and surroundings for a flimsy, drab hospital gown and the four walls of their hospital room. They are expected to conform to hospital policies and routines. It is my job to preserve their identitiy and integrity as much as possible. I am an oncology nurse who was first an oncology patient. This gives me a different perspective.

I have been asked whether it is more difficult for me to take care of patients because I am a cancer survivor. Sometimes it is. Whenever there is a patient on the unit who is dying of Hodgkin's disease, I am faced with my own mortality. When a patient my own age is dying, or a patient with children the same age as my children, I am reminded of the possibilities that exist and I say a quiet prayer of thanksgiving for the 13 years of remission that I have enjoyed.

If I had my life to live over, I probably would not choose to have cancer. Yet I have to concede that having cancer has changed my life for the better in many ways. I had to take a different path than the one I set out on 13 years ago. I had turned away from a career in medicine but was drawn back into the medical community, first as a patient, then as a patient advocate, and finally as an oncology nurse. I had to experience the difficulties of obtaining treatment without medical insurance; I had to learn to be assertive and to communicate with my physicians; I had to learn to share my experiences with my patients in a way that would be of benefit to them; and I had to learn to speak out on behalf of all cancer patients to make people aware of the critical issues they face.

Recently, I was looking through my high school yearbook. Under my picture were these lines from a poem by Robert Frost:

> Two roads diverged in a wood and I . . .
> I took the one less traveled by . . .
> And that has made all the difference.

I didn't choose to have cancer. I did choose the road to travel once I knew I had cancer. And that has made all the difference.

Note

Medic Alert is a registered trademark of Medic Alert Association.

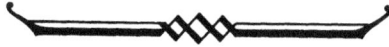

38

Adynel Wood

I truly am one of the blessed and the lucky. My childhood dream and desire to become a nurse who cares for children has come to fruition. The 35 years that I have practiced as a pediatric nurse have been fraught with challenges, opportunities, rewards, celebrations, satisfactions, and, as in all of life, some frustrations, some heartbreak, and disappointment.

In mid-1956, when I received the letter of acceptance to the diploma school of nursing to which I had applied, one of the most exhilarating periods of my life began. In September of that year I embarked on an educational journey that was the basis for realizing my goal. At that time the training consisted of university studies for one academic year, followed by clinical experiences seven days each week in the hospital-based school, plus continuing academic work on the hospital campus. I could hardly wait to experience real hands-on nursing! How I loved caring for those people! What joy I felt when they were improved enough to return home to their families, to resume their lives, and when they expressed their gratitude for my care during their recovery. And what confusion I felt when one of my patients died. I experienced sadness, discouragement, a feeling of failure and, yes, some guilt and anger that my best efforts weren't enough. During my senior year, I received permission to complete my final six months' training in pediatrics. This opportunity confirmed my desire and my God-given talent to love, to serve, and to learn from children.

After graduation I continued to gain experience as a staff nurse and later a head nurse on this 65-bed teaching unit for children. It was during this period that I met several people who eventually became significant in my professional and personal life. One of these people was a nursing student, Sandy, who was later in the pediatrics class I taught, and still later my housemate, friend, and confidante. Today, more than 30 years later, Sandy and I share wonderful memories of those times of struggle and growth. There were young physicians in training who are now in private practice or academic medicine, with whom I continue to have contact via professional, personal, and social activities. There were also children in my care whom I have subsequently ministered to in my oncology nursing practice.

It was during my tenure as head nurse that I became enamored of the eagerness and enthusiasm of the nursing students who rotated through my pediatric unit. These qualities reminded me of myself during my student days. I began to take an interest in teaching, and this aspiration became a reality for me following the unfortunate death of the nursing students' clinical instructor. I was asked to fill the position on a temporary basis while a search for a permanent instructor was undertaken. After a short period of contemplation, and with a sense of exhilaration and a bit of fear, I embarked on a brief, challenging, and most rewarding experience as a clinical instructor. I delighted in watching the students learn, participate enthusiastically in the care of the children, and grow emotionally and professionally. After a permanent replacement was hired for this teaching position, I returned to my former job as head nurse.

It soon became evident that I needed a change from the long hours, the stress, and my increasing reluctance to leave the unit. I was consumed by worries and concerns about the children when I was away. Wintering in Florida with a friend sounded like a good idea, so we packed our meager possessions and drove to Miami, where we planned to play on the beach and work just enough to survive financially. I was employed by a small pediatric hospital where there were many Cuban children who had immigrated with their families or who had been sent for chronic care for post-polio disabilities. This was a wonderful experience for me and gave me some insight into a culture previously unknown to me. The children and their families were so appreciative of the care and attention they received, were eager to learn the language and skills they needed for their lives outside the hospital, and were pleased when the "Anglo nurses" made efforts to learn their language. The Cuban missile crisis cast a pall on my delight at being in South Florida. My fear drove me back home to Memphis, where I would be near my family if or when war erupted.

After a brief period of unemployment at home, I became interested in the stories about St. Jude Children's Research Hospital, which had been opened by Danny Thomas in early 1962. I inquired about a staff position there and was disappointed to learn that all available positions were filled. I was unwilling to give up easily, however, because my initial visit there was a true spiritual experience. The spirit of love, caring, dedication, laughter, and hope permeated the hospital, and the brave and beautiful children captured my heart. A few days after that visit when I continued to be preoccupied with thoughts about the children, their families, and the staff, a voice inside insisted there was a place there for me. I called the nursing director and offered to serve as a volunteer. This offer was accepted enthusiastically, and in May 1963 I began a career that continues today—31 years later.

My volunteer service at St. Jude continued until October 1963. When a staff position became available on the evening shift and was offered to me, I eagerly accepted. This was an experience of "being in the right place at the right time" for which I am exceedingly grateful. I approached this opportunity with an eagerness and enthusiasm previously unknown to me. In 1966 it became obvious that the growing nursing staff would require the services of a staff educator, and again I accepted the position with enthusiasm and optimism. As before, I was rewarded by the positive responses of a receptive staff of young and eager nurses.

Because I had shown my eagerness, willingness, and ability to learn, to do, and to teach, in 1968 Dr. Donald Pinkel, the medical director, and Sister Lucy Ann French, the nursing director, offered to support my desire to practice in some areas of care traditionally served only by physicians. With Dr. Pinkel as my mentor, I began to do admission histories, physical examinations, and diagnostic procedures (including bone marrow aspirations and spinal taps). I began to order laboratory studies and to participate in interpreting the results, informing children and their parents of the implications and instituting therapeutic measures.

All this involved some risk-taking, for while some of my colleagues admired the courage it took to embark on this change, others openly accused me of trying to "play doctor." Still others perceived my work as an attempt to infringe upon the practice of the young physician trainees doing pediatric rotations in our hospital. Yet another group saw this as my attempt to usurp the physician's role as the planner and director of care delivery.

Through my words and my actions, I eventually convinced all concerned that my goal was to enhance care for the children and to provide the continuity that could not be given by rotating personnel. Before long, a few other nurses saw the potential for total patient–family care involvement and began to pursue similar practices. Others voiced admiration for my "pioneer spirit" but did not choose to make the commitment of time, study, and effort required to follow this path.

These innovations led to the expansion and development of my practice as a nurse practitioner in pediatric oncology. My formal nurse practitioner education followed in 1972–73. Since that time, I have participated in the development, institution, and evaluation of treatment protocols, and in the reporting of the results.

In 1973, in Atlanta, Georgia, during an impromptu meeting, three other pediatric oncology nurses and I conceived the idea of a pediatric oncology nurses' organization. We began to identify such nurses throughout the country and to establish communication with them. The responses were positive and we were chartered as a nonprofit organization in April 1976. Today, the Association of Pediatric Oncology Nurses (APON) boasts about 1,000 members from several nations. The major objectives continue to include dissemination of information that will improve treatment for children with cancer, and participation in oncology nursing research and publication.

During 1971–72, I served on the Education Committee at St. Jude. This committee was charged with the responsibility to initiate, implement, and evaluate educational programs for St. Jude staff and for residents from the University of Tennessee. During the performance of these duties, I presented a proposal to the committee, the medical director, and the hospital board that we establish a pediatric cancer nursing fellowship at St. Jude to honor Robbie Simpson, a young and dedicated member of our staff who died in 1971. The proposal was adopted and the first fellowship was awarded in 1972. I served as coordinator of the program from 1972 to 1985. The fellowship is awarded twice each year to graduate nurses employed by hospitals that admit large numbers of children with cancer. After three months of intensive training, the awardees return to their institutions with broader knowledge and experience in caring for children with cancer and their families. Recipients have come from all over the United States and foreign countries, and one has come from our own St. Jude staff. Many fellowship recipients are valuable members of the Oncology Nurses Society and the Association of Pediatric Oncology Nurses. It was this organization that recognized me as the first pediatric oncology nurse practitioner.

My heart is full of many remembrances of "my children" and their families. Volumes could be written, but perhaps a few brief stories will serve to summarize the challenges and rewards that have been mine.

One of my patients, Susan, whom I affectionately called "my baby," survived her leukemia for 20 years, despite repeated relapses. She courageously faced each new course of therapy with an attitude of hope and a commitment to try again. During one of her periods of remission she married and had a darling baby she named James. She brought this tiny miracle to see me at St. Jude. I was so proud and so humbled when she designated me "honorary grandmother"! Susan finally lost her battle, but I remain in close contact with her mother, who often visits me at the hospital. She assures me that James is a happy, active, healthy boy with warm, loving memories of his beautiful mother. Each year, on the anniversary of Susan's death, I write a note to her mother and reminisce about some of my cherished moments with Susan.

Brett was a handsome, well-built, Iowa teenager whose family raises prize cattle and owns a meat packing company. He was insistent that I visit him in Iowa to see how the family business operated. He was anxious, too, for me to have some Iowa cowboy boots. My visit finally materialized. Brett met me in his shiny new red car, took me to purchase the boots he had selected as "just right" for me, then he and his father proudly showed me the cattle and the packing plant. Shortly after I returned from that visit, Brett died. I sensed that he had willed himself to live until he could introduce me to his life in Iowa and be sure I had those boots which I still wear. I continue to correspond with Brett's family and to celebrate with his parents the activities of their children, Dana and Stan, and their three grandchildren. Brett's mother owns a travel agency. Because she knows of my wanderlust, she shares stories with me about her travel adventures with the senior citizens she accompanies on jaunts around the country. I try to keep them apprised of the Western-style functions I attend that call for the special boots as part of my attire.

Clay was the youngest son of a delightful family from Illinois. He was a bit reserved until he knew me well, and then this 8-year-old revealed himself as a chatterbox who was full of gentle mischief. While in remission and doing well, he came to St. Jude for a scheduled examination and chemotherapy, and showed me a small hangnail on his finger. After giving Clay and his parents instructions about trimming the hangnail and soaking the finger in antiseptic solution, I saw them off to an afternoon of fun before their drive home the following morning. At 4 o'clock the next morning, I awoke with a start and an intense intuition that I should call them before they left their hotel. After a momentary hesitation, I decided to trust my instinct. Clay's mother was a bit taken aback by my call, but at my suggestion, she checked and found him burning with fever. The injured finger was red, hot, and swollen, and red streaks extended up his arm. I notified the on-call physician that Clay would arrive at the hospital momentarily, and I met them there. Prompt antibiotic therapy was instituted and Clay recovered completely a few days later. Today, he is a young lawyer practicing in the Northeast and is married to a lovely woman. The happy ending to this story is the result of an unexplainable event which I believe was providential.

My very special Diego, a 7-year-old charmer from Bogotá, Colombia, arrived at St. Jude with his beautiful mother in 1990. Neither of them spoke a word of English, but within a couple of months he was conversing easily with staff and other patients and literally winning the hearts of everyone he met. Immediately after he achieved remission, he entered public school in Memphis, made honor roll consistently, became an avid Ninja Turtle fan, and wowed the city with his soccer skills. Diego's remission ended two years later. After a failed bone marrow transplant, he died on July 13, 1992. His family and I maintain an intimate friendship and reminiscence about Diego's beautiful faith, his love and concern for others, his boyhood antics, his talent at soccer, and his charming personality.

These children and their courageous families are the substance that makes this difficult job meaningful, rewarding, and worth the effort. Over my desk, in a place of prominence, is a quote from Faith Baldwin that sums up my feelings: "Life has spared those mortals much and cheated them of even more who have not kept a breathless vigil at the bedside of some Beloved Child." I draw comfort from the knowledge that I have been neither "spared" nor "cheated," for I have kept a "breathless vigil at the bedside" of many "beloved children." A part of each of these children lives in my heart and is an integral part of my past and of my hope for the children of the future. My prayer and my dream is that the past and present research efforts will result in the eradication of this scourge called cancer so that tomorrow's children will be spared.

Many more of our battles were lost in the early days, when our pharmacologic armamentarium was considerably more limited. In those days our radiation therapy equipment and techniques were less sophisticated; the diagnostic evaluations used routinely today were not available; nutritional support was limited almost entirely to nasogastric feedings; infectious diseases such as chicken pox, pneumocystis pneumonia, and various fungal infections were frequently fatal; and the long-term survival rate for children with leukemia was about 20 percent. It's nearly impossible to convey the feelings I have now, knowing that I have been part of the team that has made a difference in the lives affected by this disease. Today, 70 to 75 percent of children with the most common form of leukemia can be cured. This improved outlook is what makes it worthwhile for me to continue as an active participant in the battle against cancer.

As in many professions, and in life, I have had periods of joy, excitement, peace, serenity, hope, and faith, and periods of despair, doubt, depression, discouragement, and a desire to give up. It has been necessary for me to rely on the support, encouragement, and love of God, family, and friends to survive some of the difficult periods. I have been fortunate to have all these resources available to me, and I have made slow but sure progress in learning to accept help when it is offered. In 1980, at the Tennessee Nurses' Association convention in Gatlinburg, Tennessee, I was awarded the first annual Nurse of the Year Award. This fact may serve to demonstrate that good nurses will always have times of doubt, but will seek the support they need to give their best.

Activities outside the hospital provide some healthy distractions that refresh and renew me so that I resume my work with a renewed vigor and enthusiasm. I spend some time every day in quiet meditation and prayer and am convinced that this is fundamental to my emotional, spiritual, and physical health. Reading novels is a favorite evening pastime, and history, biography, adventure, and travel are among my usual interests. I enjoy visiting historic sites and learning the lifestyles, mores, and religions of people of different cultures. Some of my most memorable experiences include my trips to Australia, Central America, Japan, the British Isles, the Greek Islands, Caribbean islands, most of Western Europe, Canada, and many areas of the United States. In these travels and at professional meetings I have been privileged to meet people from all walks of life and have maintained many friendships, so that at every destination I have acquaintances whom I enjoy contacting. Closer to home, I enjoy gardening. I draw closer to my God via my contact with the dirt, the flowers, and the trees, and listening to and watching the birds and small animals as they carry on their business of living and raising their young in ongoing cycles.

For several years, I had the privilege to serve on the board of directors and as a builder with Habitat for Humanity. It was quite inspiring, enlightening, and rewarding to work with the generous, caring people in this organization. They build houses for those who have limited incomes but who need and desire an improved environment for their families. What a delight to see the finished product and the radiant smiles of the recipients when they are presented the keys to their own new houses.

Other volunteer work has given me a welcome diversion and a sense of accomplishment and community spirit. For example, I participate in the Peer Assistance Program of the Tennessee Nurses' Association, which provides support and encouragement to nurses who are recovering from drug and/or alcohol dependence. My role is primarily that of a concerned listener, encouraging and guiding nurses to appropriate support groups and advocating for them when they return to their work places. It is so gratifying to see nurses whose lives have been devastated by the disease of addiction begin their recovery, make progress, and return to their lives and families. These nurses find their lives happier and more meaningful and they return to professional practice with more vigor, clearer eyes and minds, and a renewed sense of being worthwhile, contributing members of society.

One of the volunteer projects I found to be light, fun, exciting, and educational was the work I did with a local professional theater group. Early on, I painted and helped build sets, cleaned the stage and theater and helped to collect furnishings and costumes for the productions. Later I served on the board of directors and even acted in a scene to promote season ticket sales. I played Nurse Ratchett in *One Flew Over the Cuckoo's Nest*. That experience quickly taught me that an acting career was not in my future.

For a couple of years I volunteered as a therapist's assistant in an outpatient treatment program for adult children of alcoholics. Again, my rewards were many and included an insight into the life experiences and subsequent behaviors of people with such a background. I learned a lot about the strength, courage, and faith that these people possessed or developed and nurtured. This was another opportunity to appreciate and respect the basic need and desire of people to live in happiness, joy, and freedom, and their willingness to accomplish this through hard work and accepting help from others.

My church community has a wonderful outreach program for inner-city residents, and I felt a strong desire to make some contribution. Since my pickup truck was ideal for transporting large insulated containers, I delivered Meals-on-Wheels to the elderly and handicapped. What gifts I received from these people! Sometimes I was the only visitor they had for the day and occasionally for an entire week. I was given a relatively short route, so I often took time to talk with my clients, make phone calls for them, and bring in their mail, which I sometimes read to them. On a couple of occasions I found people in crisis and was able to summon the help they needed. The smiles, the hugs, the stories about their families, and even the updates on the soap operas were all gifts that brightened my days.

Another outreach job I loved was teaching some of the inner-city children to swim. A generous parishioner offered us the use of his pool and we drove the children in the church van to his home for a couple of hours every week. It was so gratifying to see some of those children the first time they summoned the courage to jump into the pool and let their faces get wet. And a few really did learn to swim!

Those volunteer activities, my church affiliation, my family commitments, and my enjoyment of theater, music, baseball, golf, and quiet times with books or in the park have helped to offset the intensity of my professional life and afford me a more balanced appreciation of life in its varied aspects.

Through the years I have written a number of articles about pediatric oncology nursing and nurse practitioners in particular. *Nursing Outlook*, in February 1971, published a letter to the editor in which I proposed, defended, and advocated this area of practice for nurses, in order to improve the quality of care for children with cancer. It was also an opportunity to predict that the need for specialized pediatric oncology care would be filled, and my contention was that nurse practitioners were the people to do it best.

In 1978 I published an article in *Pediatric Nursing* that described my practice and its implications for other nurses who might wish to pursue a similar career. In this article I focused on the immediate and long-term care plans for children with cancer; on their physical, emotional, and spiritual needs; their adjustment to absences from home, family, and friends; the special tutoring school-age children might need to keep from falling behind, and the eventual impact of the cancer diagnosis on the patient's employability, insurability, and recognition as a contributing member of society.

Nursing Clinics of North America published a symposium on Cancer in Children in March 1976. For this, Shirley Stagner and I wrote the chapter, "The Child with Cancer on Immunosuppressive Therapy." The symposium was written by members of APON and became required reading in a number of nursing education programs. In 1980, at the Fifth Annual Congress of the Oncology Nurses Society, I presented one of the first reports on the problem of skin rashes occurring after long-term therapy with Mercaptopurine and Methotrexate.

I have been co-author of many articles reporting innovative treatment protocols, including early randomized studies of "prophylactic" central nervous system therapy for children with leukemia, early trials of epipodophylotoxins and cytosine arabinoside for refractory leukemia, and studies of somnolence syndrome in children with leukemia after CNS irradiation. Currently, I am participating with Dr. Gaston Rivera in a study to determine whether hemopoietic growth factors can alter the degree and/or duration of neutropenia in children receiving intensive induction therapy for leukemia. I am also investigating, with Dr. Melissa Hudson and her team, the late effects of chemotherapy and radiation therapy given to children with leukemia.

Through the years I have lectured at medical and nursing schools and given numerous talks at conferences, seminars, and workshops about cancer therapy, its outcomes, and potential long-term effects. I have spoken to professional and lay groups about my experiences as a nurse practitioner—the challenges, the heartbreaks, the rewards, and the dreams for the future.

Over the past 25 years, there have been several stories printed about me in various publications, including St. Jude's own *Partners in Hope* and *The St. Jude Journal*; *Memphis Magazine*, whose feature article was about Marlo Thomas, the work at St. Jude, and the story of my involvement with the children; *Hospital News of Greater Memphis* on the occasion of my twenty-fifth anniversary at St. Jude; and *Star*, one of the supermarket tabloids. In each of these stories I have attempted to focus on the work I do as my "calling" or my "mission" in life. I've been tempted to give up and admit that I've had enough. But each time these thoughts occur, they are offset promptly by memories of the better days: the days when the children laugh, when they hug me, when they tease me, when their parents thank me, when we share in victories—large and small— and even when we lose the battle and share some tears together.

What does it mean to be a pediatric oncology nurse? It means happiness and hard work, it means victories and defeats, it means laughter and tears, it means courage and despair. For me, it means the realization of childhood dreams and aspirations, balanced by the struggle to accept defeat and let go on some occasions. It means that lots of prayers are answered, while many questions remain unanswered. Perhaps the answers are none of my business, perhaps I'm not asking the right questions, or most likely, my assignment is to love, to trust, to be patient and kind, and leave the rest to God.

The suggestions I often pass along to younger nurses who are making career decisions include these: pray about it; spend some time in a pediatric oncology unit and watch and listen; try it for a while; and most important, take care of yourself so you are mentally, physically, and spiritually healthy enough to help others. I believe that soon you will *know*. It takes a very special love and desire to do this work, and the rewards defy description.

What a wonderful experience it has been for me to write this. I've taken time out to search through pictures, letters, cards, newspapers, magazines, and have had hours of happy reflection and moments of poignant memories. I've seen smiling faces that are no more except in my heart and I've read letters from "my children" and their parents about their work, their marriages, their children, and their joy in living. Would I do it again? Yes, without a moment's hesitation.

39

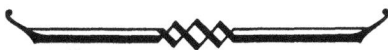

Connie Henke Yarbro

As far back as I can remember, I always wanted to be a nurse. My mother was a nurse and I guess she was my role model as I grew up. She was a housewife and mother with an active career as a registered nurse. When I was a child she worked night shifts and days in a physician's office. When I was in fifth grade she started working for the Visiting Nurses Association. She took my brother and me to school every morning and sometimes she would stop off along the way to see a patient. I remember those cold snowy mornings in northern Illinois when my brother and I would wait in the car for her return. One patient I remember in particular had diabetes and for a time she stopped every day to give an insulin shot. She would always update us on the patient's progress. That was my first contact with nursing care for a real patient. There were many other patient visits and check-ups on our trips to and from school. Each time we learned more about patient care. Becoming a nurse was natural after that.

Something else that influenced my life was helping my mother and grandmother take care of my grandfather at home. Now that I look back, I realize that he probably had Alzheimer's disease. He was bedridden for several months and I helped my grandmother take care of him until he passed away. I think this caused me to accept death as a natural part of life. Being with my grandfather when he died (I was 12 years old then) probably influenced how I later came to deal with dying patients.

It was probably no surprise that I developed an inner desire to be a nurse "just like my mom." I even decided to go to the same school of nursing that she had graduated from. It is a cliché, but it is true that in those days, most girls had three career choices: nurse, school teacher, or secretary. There were no college programs in nursing nearby and besides, my parents could not have afforded such a program even if one were available. So I applied and was accepted to the diploma program at Moline Lutheran Hospital School of Nursing where my mother had trained.

After graduation and before I started doing cancer nursing, I worked for about a year in each of the following areas: coronary care, respiratory care, orthopedics, IV team, and emergency room. During those years I remember caring for cancer patients as a part of the general care that was provided to the mixture of patients admitted to the hospital. When a patient was to receive 5-Fluorouracil (and that's what most patients got back then because there was not the large armamentarium of antineoplastic agents available today) the doctor would order an IV to be started and he would come to the unit, mix the drug, and give it. Drugs like 5-Fluorouracil and nitrogen mustard were exotic and foreign to most nurses in those days.

I remember taking care of one patient in particular when I was evening charge nurse on an orthopedic unit. She was a wonderful woman who had metastatic colon cancer and I have no idea how she ended up on our unit but she stayed with us for *months*. She had a colostomy. She required round-the-clock pain medications and sometimes the doctors would let her go home for weekend visits. She knew she had a terminal disease but her one remaining goal in life was to see her only child graduate from high school. We all kept hoping along with her that she would live to experience that important event. She did not. There were many other cancer patients that I took care of in those early years and, looking back, I don't think I viewed them any differently than patients with other diseases. I don't think I ever thought of cancer as a "death sentence," as common as that view was, but perhaps I just didn't give it much thought.

I knew that I loved nursing but never settled in one area. I was always looking for new challenges and changes and maybe that is why I kept moving on to different areas of nursing. As a matter of fact, after a year of working in the emergency room at the University of Alabama (UAB), I was ready for a change. I often thought about writing a book on the experiences I encountered as a trauma nurse in that university emergency room. It was an incredible learning experience but I missed having the opportunity to get to know and interact with patients and their families. Just as I was debating about moving and going back to school, I heard about a new position at UAB in their newly established cancer program.

It was 1971 and the National Cancer Act had just been enacted. Many new cancer programs were being established at university hospitals across the country. The advertised position was for a nurse to coordinate a statewide chemotherapy program. I remember thinking, "What have I got to lose, I'm looking for something different," so I applied for the position.

I remember quite vividly my first interview with Dr. John Durant, director of the hematology division at UAB. He proceeded to explain that this was a new grant program funded by the National Cancer Institute

(NCI) with the purpose of establishing a system so that patients with Hodgkin's disease and lymphomas, and children with acute leukemia who received their initial therapy at the medical center, could return to their primary physician for follow-up care and continued treatment. It would be the responsibility of the nurse to follow the patients, provide their chemotherapy treatments in their communities, collaborate with the primary physicians, and teach the nurses in the communities about the patients' treatments, side effects, and supportive care. I remember leaving that interview and thinking, "I sure would like that job! What a challenge! How exciting!" I also knew several other colleagues who interviewed for the position, and I was thrilled when several weeks later I was called back for a second interview and offered the position.

That day I began, unknowingly, my long and rewarding journey in oncology nursing—a journey that has constantly challenged me in a specialty that I dearly love and have never had the desire to leave. There is something distinctive about cancer patients. I was then and I remain amazed at their strength and the way they cope with life and the fear of death. I was providing care to them and they were teaching me so much about living.

After I was hired, I remember spending a lot of time reading about Hodgkin's disease, lymphoma, and acute leukemia. There was so much to learn—drugs I had never heard of, new tests that were unfamiliar, research protocols to learn, and all of the potential side effects and problems that could occur. I went with the oncologists on rounds, saw patients in the outpatient clinic, and learned how to administer chemotherapeutic agents.

As I was gaining experience in oncology I was also traveling throughout the state of Alabama telling physicians about the program. Patients were entered on treatment and after their initial therapy I would work with their primary physicians and administer their chemotherapy in their doctors' offices. We established a computerized program to collect data and a system to report the blood counts before visits were made in the rural areas. Many nurses in the community did not want to have anything to do with cancer drugs; even some of the physicians were afraid. Often I had to meet the patients in the emergency rooms at their hometown hospitals where I mixed the drugs, delivered the treatment, and did patient teaching.

In 1972 Dr. Durant received a $5 million federal grant to officially establish the cancer center. Our world of two examining rooms in the basement of the UAB hospital and one little room where the lab work was done with one chair to administer the chemotherapy was soon to change to a separate building with many treatment rooms, a modern radiation therapy facility, research laboratories, and eventually an attached inpatient ward and research unit.

It was an exciting time as an oncology nurse. There was so very much to do and so very much to learn. Cancer research and care were literally exploding across the land. While I was not the first to practice cancer nursing at UAB, I was the first to call herself an oncology nurse. I had no role model to follow and the role of the oncology nurse was not well defined. I often asked myself what was the best way to care for the multitude of problems encounted by my patients and families. It is probably hard for the younger nurses today or those new to oncology nursing to imagine what it was like in the early 1970s. There were no patient or staff education materials available. If you tried to find someone to explain how to reconstitute or administer a chemotherapy agent, you couldn't—nobody knew. Those were not the days of biological safety cabinets or pharmacies that did all the mixing for you.

In 1973 I attended the first national cancer nursing conference in Chicago sponsored by the American Cancer Society. At this conference I had a chance to meet a few nurses who had the same problems and fears and frustrations that I had. *Now I knew I was not alone!* I described this unique experience in an article I wrote on the history and early days of ONS (Yarbro, 1984). It was at this time that a small group of us began discussing the concept of a national organization for oncology nurses. These early deliberations subsequently led to the establishment of the Oncology Nursing Society (ONS). Those initial days of ONS were a highlight of my professional career.

During the decade of the 1970s at the UAB Comprehensive Cancer Center (1971–1979), my professional career as a cancer nurse evolved. The statewide chemotherapy program was off the ground and as the cancer center grew I became oncology nursing coordinator of the comprehensive cancer center and director of nursing services for the division of cancer control. During these years, I had many fortuitous opportunities to start, participate in, and coordinate numerous activities related to patient care, research, and nursing education.

Patient Care

Much was happening in the sphere of patient care. It seemed as though every day there was a new protocol, a new drug, more unique side effects to contend with. Of course the patient population continued to increase. It was frustrating to help patients deal with their side effects when so little was known about alleviating or preventing them. The antiemetic regimens that we know today did not exist. It was a challenge to encourage the patients (especially those who were curable such as the younger population with Hodgkin's disease) to continue their treatment when the patients wanted to stop. After several courses of chemotherapy patients were told that they had no evidence of disease but still needed to finish all their courses of therapy. It was frustrating and tragic to have a patient cease therapy and subsequently relapse. I remember one young man in particular who came very close to stopping his ABVD regimen but with our encouragement and support he continued. One of the residents even obtained some marijuana from the police department to see if it would help the nausea and vomiting. Today that patient is free of disease and married with adopted children. It is that kind of success story that makes the work and frustration worthwhile.

Today patient support groups are widespread and groups are available for many different types of cancer. In the early days we had to invent our own. One of our major projects was the development of our first patient support group. We did it by helping the patients themselves to develop their own program. They named their group TOUCH (Today Our Understanding of Cancer is Hope) and they proceeded to develop chapters of the group throughout the state.

Research

During 1976–1977, I worked with Marilyn Cain, our rehabilitation coordinator, on a study to identify the nonmedical needs of a sample of cancer patients in our outpatient clinic. We devised an instrument to assess these needs in order to stimulate interest and give attention to the psychosocial consequences of cancer. We were concerned with their quality of life and their coping mechanisms. Our study, "Living with Cancer: A Random Sample of 50 patients in a Hematology Oncology Clinic" (Cain & Henke, 1978), was one of my first ventures in the research process. We did not know it at the time, but our quality of life instrument would subsequently be considered one of the first such instruments to be developed.

Research has always been the foundation of oncology care. One cannot work in a major academic setting without being surrounded by the constant development and implementation of research studies and clinical trials. This was not always the case. I watched the transition from the time when "a little 5-FU or nitrogen mustard" was the standard treatment, to the complex protocol-dominated clinical milieu of today in which almost every patient is entered on a clinical trial. I had the opportunity to participate in an early research study on the use of clinical algorithms for our statewide chemotherapy outreach program and was project manager for a simulated computer network protocol information system on Hodgkin's disease for cooperative multi-institutional clinical trials. Included in our support were funds for facsimile machines to be placed in cooperating physicians' offices. Although FAX machines are common today, in the 1970s they were very expensive, large, bulky machines and everyone was leery as to their productive use. (I think some people even doubted their accuracy.) Computers were still those big machines that took up a whole separate room.

In 1976 Dr. Durant, who was chair of the Southeastern Cooperative Cancer Study Group (SECSG), appointed me chair of the newly established nursing research committee. The first committee meeting took place in St. Louis where a small group of us identified goals and projects. Our committee was "ahead of the times" since no other cooperative group had a nursing research committee and many of them did not form such committees until years later. This was another occasion when I was lucky enough to get involved in an activity on the ground floor. Our nursing research committee proceeded to submit a bylaw amendment to the SECSG board that would permit nurses to be members of the group and the committee to be a standing committee. We were accepted as members, a nurse was appointed as a member of each disease committee, the nursing research committee reviewed new protocols under development, and several of us actually developed nursing research companion studies that were approved by NCI. I remember the first study that Deborah Mayer and I submitted. The staff at NCI had no idea what to do with it! Maybe our studies passed the NCI process more rapidly in those days because they did not have a process that required all the red tape that exists today.

Nursing Education

There was a real need for nursing and staff education regarding cancer care as cancer centers were developing. This has become an ongoing aspect of my career. I taught several quarterly classes to adult health nursing students and in the family practitioner program. However, my big challenge came when I wrote and submitted a grant to NCI for an oncology nurse practitioner program. This grant was funded and I served as project co-director with Judy Holcombe at the school of nursing. It became a learning experience for me because I entered the world of curriculum development and grant writing. We had three students the first year. The grant accomplished its goals but we did not renew it because NCI changed its focus to the master's fellowship program in oncology nursing. When I look back, however, I can see that the oncology nurse practitioner program was a necessary preliminary step on the way to recognition of the importance of the master's degree, and yet another example of something that was "ahead of the times."

Oncology Nursing Society

I must elaborate on my early ONS days, because, after all, ONS has consumed a good portion of my life for quite a few years. I have loved every minute of it, even the times of struggle and frustration because there was always a positive end result in even the most difficult times.

While our activities during 1973 and 1974 laid the groundwork, the culmination came in May of 1975 at the ASCO meeting in San Diego, when it was decided to establish a formal national organization. As many know, the initial four officers selected and charged with incorporation were Lisa Begg Marino, president (Chicago); Cindi Mantz, vice-president (St. Louis); Daryl Maass, secretary (New York); and me as treasurer. We left San Diego with a firm determination to make our dream a reality. At that time I am not sure any of us had a vision of what ONS would be 20 years later. Our time was spent trying to meet the needs of cancer nursing in the 1970s. Subconsciously we must have been thinking of the future because we spent a lot of time developing the purposes of ONS and the subsequent goals that guided us in the development of standards, education, and the promotion of nursing research.

I remember the hesitation with which I accepted the appointment as treasurer, not just because of the responsibilities and the work it would require, but because of the unknown. At that time, I had no idea of the enormous amount of work that would have to be done or of the problems that would be encountered in the unexpected and tortuous struggles of national cancer and national nursing politics. However, I went back to Birmingham, established a bank account, worked with the cancer center's bookkeeper, and learned how to budget. I set up the ledgers and maintained the ONS accounting system with paper and pencil. Of course it was easier then because we had no money. Early on, the cancer center purchased the equipment and supplies that I needed until the membership dues came rolling in.

By that October we had over 200 members and my dining room table was covered with ledgers, checks, and membership cards. It was before the days of home computers and I wrote every membership card and envelope out by hand. I was probably considered a "tightwad" in those days because I had a hard time spending any of the money coming in. The ONS officers used their institutional resources for meetings, phone calls, and everything else that was "reasonable." However, after the first year we had a budget, reimbursement policies and forms, and eventually a system whereby committees could establish their budgets for board approval. One of my early goals was to maintain a savings account equal to the yearly expenses in case we ran into "hard times." I would like to think that my frugality and monitoring of expenses played a small part in leading to the financial stability of ONS today. Serving as ONS treasurer was a splendid learning experience. It had been such a challenge laying the groundwork that I felt confident in 1978 when I turned the books over to the new treasurer, Pearl Moore. I also remember thinking that she was so lucky, because she was going to have a computerized system of accounting—what progress!

Even though I ended my three-year term as treasurer, my involvement did not end. I will never forget the year 1979—a banner year for me! Within just a month and a half, *six short weeks*, I chaired the 1979 ONS Congress, was elected ONS president, graduated with my B.S.N., left my job at the University of Alabama, moved to Columbia, Missouri, got married, and had my first board meeting as ONS president. How is that for stress?!!

In those days, the ONS president also served as chief executive officer since we had no full-time administrative help. At my first board meeting as ONS president we decided to advance from a post office box to a small headquarters office in Pittsburgh with Nancy Berkowitz as part-time administrative assistant. Even though we now had a home, my spare bedroom became the second home of ONS. So much happened during my four years as ONS president that I could write a separate chapter on that experience alone. There were struggles and frustrations but the excitement and progress far outweighed any of the problems. Thanks to the constant eager volunteer efforts of so many members, a lot began during those years that continues today. We developed practice and education standards, local chapters, chemotherapy guidelines, a certification task force that led the way to formal certification, and the first research grants and awards for our members. Every committee expanded its activities and the first long-range plan was started.

Several monumental moments stand out so vividly that I must tell about them. Much occurred at the four annual business meetings over which I presided as president. Believe me—and as many of you may remember—*they were not boring*. The issues that arose again and again where emotions dominated the discussions (though reason ultimately prevailed) included the entry level into practice, the Equal Rights Amendment, and associate membership, to name only three. Through all of this, however, it was the active input of members and the beginning of the tradition whereby members manage and direct the organization that shaped the ONS of today.

In addition, there were two goals I envisioned that I believe were especially important for the society. First was the establishment of the Oncology Nursing Foundation in 1981. To me the foundation was an investment in the future of our profession. I remember presenting this idea to the board and being afraid that they would neither support this effort nor understand its importance. However, they were very supportive and let me proceed. I think the foundation was a fairly new concept at that time and it was a real challenge to educate the members as to its purpose and potential. I always said and still do, "If only each member would give ten dollars a year, just think how it would help the foundation expand the awards and research endeavors." Today, ten dollars from 25,000 members is a quarter of a million dollars a year! A lot has happened with the foundation since 1981, many new awards and programs, more annual givers, but it would still be great if we could get *every* member to give just ten dollars per year.

The second goal I felt strongly about was the establishment of a full-time executive director position. If we were going to continue to grow, the next president and board should be free to concentrate on goals, policies, and activities and not be encumbered with the day-to-day business. So an administrative task force was established and this initiative was pursued. I was fortunate that when I became president in 1979, my husband John was very supportive of my professional endeavors and I was able to let my ONS activities consume my life. By the time I left office in 1983, we had hired Pearl Moore to be the executive director of ONS.

I have often said that in the 1970s ONS was a special dream—a dream that became a reality. The pioneers in the earlier years, the 1940s and 1960s, sowed the seeds and laid the foundation. I am proud and privileged to have been one of those allowed to place the cornerstone of a structure that will influence the course of cancer care long after the trailblazers are gone and forgotten. However, my pioneering days did not end with my presidency of ONS. I continued to expand my horizons and contributions to the specialty of nursing that still today is a significant part of my life.

Continued Involvement as an Oncology Nurse

After leaving the office of ONS president, I remained active as chair of the Oncology Nursing Foundation and served as an oncology nursing consultant nationally and internationally. I have enjoyed the opportunity of meeting so many nurses from around the world and observing cancer nursing care worldwide. In 1985 I launched *Seminars in Oncology Nursing*. Numerous medical specialties had a review journal related to their specific areas and I felt there was a need for a nursing journal to address specific topics related to cancer nursing. Today the journal is ten years old and the topics that need to be addressed are endless. I became a self-taught editor (as I taught myself so many other endeavors) but what has been most rewarding is providing a chance for other oncology nurses to learn the process of editing. Over the past ten years I have helped over 40 guest editors learn the editorial process and have worked with over 300 contributing authors who are experts in specific specialty areas in oncology nursing. I have learned a lot about writing, editing, and the mechanisms of publishing, which in itself could be another chapter of my life to write about. Venturing into the world of editing books has been another challenge and a rewarding opportunity that was an outgrowth of journal editing. I am particularly proud to be one of four editors of *Cancer Nursing: Principles and Practice*, now in its third edition. I often wonder what life would be like without deadlines.

Recently I have represented the United States on the board of directors of the International Society of Nurses in Cancer Care. This young organization brings together leaders in cancer nursing from nations around the globe to share their experiences at an international conference every two years.

Mentors and Mentoring

When I think about mentors, several people come to mind who have played a key role in the various chapters of my life. My first mentor, of course, was my mother, but over the years I have had other mentors, other "wise and trusted counselors and teachers." During the 1970s I remember Dr. Durant as a wise counselor and teacher who taught me about cancer and cancer treatment. He believed in me, supported my professional growth, and taught me a lot about collaboration between medicine and nursing. I don't think I ever remember him saying "no" to a new idea or project that I suggested. When I was asked to write a chapter for a nursing textbook on the adult with acute myelogenous leukemia (my first endeavor at writing), I was scared. But he encouraged me and reviewed this work.

Several nurses were mentors as well. One was a mentor at a distance that I looked up to as a role model, Renilda Hilkemeyer. My first direct contact with Renilda was in 1973 when we were both on a cancer nursing program in Baton Rouge, Louisiana. This was my first speaking engagement and I was really nervous, not only about giving the talk but also about being on the same program with this "famous" person in cancer nursing. Everything went smoothly and I was delighted to have the opportunity to meet her. But I was even more excited when one evening several months later I received a call from Renilda asking me to speak on the statewide chemotherapy program at a nursing session at the American Cancer Society and NCI national conference on the advances in cancer management in New York in November of 1974. Speaking locally was one thing but this was "the big time." I felt honored that she had thought of me. She was a role model for me; I admired her work and contributions to cancer nursing.

Bettie Jackson, R.N., Ed.D., who was on the faculty at the UAB School of Nursing, was another wise counselor and teacher. In my involvement with the school of nursing our paths crossed. She was active in an enterostomal therapy organization and was always encouraging her students and colleagues to get involved in professional activities and to publish. She provided me with a lot of insight into the profession and if I had a new idea she was always there as a sounding board providing the necessary encouragement.

As the years have passed, my life has been blessed with many role models and mentors and nurses that I continue to admire and respect for their many achievements. I feel fortunate to have had the opportunities to work with such talented people. I can best thank those who helped me by helping others. It is a privilege mentoring nurses to serve as editors and writers. And in my job as Director of Nursing Resource Development at Memorial Medical Center I encounter a cadre of nurses who I have been able to help support in their professional development. It is exciting. It is fun. However, I cannot let these pages slip by without acknowledging a major force in my life—my husband. John has not only been a husband, but a friend, mentor, counselor, and a wise teacher who has taught me a lot about writing and editing. I, in turn, have taught him a lot about cancer nursing. Our professional lives are so intertwined with our personal lives that we are constantly bouncing ideas off each other and discussing the issues of cancer care. Balancing a career and personal life seem to go hand in hand with us.

The past 27 years as a nurse and 23 years as an oncology nurse have passed by so very quickly. I cannot imagine not being a nurse or not being involved in cancer nursing. I am presently attending graduate school and continue to think of so many things I would like to do from a professional nursing perspective. It is a joy to recall the memories of the past years, the patients and families I have been involved with and the sorrows and happiness that we have shared. It is a joy to see the continued growth of ONS, the impact that oncology nurses are making on cancer care, and the advances in oncology nursing research. And most of all, it is a joy to know that oncology nurses do "make a difference."

References

Yarbro, Connie Henke, "The Early Days: Four Smiles and a Post Office Box," *Oncology Nursing Forum* 11(1), (January/February 1984):79–85.

Cain, Marilyn and Connie Henke, "Living with Cancer: A Random Sample of 50 Patients in a Hematology/Oncology Clinic," *Oncology Nursing Forum* 5(3) (1978):4–5.

www.ingramcontent.com/pod-product-compliance
Lightning Source LLC
Chambersburg PA
CBHW060743220326
41598CB00022B/2314